# THE HISTORY OF SCURVY AND VITAMIN C

Also by Kenneth J. Carpenter

*Pellagra* (1981)

# THE HISTORY OF SCURVY AND VITAMIN C

### KENNETH J. CARPENTER

*Professor of Nutrition*
*University of California, Berkeley*
*Formerly Fellow of Sidney Sussex College*
*and Reader in Nutrition, University of Cambridge*

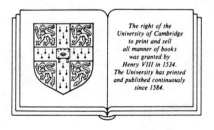

## CAMBRIDGE UNIVERSITY PRESS

*Cambridge*
*London   New York   New Rochelle*
*Melbourne   Sydney*

Published by the Press Syndicate of the University of Cambridge
The Pitt Building, Trumpington Street, Cambridge CB2 1RP
32 East 57th Street, New York, NY 10022, USA
10 Stamford Road, Oakleigh, Melbourne 3166, Australia

First published 1986

Printed in the United States of America

*Library of Congress Cataloging-in-Publication Data*
Carpenter, Kenneth J.
The history of scurvy and vitamin C.
Bibliography: p.
Includes index.
1. Scurvy – History.  2. Vitamin C – History.
I. Title.  [DNLM:  1. Ascorbic Acid – history.
2. Scurvy – history.  WD140 C295h]
RC627.S36C36  1986  616.3'94'009  85-25464
ISBN 0 521 32029 1

*British Library Cataloging-in-Publication applied for*

# Contents

# Illustrations

# Preface

If we exclude straightforward famine, scurvy is probably the nutritional deficiency disease that has caused most suffering in recorded history.

This book sets out to describe the work of a relatively small number of people who tried to understand the cause of this strange disease and to find the means of its prevention and cure. It is a story that can be followed without any special background in science, and illustrates the historical development of a scientific approach to a practical problem. We see the repeated assertion of theory after theory, which at first seemed only to impede progress, but eventually led to a dramatic success. We also see a succession of eminent people playing the roles of heroes or villains in this story, sometimes with surprising casting.

No attempt has been made to catalog every outbreak of scurvy, or to delve into either the detailed changes seen in the tissues of a sufferer or the exact biochemical functions discovered for the vitamin that finally emerged. Rather, the book sets out to record the arguments and the logic, and the observations on which they were based, that led to the various theories, and finally to the isolation and synthesis of vitamin C (ascorbic acid).

I have also tried to summarize the modern claims made for the use of ascorbic acid at very high levels, and the most important evidence for and against the practice, without giving any personal opinion in the matter.

Any writer on a subject such as this is in debt to, and becomes filled with respect for, the work of earlier scholars. In this field, James Lind in the eighteenth century and Hirsch and Mahé in the nineteenth century have given us examples of the objective reporting of other people's observations and conclusions. Of the writers in this century, I have felt particularly indebted to Keevil, Lloyd, and Coulter for their four-volume work, *Medicine and the Navy 1200–1900*, to Stewart and Guthrie for their bicentennial edition of Lind's 1753 *Treatise*, to R. E. Hughes for his reassessments of old remedies, and to Surgeon Vice-Admiral Sir James Watt for his writings on the medical problems of eighteenth-century exploration at sea. In a book of this kind, one cannot keep telling the reader that one agrees with another reviewer's interpretation of a primary source; in my effort to avoid this, I am aware that I may have given the reader a distorted view, by citing others mainly when venturing to disagree with them on a point.

Again, collecting material for this book has taught me to appreciate even more the work of many generations of scholars, librarians, and donors, who have built up our present library resources so that it is now possible to have such ready access to past writing. I am particularly indebted to the University of California Library system with its excellent Interlibrary Loan Service and to the Wellcome Institute for the History of Medicine, the Royal Society of Medicine in London, and the Scott Polar Institute in Cambridge for advice and the use of their libraries.

I am most grateful to Dr. John Heilbron and his colleagues for providing a congenial working environment for this project in the Office for the History of Science and Technology at Berkeley. My wife, Antonina, has helped me in translating from Latin, and my colleagues, Marc Schelstraete and Janet Eatherton, in translating from Dutch and Danish, respectively. Others who have gone out of their way to provide specific points of information include Professor H. H. Draper of the University of Guelph, Dr. D. H. Hornig of Hoffman-La-Roche, Basel, and Dr. S. Nagy of the Florida Department of Citrus. Finally, Gwen McIntosh cheerfully did the major work of putting the handwritten manuscript and bibliography, with its successive revisions, onto a word processor.

To reduce the bulk of footnotes, I have used the same footnote number more than once within a chapter if a single note documents more than one item.

# 1

## The explorers' sickness (1498 – 1700)

At the end of the Middle Ages, sailors began to make ever more daring voyages out from Western Europe. This could be explained, in part, by technical developments in the design of the ships that allowed them to sail at a greater angle from the direction of the wind, and in methods of navigation with a more reliable compass.[1] There were also strong commercial inducements to find a sea route that would eliminate the middlemen in the overland trade of silk and spices between Europe and the Far East. The new activity also seemed to reflect a new spirit of adventure and curiosity evident in this period of renaissance.

### Portuguese and Spanish expeditions

From 1440 on, Portuguese sailors had been exploring the west coast of Africa, getting successively farther south, and finally rounding its southern Cape in 1487.[2] Ten years later, Vasco da Gama led an expedition designed to go by this route all the way to the Indies. The fleet of four ships, with a total of about 140 people on board, left Lisbon on July 9. By January 24 of the new year 1498, they had rounded the Cape and reached a river mouth on the southeast coast of Africa. They spend a month there cleaning the ship hulls and refitting a mast. Da Gama notes that "many of our men fell ill here, their feet and hands swelling, and their gums growing over their teeth so that they could not eat." They ran up the eastern coast, and on April 6, while beached at night, two boats manned by Moorish traders approached, one laden with fine oranges "better than those of Portugal." Two of the moors remained on board, accompanying them that day to Mombasa. "In front of the city there lay numerous vessels all dressed in flags. . . . Anxious not to be outdone we even surpassed their show, for we wanted in nothing but

---

[1] Quinn (1977), Chap. 4.    [2] Newby (1975), 62–81.

1

men, even the few we had being very ill." By April 12, "it pleased God in his mercy that . . . all our sick recovered their health for the air of this place is very good." [3]

On the return journey across the Arabian Sea, they were hindered by "frequent calms and foul winds," and were twelve weeks at sea (October to December, 1498). The sailors "again suffered from their gums; their legs also swelled, and other parts of the body, and these swellings spread until the sufferer died, without exhibiting symptoms of any other disease." As on the previous occasion, thirty men died, and only seven or eight were fit enough to navigate each ship.

In another two weeks there would have been no men at all to navigate the ships . . . all bonds of discipline had gone . . . we addressed vows and petitions to the Saints . . . it pleased God in his mercy to send us a wind which, in the course of six days, carried us within sight of land . . . at this we rejoiced as . . . we hoped to recover our health there as we had done once before. . . . On Monday, the 7th of January we again cast anchor off Mitindy. . . . the Captain-Major sent a man on shore to bring off a supply of oranges which were much desired by our sick.[3]

There is no further description of sickness in the later part of the voyage, just a comment, as they rounded the Cape of Good Hope, that "those who had come so far were in good health and quite robust." But they were no more than half of the original complement. What can we conclude from this record? First, it seems that the sickness they encountered had been quite outside their previous experience; nor do they relate it to anything they had read. It would also seem that, by the time of its second appearance, the crew were convinced that the oranges that they had eaten on the earlier occasion were powerful curatives, because they were specifically asking for them. On each occasion apparently, the sickness appeared only after they had been ten weeks at sea. Finally, the captain was convinced that landing places differed significantly in the quality of their air and that this could vitally affect his men's health.

At least one modern writer has suggested that the value of oranges and lemons in preventing scurvy was already known in the fourteenth century, and has cited a Spanish medical tract from that period. The reference, which appears in a section entitled "On foods and remedies which preserve the body against pestilential maladies," has been translated as follows: "One should use in all foods much vinegar, sorrel, juice of oranges and lemons and other acid things which are most beneficial." [4] However, the translators make it clear in another paper that this tract is specifically written as advice for people trying to avoid the Black Death (bubonic plague) that was sweeping through Europe at that time.[5]

---

[3] Ravenstein (1898), 20–1, 35, 39, 89, 93, 124.    [4] Winslow & Duran-Reynals (1949), 80.
[5] Winslow & Duran-Reynals (1948), 747.

After the return of da Gama, the Portuguese rapidly organized further expeditions, using the same sea route, and founded trading colonies at Goa in India (1510) and Malacca in Malaysia (1511), establishing their influence in the Moluccas and finally colonizing Macao, an island off the Chinese coast (1557). The published narrative of the first of these expeditions, led by Cabral, notes briefly that some were sick with *"amalati de la boccha"* (literally "the curse of the mouth") by the time they reached Mombasa. Here they obtained "sheep, hens, geese and lemons and oranges, the best in the world and the oranges made them well again." [6] It seems that they were never able to eliminate the high risk of sickness and mortality on these voyages. In 1579, Thomas Stevens, who was a passenger on one of the regular voyages from Lisbon to Goa wrote home:

. . . by reason of the long navigation, and want of food and water, they fall into sundry diseases, their gums wax great, and swell, and they are fain to cut them away, their legs swell, and all the body becometh sore, and so benumbed, that they can not stir hand nor foot, and so they die for weakness, other fall into fluxes and agues, and die thereby . . . ; yet though we had more than one hundred and fifty sick, there died not past seven and twenty; which loss they esteemed not much in respect of other times. [7]

On this voyage they were 202 days at sea, and did not call at Madagascar. A paymaster's report from Goa in 1634 states that of 5,000 soldiers embarking from Lisbon in the previous five years, less than one-half survived the voyage. [8] This was due, in part, to shipwrecks as well as to sickness.

In the same period as de Gama's voyage, Christopher Columbus, in his voyages from Spain, had been endeavoring to reach the Indies by sailing to the west. These voyages, in fact to the Caribbean area, were much shorter. He was never at sea for as long as twelve weeks at a time, and his crews are not generally thought to have been attacked by the new sickness, although two writers in this century have said that Columbus's second voyage had some such trouble. [9] The only possible, and indirect, allusion that I have seen in the physician's account of the expedition refers to their being visited by Carib Indians "who come loaded with 'ages,' a sort of turnip, very excellent food, which they cook and prepare in various ways. This food is very nutritious, and has proved of the greatest benefit to us all after the privations we endured when at sea, which in truth were more severe than man ever suffered." [10] But even this passage in another version appears much less serious:

They all bring yams, which are like turnips and very good food, and we prepare them for eating in a variety of ways. They are so nourishing that we are all greatly

---

[6] Greenlee (1958), 65.    [7] Hakluyt (1927), *IV*, 238.    [8] Boxer (1959), 17n.    [9] Morison (1939), 11; Moll (1944), 68.    [10] Fernandez de Ybarra (1907), 452.

restored by them, for we have been living on the smallest possible rations during our months at sea. . . . it was only prudent that we should limit our consumption in order to have enough to keep alive however long the voyage might last.[11]

Certainly, if there was any disease problem while they were at sea, it must have been unimportant in comparison with the malaria and other fevers that plagued them in the islands.[12]

Because Portugal had seized control of the eastward route to the Indies, Spain tried again to reach them by a westward route going around the southern part of the American continent. The next very long, pioneering voyage was that led by Magellan in 1519. Magellan himself was Portuguese and had gained his experience in Portuguese expeditions, but was then in disgrace at home and had transferred his allegiance to Spain. His five ships left Seville in August 1519. After fifteen continuous weeks at sea, including a stormy navigation of the "Straits of Magellan" and a long journey into the ocean that he named "Pacific," they were in a desperate state, but "above all other calamities this was the worst: in some men the gums grew over the teeth, both lowers and uppers, so that they could not eat in any way and thus they died of this sickness; nineteen men died and . . . 25 – 30 became sick, some in the arms, in the legs or other places, so that few remained healthy."[13] However, their condition differed from that of the men in da Gama's expedition, because they were short of any kind of food, and chewing on leather or swallowing sawdust in their desperation.

Finally they reached the island of Guam and were able to obtain rice and fruit, on March 9. Ten days later they were in the Philippine Islands, and the sick were put to shore to enjoy exotic fresh foods that included bananas and coconuts. Magellan himself was killed in the following month. After making friends with the Sultan of Cebu Island, he offered to show his friendship by helping to attack any of his neighboring enemies. It was an ill-organized, amphibious operation on Mactan Island, and Magellan and seven of his crew died, bravely covering their men's retreat to their boats. A few days later, twenty-five more from his party were captured on Cebu by the Sultan's treachery, and the survivors escaped in two ships. After visiting the Spice Islands (i.e., the Moluccas) which were the target of their voyage, one ship continued the circumnavigation and finally reached Seville again on September 8, 1522. Despite the appalling losses, the value of the cargo of cloves in the one ship meant that the voyage had been commercially profitable to its sponsors.[14]

Three years later, Spain sent out a more ambitious expedition, with seven ships and 450 men, on the same voyage.[15] This time more of the ships returned. The flagship reached the Spice Islands, but in the last leg of the voyage across the Pacific the Admiral and 4 of her crew of 150 died. The

[11] Cohen (1969), 153.    [12] Moll (1944), 68–9, 507.    [13] Nowell (1962), 123.    [14] Morison (1974), 415–32.    [15] Ibid., 474–98.

contemporary record of the voyage says only that they had "weakness and sickness" with deaths continuing over many weeks.[16] In the Islands, the Portuguese, who were then well established, captured and burned the flagship. Spain then conceded that the Spice Islands were in the Portuguese "hemisphere," but they remained in the Philippines, trading with them by galleon from their colonies on the west coast of America.[15] This still involved a long, trans-Pacific voyage that was never freed from serious sickness, as is mentioned in the following account written seventy-five years later.

In 1602, Father Antonio de la Ascension, a would-be missionary of the Order of Barefoot Carmelites, was the diarist in an expedition from the south of Mexico exploring the coast of what is now Baja California and the State of California. Even though they had repeatedly been ashore and bartered for provisions with curious Indians, both officers and men began to suffer from disabling sickness. He said that it was the same illness that attacked

every year those who sail from the Philippines to New Spain [Mexico] and come in sight of the neighborhood of Cape Mendocino or in that latitude. . . . It is this which causes the death of almost all those who die on that route, there being years when hardly a person is left on the ships to manage the sails. . . . From the latitude of 30° upward, on those who are going . . . to Cape Mendocino, a very sharp, subtle and cold wind blows. . . . It must carry with it much pestilence, and if in itself the air is not bad, it produces with its subtlety and coolness some corruption of bad humors, especially in persons worn out and fatigued with the hardships of the navigation. The first symptom they notice is a pain in the whole body which makes it so sensitive to touch. . . . After this, all the body, especially from the waist down, becomes covered with purple spots larger than great mustard seeds. Then from this bad humour some strips or bands come behind the knee joints, two fingers and more wide like wales [weals]. . . . These become as hard as stones, and the legs and the thighs become so straight and stiff with them that they cannot be extended or drawn up a degree more than the state in which they were when attached. . . . The sensitiveness of the bodies of these sick people is so great that . . . the best aid which can be rendered them is not even to touch the bedclothes. . . . the upper and lower gums of the mouth in the inside of the mouth and outside the teeth, become swollen to such a size that neither the teeth nor the molars can be brought together. The teeth become so loose and without support that they move while moving the head. . . . With this they cannot eat anything but food in liquid form or drinks, . . . they come to be so weakened in this condition that their natural vigor fails them, and they die all of a sudden, while talking. Of this disease die those who come from China as well as did more than forty of this fleet, but Our Lord, Jesus Christ, was pleased that all passed away after having confessed and received extreme unction.[17]

Because conditions were so bad on this expedition, when they had reached Monterey (36°30′ N and were well short of their objective of

---

[16] C. Markham (1911), 50–3.     [17] Wagner (1929), 244–6.

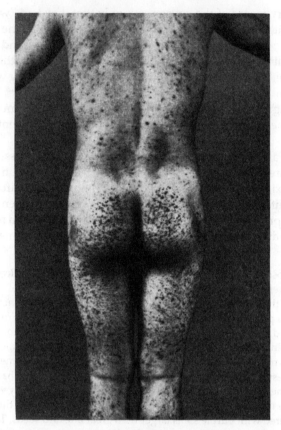

A sufferer from scurvy showing "the body, specially from the waist down, covered with purple spots," as described by Father Antonio de la Ascension in 1602.
Photograph of a Russian soldier in World War I. (From Aschoff & Koch, 1919,
p. 10.)

reaching at least 40° N), they headed south for home. When they had
retreated as far as Mazatlan, what they regarded as a miracle occurred:

As the sickness was so pestilential and inflammatory, all had lost confidence in being
able to regain their strength during the rest of their lives. When they arrived here,
nothing was heard on the ship but pitiful lamentations, and calls upon Our Lady, the
Virgin Maria del Monte Carmelo. . . . As a pious mother, she . . . came to their
relief in such a way that, in the nineteen days the ship remained here, almost all
recovered their health and strength, and the most crippled arose from their beds, so
that when the *Capitana* sailed from this port for Acapulco all could assist in manag-
ing the sails and keep watch and guard, as they had done on the outward
voyage. . . . health came not by doctors or surgeons, medicines or other drugs from
the pharmacies, or by any human remedy understood to be a medicine usually given
in this disease. If there was any human relief it was, in one case, the fresh and

substantial food which was given them by the good efforts of the General and the *alcalda major* of that province, and in the other a miraculous one, which brought health in a visible manner, namely, the eating of a little fruit found in those islands in great abundance at this season and which the natives call *jocoistles.* In other parts they call them *mancanillas.* . . . The pulp is white, . . . slightly sweetish, with a touch of acid, which gives it a very good flavor. It has a cleansing and astringent virture, and besides is a recognized antiseptic. It produces all these effects with noteworthy pleasure and suavity, and, taking the swelling out of the gums, contracts and fortifies them. With this the teeth become tightened and fast. If this fruit had not produced this effect, the fresh food which came could not have been eaten or passed into the stomach.

The way that the virtue of this little fruit came to be known was this. When some soldiers went to the island with the Father Comisario, to say mass and bury some dead, a corporal anxious to try things of the country, plucked one and cutting it in half with a knife and separating the skin from the pulp, put it into his mouth with difficulty, as best he could. He tried to chew it to see what flavor it had, and found it of good taste. He soon commenced to throw out of his mouth much fetid blood. . . . He then continued eating others, and each time he found himself better able to eat them. When he returned to the ship, he took a bunch with him. His shipmates commenced to try it, and went again to the island and brought a quantity of the fruit, and found themselves much improved. When the General returned from his journey inland to bring fresh food, they began to eat what had been brought with good spirit, at which he was much amazed and gave thanks to Our Lord, Jesus Christ, and His Blessed Mother. He arranged that fresh bread, hens, calves, kids and fruits should be brought each day, so that they were cured and recovered their health inside of nineteen days, as I have stated.[18]

The modern editor of this journal suggests that the fruit came from the cactus *Opuntia imbricata.* Although southern California has come to be associated with the large-scale production of oranges and lemons, these fruit were not native, and the citrus industry was established only after 1850.[19] It is again interesting that although we can now see that this sickness had been the common experience of long-distance voyagers for at least 100 years, Father Antonio regarded it as a local phenomenon brought on by some unique quality of the air off the central California coast.

## The French and English in North America

When it became clear that the Portuguese and Spanish had, between them, secured the two southern routes to direct and profitable trade with the Far East, the French tried to find a northern route. An expedition setting out in 1523 explored much of the eastern coast of North America and established that it was indeed a thick, continuous land mass separating them from the

---

[18] Ibid., 260–1. Buño (1953) reproduces another, very similar account of these experiences; also Lind (1772), 332–8.    [19] Lorenz (1957), 473.

East.[20] A second expedition, under Jacques Cartier, left in 1534 with the aim of trying to find a route that would lead them across the continent, beginning with a navigation into the St. Lawrence estuary. After a summer's reconnaissance, he returned safely to Saint-Malo, and immediately received support and royal approval for a further voyage. In the following May, he left with 112 men in three ships victualed for fifteen months. This time they took their ships up the Saint Lawrence River as far as the present site of Quebec, and some of them explored as far as the site of Montreal.[21] By then (late September), it was too late to return home; they were faced with wintering where they were, and built a stockade on an island in the river bed. From mid-November until mid-April 1536, their ships were frozen in. The following is a summary of their account:

In the month of December we received warning that the pestilence had broken out among the people of Stadacona [i.e., the local American Indians] to such an extent, that already, by their own confession, more than fifty persons were dead. Upon this we forbade them to come either to the fort or about us. But notwithstanding we had driven them away, the sickness broke out among us accompanied by most marvellous and extraordinary symptoms; for some lost all their strength, their legs became swollen and inflamed, while the sinews contracted and turned as black as coal. In other cases the legs were found blotched with purple-coloured blood. Then the disease would mount to the hips, thighs, shoulders, arms and neck. And all had their mouths so tainted, that the gums rotted away down to the roots of the teeth, which nearly all fell out. The disease spread among the three ships to such an extent, that in the middle of February, of the 110 men forming our company, there were not ten in good health so that no one could aid the other, which was a grievous sight considering the place where we were. For the people of the country who used to come daily up to the fort, saw few of us about. And not only were eight men dead already but there were more than fifty whose case seemed hopeless.

There died Phillip Rougemont, aged some twenty-two years, a native of Amboise. And because the disease was a strange one, the Captain had the body opened to see if anything could be found out about it, and the rest, if possible, cured. And it was discovered that his heart was completely white and shrivelled up, with more than a jugful of red date-coloured water about it. His liver was in good condition but his lungs were very black and gangrened; and all his blood has collected over his heart; for when the body was opened, a large quantity of dark, tainted blood issued from above the heart. His spleen for some two finger breadths near the backbone was also slightly affected, as if it had been rubbed on a rough stone. After seeing this much, we made an incision and cut open one of his thighs, which on the outside was very black, but within the flesh was found fairly healthy. Thereupon we buried him as well as we could. May God in His holy grace grant forgiveness to his soul and to those of all the dead.

After this the disease increased daily to such an extent that at one time, out of the three vessels, there were not three men in good health, so that on board one of the ships, there was no one to go down under the quarter-deck to draw water for himself and the rest. We were also in great dread of the people of the country, lest they

---

should become aware of our plight and helplessness. And to hide the sickness, our Captain, whom God kept continually in good health, whenever they came near the fort, would go out and meet them with two or three men, either sick or well, whom he ordered to follow him outside. When these were beyond the enclosure, he would pretend to try to beat them, and vociferating and throwing sticks at them, would drive them back on board the ships, indicating to the Indians by signs, that he was making all his men work below the decks; and that it would not do to have them come and loaf outside. This the Indians believed. And the Captain had the sick men hammer and make a noise inside the ships with sticks and stones, pretending that they were calking. At that time so many were down with the disease, that we had almost lost hope of ever returning to France.

From the middle of November until the fifteenth of April, we lay frozen up in the ice, while on shore there were more than four feet of snow, so that it was higher than the bulwarks of our ships, below hatches and above, there was ice to the depth of four finger breadths. And the whole river was frozen where the water was fresh up to beyond Hochelaga. During this period there died to the number of twenty-five of the best and most able seamen we had, who all succumbed to the aforesaid malady. And at that time there was little hope of saving more than forty others, while the whole of the rest were ill, except three or four. But God in His divine grace had pity upon us, and sent us knowledge of a remedy which cured and healed all.

One day our Captain caught sight of a band of Indians approaching from Stadacona, and among them was Dom Agaya whom he had seen ten or twelve days previous to this, extremely ill with the very disease his own men were suffering from. The Captain, seeing Dom Agaya in good health, inquired of him what had cured him of his sickness. Dom Agaya replied that he had been healed by the juice of the leaves of a tree and the dregs of these, and that this was the only way to cure sickness. Upon this the Captain asked him to show it to him that he might heal his servant who had caught the disease when staying in Chief Donnacona's wigwam at Canada, being unwilling that he should know how many sailors were ill. Thereupon Dom Agaya sent two squaws with our Captain to gather some of it; and they brought back nine or ten branches. They showed us how to grind the bark and the leaves and to boil the whole in water. Of this one should drink every two days, and place the dregs on the legs where they were swollen and affected. According to them this tree cured every kind of disease. They call it in their language *Annedda*.

The Captain at once ordered a drink to be prepared for the sick men but none of them would taste it. At length one or two thought they would risk a trial. As soon as they had drunk it, they felt better which must clearly be ascribed to miraculous causes; for after drinking it two or three times, they recovered health and strength and were cured of all the diseases they had ever had. And some of the sailors who had been suffering for five or six years from the French pox were by this medicine cured completely. Then there was such a press for the medicine that in less than eight days a whole tree as large and as tall as any I ever saw was used up, and produced such a result, that had all the doctors of Louvain and Montpellier been there, with all the drugs of Alexandria, they could not have done so much in a year as did this tree in eight days; for all who were willing to use it, recovered health and strength, thanks be to God.[22]

---

[22] Biggar (1924), 204–15. This is a more complete version than that used by Major (1932), 552.

From this dramatic account it seems clear that Cartier had not previously ever heard of such a disease, even though he had been on previous expeditions to Newfoundland and Brazil. It is also interesting that he regarded it as contagion, coming from their contact with the native Indians who were the first to show it. There has been a continuing controversy as to the identity of the tree which the Indian chief had called *"Annedda."* Jacques Rousseau made a careful review of all the possibilities; his conclusion is that it was probably the white cedar, *Thuja occidentalis*, and that this was brought to Fontainebleau from Canada in 1542 and named *arbor vitae* (tree of life), though the reason for this name was soon forgotten.[23] In 1542–43, another party of 200 French people, under the nobleman Roberval, wintered in almost the same spot. His account states: "In the end many of our people fell sick of a certain disease in their legs, loins and stomach, so that they seemed to be deprived of their limbs, and there died as a result about fifty."[24] There is no mention of their even trying the treatment that Cartier had found to be so successful only seven years previously.

For the next 100 years, the story was much the same.[25] Monsieur de Monts's party of eighty spent the winter of 1604–5 on another island, this time in the mouth of the St. Croix River (which now divides the state of Maine, in the United States, from New Brunswick, Canada, and is some 200 miles southeast of Cartier's island on the St. Lawrence), and thirty-six died. The chronicler, Monsieur Lescarbot, described the disease from which they were all suffering.[26] It was at that time called *mal de terre* (land disease), and, as he said, the description is virtually identical to that given by Cartier; *however*, the natives in that region had no knowledge of the annedda tree, and no other remedy could be found. "Our surgeons could not help, suffering themselves in the same manner as the rest."[27]

Those who survived until spring all then recovered, and in summary, Lescarbot speculated that

. . . there is here another bad quality of the air by reason of Lakes . . . and great rottenness in the Woods during the rains of Autumn and Winter . . . the winds do participate with the air, . . . and in the quality have great power over the health and sicknesses of men. . . . The seasons are also to be marked in this disease . . . as the growing heat of the Spring maketh the humours closed up in the Winter to disperse themselves to the extremities of the body, and so cleareth it. . . . I would add willingly to the aforesaid causes bad food, this sicknesse proceeding from an indigestion of rude, gross, cold and melancholy meats, which offend the stomache, I think it good . . . to accompany them with good sauces, be it of Butter, Oil, or Fat, all well spiced, to correct as well the quality of the meat, as of the body inwardly waxen cold. . . . He that shall eate good Capons, good Partridges, good Ducks, and good Rabbits, may be assured of his health, unless his body is of a bad

[23] Rousseau (1953), 117.    [24] Hakluyt (1928), *IX*, 459.    [25] Biggar (1901), 18–62; Heagerty (1928), 1–15.    [26] Purchas (1906), *XVIII*, 236–42. (This is a new edition of Purchas's seventeenth-century translation.)    [27] Grant (1907), 54.

constitution. . . . The young buds of herbs in the Spring time be also very sover-eign.

But one singular preservative against this perfidious sickness, is . . . to rejoice oneself, and do good, and to take pleasure in one's owne works. They that have done so, in our company, have found themselves well by it: contrariwise some always grudging, repining, never content, idle, have been found out by the same disease. It resteth necessary for the accomplishment of mirth, for every one to have the honest company of his lawfull wife: for without that, ones minde is always upon that which one loves and desireth; the body becomes full of ill humours, and so the sickness doth breed." [26]

It seems characteristically French that Monsieur Lescarbot should empha-size the importance of good morale in the maintenance of physical health, and that this required feminine companionship and meat served up with good sauces.

Monsieur de Champlain, who had been with de Monts's expedition, led another party that wintered at Quebec in 1608–9. Again there were deaths from *"mal de terre,"* which included the party's surgeon. His opinion was that "eating excessively of salt food and vegetables, which heat the blood and corrupt the internal parts" was the main cause, but that the cold of winter and the vapors arising from windy cleared land were secondary factors.[28] The disease attacked "one who was well clothed and housed and took particular care of himself as readily as one whose condition is as wretched as possible." He went on to say that it was the same disease that attacked sailors going to the East Indies, and that "some time ago the Flemish . . . found a very strange remedy, which might be of service to us, but we have never ascertained the character of it."

This last statement may relate to the experience of Francois Pyrard, who recorded the voyage of two French ships to the East Indies in 1602–3. For part of the outward journey they were in company with a Dutch ship. When they reached Madagascar, the French had a great number sick of "mal de terre" and the Dutch none.[29] He wrote that he "does not know why we French call it 'le mal de terre' [land sickness] for it comes at sea and is cured on land." (A recent suggestion is that "mal de terre" was an abbreviation of "mal de Terre-Neuve" [disease of Newfoundland], because it was suffered by early French fishermen working off that coast.[30]) Pyrard gave a detailed description of the disease, including the comment that "during this sickness a sore never heals or closes up," and that autopsies showed the brain to be black and tainted, the lungs dry and shrunk like parchment held to the fire, and the liver and spleen immoderately large and black. He also gave a list of conditions that brought it on ("great length of a voyage, want of cleanliness, sea air, the corruption of water and victuals"), and added that "it is very contagious even by approaching or breathing another's breath." At another

[28] Ibid., 147–8.   [29] Gray (1887), *I*, 31.   [30] Grmek (1966), 515.

point he said: "There is no better or more certain cure than citrons and oranges and their juice: and after using it once successfully everyone makes provision of it to serve him when in need." [31]

The English colonies being established on the east coast of America in the early 1600s had less severe winters than had been experienced by the French in Canada, but they still had serious health problems in the early years. In Massachusetts, it was said in 1628 that "for want of wholesome diet and convenient lodgings, many die of scurvy and other distempers." [32] In the journal for the following year, we read that, of the sixty who made up the first group in the founding of Plymouth, one-half died of scurvy, but none of those more recently arrived had died from it, and that after "this ship came, which brought store of juice of lemons, many recover speedily." [33] Lord De La Warre, who had been put in charge of the plantation (colony) of Virginia, returned home unexpectedly in 1611. His explanation to his sponsors was that he had been forced to do so by ill health. On his first arrival in Jamestown, he was "welcomed" by a violent ague (malaria?), which would come and go; then he had dysentery, followed by cramps and gout: "These making my body through weakness unable to stir . . . drew upon me the disease called the scurvy." His friends told him that "wanting [lacking] both food and physic fit to remedy such extraordinary diseases," he should go to the West Indies to recover. "There I found help for my health, by means of fresh diet, and especially of oranges and lemons . . . an undoubted remedy for that disease," but his friends still advised him that, before returning to Virginia, he should seek to recover his strength completely "in the natural air of my country." [34] One can imagine that worse things happened to less privileged men, but their story has gone unrecorded.

## British experience at sea

We have not, so far, referred to any British experiences at sea. The first exploration of the Newfoundland coast had been achieved by a British expedition under the leadership of an Italian, John Cabot, in 1497. [35] We have few details of the voyage; it was short, and there is no reference to serious sickness. In the first half of the sixteenth century, there were regular expeditions to the Newfoundland coast with the aims of fishing and general exploration, but they are referred to in passing, rather than recorded in detail.

The first really long-distance voyage of great interest was Sir Francis Drake's circumnavigation (1577–9) that extended to California. Only the flagship (the *Pelican*, renamed the *Golden Hind* in mid voyage) completed

[31] Gray (1887), *I*, 48; *II*, 390–1; see also Martin (1604), 128–30.    [32] Arber (1879), 485.    [33] Ibid., 576–7.    [34] Purchas (1906) *XIX*, 85–7.    [35] Morison (1971), 157–209.

the voyage. The impression from general histories is that Drake had no health problems. It is true that he had no deaths, but it does seem from the more detailed record that his men were repeatedly weakened and sick, but then "refreshed" again before this reached a crisis point. The voyage followed roughly Magellan's route to the Pacific.[36] When they were lying off the Brazilian coast at the mouth of the River Plate, it was decided to leave one ship behind to reduce work: "Some of our men being sick . . . and any diseased men might have more energy to recover themselves."[37]

Within the Straits they spent two days at an island where they found herbs growing wild, ". . . thyme, marjeron, alexander, scurvy grass etc. . . . whereby we received great help both in our diet and physic to the great relief of the lives of our men."[38] On entering the ocean which Magellan had found "pacific," they were battered by storms for fifty-six days and blown further south. Finally they were able to anchor at Henderson Island for two days.[36] The ship's chaplain records: ". . . the Lord having given us this breathing time . . . we set ourselves in order to go ashore to see what good things the place would yield us for the sustaining of our poor and feeble bodies, for our diet had been most pinching to nature in this time."[39] The main narrative then tells us that "our men began to receive good comfort, especially by the drinking of one herb (not much unlike that herb we commonly call Pennyleaf), which purging with great facility, afforded great help and refreshing."[40]

After their voyage north to California, and then a westward crossing of the Pacific, they were again "sickly, weak and decayed," and, when refreshing themselves in the Celebes, they refer to their enjoyment of especially large crayfish, "being a very good and restorative meat, the special means (as we conceived it) of our increase of health."[41] Finally, on the way back to England, on the west coast of Africa they found "oysters and plenty of lemons, which gave us good refreshing."[42] Drake later led several shorter expeditions to the West Indies, took a leading part in repulsing the Spanish Armada, and died in an epidemic of fever in a West Indies fleet in 1596.[43]

In 1582, an expedition led by Edward Fenton was beaten back from the Straits of Magellan by adverse storms and returned home. Richard Hakluyt, in his *Principall Navigations* published in London in 1589, records that when in sight of home two men died of the "skurvie."[44] This is one of the first appearances of the word in an English publication. The diary of the expedition's Secretary has recently been published; he noted, at the start of the voyage, "the more exercise within reason the better, for if you once fall to laziness and sloth, then the scarby is ready to catch you by the bones and will shake out every tooth in your head."[45]

---

[36] Morison (1974), 634–62.   [37] Penzer (1926), 113.   [38] Ibid., 130.   [39] Ibid., 134.
[40] Ibid., 32.   [41] Ibid., 74–5.   [42] Ibid., 84.   [43] Creighton (1891), 591.   [44] Hakluyt (1589), 672.   [45] Donno (1976), 110.

Thomas Candish (or Cavendish) led another circumnavigation, setting out in 1586 and following a similar route. On November 9 (i.e., on first reaching the Brazilian coast), one man "died of the disease called scorbuto which is an infection of the blood and liver";[46] Three weeks later, another died of the same disease, but there is no mention of any further cases. It seems that they were relatively fortunate with their weather even in the Straits, which they traversed in mid summer (i.e., January). Their journal refers repeatedly to the value they attached to fresh fruit, which they obtained on at least seven occasions. They also enjoyed the potatoes that were among the many things that they pillaged from Spanish settlements in South America.[47] They reached home in 1588 in time to hear the welcome news of the defeat of the Spanish Armada.

With the defeat of Spain, British sailors started on new adventures. The first, led again by Thomas Candish, was disastrous. They missed the best season for passing through the Straits, the ships were separated, and Candish died on the way back across the Atlantic. John Davis's ship, the *Dainty*, got through the Straits only to be driven back, and the crew rested on the Argentine coast; the narrator went on: "In this place we found a herbe called scurvygrass, which we fried with eggs, using train oil instead of butter. This herbe did so purge the blood, that it took away all kinds of swellings, of which many died, and restored us all to perfect health of body, so that we were in as good a case as when we came first out of England." [48] "Scurvy grass" can mean the spoonwort *Cochlearia curiosa*, or *officinalis*, or cresses such as *Cardamine glacialis* and *hirsuta*.[49] Train oil was obtained by boiling the carcasses of seals and skimming it off.

While in the same harbor, they killed and dried 20,000 penguins. A storm blew up, and they finally embarked only (!) 14,000. They planned to make their stock of food last them for a six-month voyage home; it worked out to include a ration of 1¼ penguins per head per day. Unfortunately, as the sailors went through the Tropics, the inadequately dried and salted birds began to corrupt and harbor loathsome-looking worms. After crossing the Equator,

the men began to fall sick of a monstrous disease: for in their ankles it began to swell, from thence in two days it would be in their breasts, so that they could not draw their breath, and then fell into their cods, and their cods and yardes did swell most grievously and most dreadfully to behold, so that they could neither stand, lie, nor go. Whereupon . . . divers grew raging mad, and some died in most loathsome and furious pain. . . . To be short, all our men died except sixteen of which there were but five able to move.[50]

---

[46] Hakluyt (1589), 809. The quotation is omitted from later editions.    [47] Hakluyt (1927), *VIII*, 206–54.    [48] A. H. Markham (1980b), 122.    [49] Hedrick (1909), 140–1, 181–2.    [50] A. H. Markham (1880b), 126–7.

Davis and the survivors just managed to bring the ship to the Irish coast and run her ashore. Obviously this disease was not scurvy. It has been suggested that it was caused by a parasitic infestation or, more probably, that it was a form of beriberi.[51] We shall have to return to the relationship between scurvy and beriberi in a later chapter.

Sir Richard Hawkins led another expedition in 1593. He had been a leader in the fight against the Armada, and both his father and grandfather had been famous sea captains. Twenty years after his return, he published his "observations" on the voyage; this is an elder's book of advice rather more than a detailed record of the voyage. They had sailed out of London in April, but were held up in Plymouth until mid-June. In about mid-August, they were near the Equator, without having made any landing en route, and scurvy began to appear in the crew. Because of contrary winds, it was not until mid-October, and with only four men still healthy, that they were able to go ashore – at Santos in southern Brazil. There, under a flag of truce the Portuguese allowed them to trade cloth for oranges and lemons.

There was great joy amongst my company; and many, with the sight of the oranges and lemons, seemed to recover heart. This is a wonderful secret of the power and wisdom of God, that hath hidden so great and unknown virtue in this fruit, to be a certain remedy for this infirmity; I presently caused them all to be divided amongst our sick men, which were so many, that there came not above three or four to a share.[52]

Hawkins then considered the diseases at some length: "The signs to know this disease in the beginning are divers: by the swelling of the gums, by denting of the flesh of the legs with a mans finger, the pit remaining without filling up in a good space. Others show it with their laziness: others complain of the crick of the back, etc., all which are, for the most part, certain tokens of infection."[53] He suggested that it was most prevalent in the Tropics and that Englishmen were particularly susceptible because they were not adapted to the climate, and the natural heat of the stomach was now dispersed through the body, "the stomach finding less virtue to do his office." This combined with the "greater force for digestion" required for meats preserved with salt, meant that the stomach was not distributing properly digested material, with the result that "all the body is unlusty, and unfit for any thing, and yieldeth to nothing so readily as sloathfulnes."[52]

To prevent its appearance at sea he recommended keeping the ship clean, sprinkling vinegar, and burning tar; feeding upon as few salt meats in the hot country as may be; ensuring that the crew have dry clothes; keeping the company at work, or "dancing," and providing a breakfast of bread and diluted wine so "that the pores of the body may be full when the vapours of the sea ascend up."[54]

He added (with some spelling changes):

[51] Creighton (1891), 593.    [52] Hawkins (1847), 80–2.    [53] Ibid., 56–7.    [54] Ibid., 58–9.

# OBSERVATIONS

OF

## S<sup>IR</sup> RICHARD HAVV-
KINS KNIGHT, IN HIS
*VOIAGE INTO THE*
South Sea.

Anno Domini, 1593.

❊❊❊❊❊❊

BEING betwixt three or foure degrees of the equinoctiall line, my company within a fewe dayes began to fall sicke, of a disease which sea-men are wont to call the scurvey:

The signes to know this disease in the beginning are divers: by the swelling of the gummes, by denting of the flesh of the leggs with a mans finger, the pit remayning without filling up in a good space. Others show it with their lasinesse: others complaine of the cricke of the backe, etc., all which are, for the most part, certaine tokens of infection.

The seething of the meate in salt water, helpeth to cause this infirmitie, which in long voyages can hardly be avoyded: but if it may be, it is to be shunned; for the water of the sea to man's body is very unwholesome. The corruption of the victuals, and especially of the bread, is very pernicious; the vapours and ayre of the sea also is nothing profitable, especially in these hot countries, where are many calmes.

The best prevention for this disease (in my judgement) is to keepe cleane the shippe; to besprinkle her ordinarily with vineger, or to burne tarre, and some sweet savours; to feed upon as few salt meats in the hot country as may be; and especially to shunne all kindes of salt fish, and to reserve them for the cold climates; and not to dresse any meate with salt water, nor to suffer the companie to wash their shirts nor cloathes in it, nor to sleepe in their cloaths when they are wett.

The second antidote is, to keepe the companie occupied in some bodily exercise of worke, of agilitie, of pastimes, of dauncing, of use of armes; these helpeth much to banish this infirmitie. Thirdly, in the morning, at discharge of the watch, to give every man a bit of bread, and a draught of drinke, either beere or wine mingled with water , that of the pores of the bodie may be full, when the vapours of the sea ascend up.

That which I have seene most fruitfull for this sicknesse, is sower oranges and lemmons, and a water which amongst others (for my particular provision) I carryed to the sea, called Dr. Stevens his water, of which, for that his vertue was not then well knowne unto me, I carryed but little, and it tooke end quickly, but gave health to those that used it.

The oyle of vitry is beneficiall for this disease; taking two drops of it, and mingled in a draught of water, with a little sugar. It taketh away the thirst, and helpeth to clense and comfort the stomache. But the principall of all, is the ayre of the land; for the sea is naturall for fishes, and the land for men. And the oftener a man can have his people to land, not hindering his voyage, the better it is. I wish that some learned man would write of it, for it is the plague of the sea, and the spoyle of mariners. Doubtlesse, it would be a meritorious worke with God and man, and most beneficiall for our countrie; for in twentie yeares, since that I have used the sea, I dare take upon me to give accompt of ten thousand men consumed with this disease.

Excerpts from Sir Richard Hawkin's observations at the end of the sixteenth century, in relation to scurvy – which, from his description, was probably combined with beriberi.

That which I have seen most fruitful for this sickness, is sour oranges and lemons, and a water which amongst others (for my particular provision) I carried to the sea, called Dr. Stevens' water, of which, for that its virtue was not then well known unto me, I carried but little, and it took end quickly, but gave health to those that used it. The oyle of vitry is beneficial for this disease; taking two drops of it, and mingled in a draught of water, with a little sugar. It taketh away the thirst, and helpeth to clense and comfort the stomach. But the principal of all, is the air of the land; for the sea is natural for fishes, and the land for men. And the oftener a man can have his people to land, not hindering his voyage, the better it is. I wish that some learned man would write of it, for it is the plague of the sea, and the spoil of mariners. . . . in twenty years, since that I have used the sea, I dare take upon me to give account of ten thousand men consumed with this disease.[55]

"Oyle of vitry" (or oil of vitriol) is, of course, sulfuric acid, made at that time by distilling ferrous sulfate.[56]

## British trading voyages to the East Indies

For all his belief in the special, curative virtues of oranges and lemons, Hawkins apparently had no idea of carrying them as preventives. But we do hear of this in the 1601 expedition with Sir James Lancaster as its General. This was the first sent out by the English East India Company to trade with Sumatra, and it followed the eastward route via the Cape of Good Hope. Lancaster had led a previous private expedition on this route in 1591, and cases of scurvy had appeared, as was to be expected, before they reached the Cape.[57] In the new expedition they had a very slow voyage, being at sea some twenty-nine weeks before reaching it. The journal reads:

. . . by this time very many of our men were fallen sick of the scurvy in all our ships, and unless it were in the general's ship only, . . . our weaknesses of men was so great that in some of the ships the merchants took their turns at the helm, and went into the top to take in the topsails, as the common mariners did. . . . the ninth of September, we came to Saldania [Table Bay at the Cape]; where the general before the rest bare in and came to an anchor, and hoisted out his boats to help the rest of the ships, for now the state of the other three was such that they were hardly able to let fall an anchor. The general went aboard them and carried good store of men and hoisted out their boats for them. And the reason why the general's men stood better in health was this; he brought to sea with him certain bottles of the juice of lemons, which he gave to each one, as long as it would last, three spoonfuls every morning, fasting; not suffering them to eat anything after it till noon. This juice worketh much the better if the party keep a short diet and wholly refrain from salt meat; which salt meat, and long being at the sea, is the only cause of the breeding of this disease. By this means the general cured many of his men and preserved the rest; so that in his ship (having the double of men that was in the rest of the ships) he had not so many sick nor lost so many men. . . .[58]

[55] Ibid., 59–60.   [56] Parkes (1830) *I*, 212: Clow & Clow (1952), 130.   [57] Foster (1940), 2.
[58] Ibid., 79.

Keevil suggested that the juice that Lancaster had brought from London had been preserved by the secret process referred to by Sir Hugh Platt in the broadsheet (advertisement) that he issued in 1607.[59] The document is of great interest, and the relevant portions are reprinted in the Appendix to this chapter. He claimed that by using "philosophical fire" (the scientific application of heat), he could preserve any kind of liquid from fermentation or other deterioration.[60] It would seem that he was using the principles of sterile "bottling" or "canning," the discovery of which is usually attributed to Nicholas Appert 200 years later. However, another writer has suggested recently that the "fire" was simply a nostrum in the form of a powder which he added.[61] In any case, Platt did not claim to have prepared the lemon juice for Lancaster, only that "the juice of lemons was found [by him] to be an assured remedy for the scurby." His claim was that such juice, by "fortifying it with his own fire, it will be lasting and durable," whereas if not so treated, it would "lose much of its first manifest nature, which it had while it was contained within its own pulp and fruit." Platt ended his sheet with the warning that, if there was no speedy acceptance of his offer, he would give up devoting himself to the public good and turn to more profitable pursuits. This seems to have been what happened, as nothing more is heard of such preservation of foods and beverages.

The Lancaster expedition spent six weeks at Table Bay "refreshing," and thus were "stronger at our departure . . . than we were at our coming out of England. . . . " After another seven weeks of sailing, "our men began again to fall sick of the scurvy," and it was "thought best to bear into the Bay of Antongile [on the northeast coast of Madagascar] to refresh our men with oranges and lemons, to clear ourselves of this disease." [62] A journal kept in another of the ships also noted that while there, they sent a boat to a nearby island: "They could get nothing there but oranges and lemons, of which we made good store of water, which is the best remedy against the scurvy." [63] "Lemon water" is the term often used in the 1600s for what we call "lemon juice." [64] They appear to have thought that when a large supply of lemons was available, they were best preserved as juice, even by the simple type of procedure that would have been practicable under their conditions.

A second expedition was sent out by the English East India Company in 1604 under Sir Henry Middleton. They sailed on March 25 and on May 16 they were at the Equator, "where many of our men fell sick of the scurvy, calenture [tropical fever], bloody flux [dysentry], and the worms; being left to the mercy of God, and a small quantity of lemon juice every morning. . . . " By July 13, when they were off the Cape, there were

at least 80 men sick of the scurvy in our ship. . . . The general commanded the tacks aboard, intending to go about the Cape [i.e., to continue the voyage without landing

[59] Keevil (1957), I, 108, 112.    [60] Platt (1607).    [61] French (1982), 60.    [62] Foster (1940), 82–3.    [63] Ibid., 124.    [64] Nixon (1937), 194–5; Creighton (1891), 602–3.

there] but our sick men cried out most lamentably, . . . made a petition to the general, most humbly entreating him for God's sake to save their lives, and to put in for Saldania, otherwise they were but dead men. The general perusing their pitiful complaint, and looking out of his cabin door, where did attend a swarm of lame and weak diseased cripples, and beholding this lamentable sight extended his compassion towards them, and granted their requests." [65]

The narrator may have intended to show the commander in a favorable light in painting this vivid picture. However, one would have expected him to have had a better knowledge of the health of his men, and to be doing everything to foster it, even from the selfish viewpoint of the safe handling of his ship, without any need for "humble entreaties."

The editor of the journal of this voyage commented that "the deficiency of lemon juice was an unfortunate oversight; Captain Lancaster has proved its importance." [66] Of course, we do not know that Middleton necessarily carried less than Lancaster, who issued a ration of three spoonfuls every morning. Other commentators have curtailed the quotation referring to Lancaster, ending after "cured many of his men and preserved the rest" and omitting "so that . . . he had not so many sick nor lost so many men." It does not seem certain that Lancaster's men were free from scurvy, only that they had *fewer* cases and *fewer* deaths than the other ships, and that *some* of the crew were still strong enough to hoist out the boats.

The Company's minutes for 1607 include "lemon water" in the supplies to be provided for future expeditions, [67] and a published letter book shows it among the victuals to be supplied for the third expedition, which sailed that year, though, strangely, it is the only item for which the quantity is unstated. The ration of cider, for example, was one quart per man per day, and 110½ tunns (barrels) were purchased. [68] Possibly the Company was uncertain as to how much was going to be available by the time of the fleet's departure. On this voyage the ships became separated in bad weather. David Middleton, in the *Consent*, reached Table Bay after eighteen weeks and recorded that "all our men in good health; only Peter Lambert the day before fell of the topmost head, whereat he dyed." [69] However, the other two ships had put into Sierra Leone at almost the same time, "grievously diseased," which is attributed in part at any rate to a shortage of water. While there they bought two to three thousand lemons on July 15, and two days later, it being a dry day, the Captain "appointed making of Lemon-water." Again on the 22nd, "we went ashore, where we made six or seven Barricos [small casks] full of Lemon-water" and "opened the Companies Firkin and Knives to buy Limes withall." [70]

There are published journals for sixteen more voyages in the period up to 1617. For eight there is clear evidence of scurvy in the outward voyage; [71, 72]

[65] Corney (1855), 6–7.   [66] Ibid., 6n.   [67] Creighton (1891), 602.   [68] Birdwood (1893), 100, 102.   [69] Purchas (1906), *III*, 51.   [70] Ibid., 506.   [71] Ibid., *III*, 74, 135; *IV*, 119, 280, 289, 502, 535.   [72] Foster (1934), 12–13.

for three more there is either positive mention of good health or else the stop at Table Bay was so short that it seems improbable that they had sick who needed to be refreshed ashore.[73] The remaining journals are very short and mainly designed as guides to navigational problems, so that the disease may have occurred but not been mentioned.[74]

The tenth expedition (1612) fared particularly badly. At Table Bay, some ninety sick men were landed from the *Dragon* and lodged in tents for eighteen days. All but one recovered rapidly; the captain attributed this to "beef and mutton, . . . fresh fish and fowl . . . fresh water and good air";[72] the ship's surgeon added "fresh salletts" (i.e., salads) to the list in his journal.[75] On the last leg of the homeward journey, "notwithstanding our short passage, having been from St. Helena but 2 months and 9 days, the one half or more of our company are laid up of the scurbute and two dead of it. Yet plenty of all victuals, bread, wine, beef, rice, oyle, vinegar, sugar, and all these even without allowance."[76] The captain attributed this misfortune to the abrupt change to much colder weather.

Creighton has cited more instances of illness from the 1620s[77] and it seems clear that scurvy remained a real hazard on the Company's voyages right through the seventeenth century. In 1630, a fleet from England landed their sick men in Madagascar "but having no oranges and lemons were not recovered but something better than they were."[78] In 1673, at the same point in the voyage, "half the fleet were disabled . . . [and] it is incredible to relate how strangely they revived in a short time by feeding on oranges and fresh limes. . . ."[79] Finally we read of a voyage in 1696 with men "falling down upon the scurvy," and, when approaching Table Bay, "most of our men were down sick and by then we had buried above thirty men."[80]

I have listed the problems on these voyages at some length because Nixon, writing in this century, quotes with approval a nineteenth-century writer who said: "We have already given an instance of the extraordinary efficacy of lemon-juice as a preventive of scurvy, in the first voyage for the establishment of the East India Company in 1600. After this it seems to have been pretty generally used"; later he said that "it is difficult to see how this knowledge of the value of oranges and lemons did not spread from the East India men to the Navy."[81] There appears to be confusion here between the value of fresh citrus fruit as a treatment for scurvy, which was generally accepted, and the usefulness of including lemon juice among a ship's victualing in the manner adopted by the East India Company. As we have seen, lemon juice of the quality supplied and in the quantities actually consumed could *not* be relied on to prevent outbreaks of scurvy in their ships.

What the actual practice was is uncertain. We have already noted that the quantity of lemon juice was left unspecified in the instructions for the 1607

[73] Purchas (1906), *III*, 90, 357; *IV*, 180.    [74] Ibid., *III*, 61, 304; *IV*, 77, 175, 214.    [75] Foster (1934), 101.    [76] Ibid., 91.    [77] Creighton (1891), 606–7.    [78] Foster (1910), 42.    [79] Crooke (1909), 58.    [80] Lubbock (1934), *II*, 462–3.    [81] Nixon (1937), 196.

expedition. Captain Keeling wrote home to the Company in 1616 when his ships had reached Saldania, and the published abstract of his letter includes the comment: "Your lemon water in that fleet stark naught [utterly worthless]."[82] However, it is not clear whether he refers to quantity or quality. One might expect that he was making this comment in connection with a high level of sickness among his men: In fact, three sentences earlier, the abstract states: "But 25 men sick in all the fleet to Saldania." This was obviously considered very good at that point for a total of 400–500 men aboard the fleet of four ships.

Woodall, the Company's consultant surgeon, wrote in his book, *The Surgion's Mate*, first published in 1617: "There is a good quantity of juice of lemons sent in each ship out of England by the care of the merchants, and intended only for the relief of every poor man in his need, which is an admirable comfort to poor men in that disease." And later, "Some surgeons also give of this juice daily to the men in health as a preservative, which course is good if they have store; otherwise it were best to keep it for need."[83]

In 1619, the minutes of the Court of Directors included instructions for "the fleet to be supplied with 15 tuns of white wine, to be drunk at the Line [the Equator] and the Cape, which is used by the Dutch to preserve men from scurvy, and will refresh the men and scour their maws [cleanse their stomachs or throats], and open and cool as well as lemon water."[84] It appears that they were looking for a way to do away with "lemon water," perhaps because the men disliked it. However, there must still have been a normal supply until 1625, because the minutes for that February noted "the demand of the woman, who serves the Company with lemon water, for 12 pence a gallon above the wonted [usual] price, pretending the scarcity of lemons." The Court decided "to send none, and hereafter to provide it out of Spain, where it is much better than here."[85]

In October of 1626, the Court of Directors debated the cause of the severe mortality from scurvy on the ships that had returned from the East that year – presumably the same ones that had been sent out without lemon juice in the previous year. "Some were of the opinion that lemon juice was very good but Mr. Styles related that tamarind was the excellentest thing"; however, there had been plenty of tamarinds on the ships, and a ship's officer had testified that the crew had all received tamarind.[86] Woodall had already referred to "the pulp of tamarinds" as an alternative antiscorbutic if lemon juice were not available,[87] and the 1621 expedition had been instructed that "at Saldania . . . search . . . be made for the drug tamerine [tamarind] which is a sovereign remedy for the scurvey or scurbuit." We know from a journal that in 1670, lime juice was being brought from the

[82] Foster (1897), *II*, 190.  [83] Kirkup (1978), 185.  [84] Creighton (1891), 603.  [85] Tickner & Medvei (1958), 43.  [86] McDonald (1954), 363.  [87] Foster (1928), 133.

West Indies to England in commercial quantities: ". . . the seas breaking into our ship and damaging a great deal of our goods . . . we lost fifty pounds worth of lime juice which ran out into the sea." [88]

## Dutch voyages to the East Indies

At this point, it seems useful to review the comparable experience of the Dutch because they had been the pioneers in challenging the Portuguese influence in the East Indies and had at first worked closely with the English as Protestant allies fighting against Catholic Spain. The Dutch East India Company sent out its first expedition in 1595, which clearly had the usual problem after entering the Indian Ocean: "They turned back to Madagascar because the scurvy was starting again and the sick people began to be many." [89] There they obtained sugarcanes, citrons, lemons, and poultry, and were amazed how "they are medicine to us." The second expedition sailed in 1598. Schoute, who has studied the Company's records says that the men on it "were served lemon juice as a preservative." [90] Nevertheless, they were glad to reach Mauritius "because scurvy [*schuerbaujck* in the original Dutch, and now *scheurbuik*] began to increase in the ships" and, again, to see Sumatra come in sight "because we had many people laid up with scurvy." [91]

As with the English Company the health record varied in subsequent voyages. Those that made the fastest trips did best, and the Dutch discovered more favorable westerly winds for the outward voyage, if they continued on east from the Cape of Good Hope, rather than going northeast at this point. [92] As an incidental result, the west coast of Australia was discovered. However, in other voyages there were many cases of scurvy and even deaths; records have been reproduced in some detail for expeditions leaving in 1631, 1647, and 1696. [93] McCord has reproduced some further descriptions of their experiences. [94]

The Dutch obviously knew the value of fruit. In their first voyage of circumnavigation (1958), scurvy was found to have cleared up in fifteen days with "a sort of sour plums" growing on an island off the coast of Brazil. [95] In the second voyage (1614), they stopped at Sierra Leona "since our crew was fast beginning to contract scurvy." In the first few days they obtained about 3,000 lemons by barter, and on the last "at a guess, some 25,000 lemons, all for a few beads and some poor Nuremberg knives." [96] Of course, even that number would provide 250 men with only one lemon per day for about three months.

[88] Lubbock (1934), *II*, 348.    [89] Rouffear & Ijzerman (1925), *II*, 10.    [90] Schoute (1937), 15.    [91] Keuning (1938), lxxxii.    [92] Tickner & Medvei (1958), 40–2.    [93] Naber (1932), *XIII*, 9; Schoute (1937), 16–7.    [94] McCord (1971), 488–91.    [95] Harris (1705), *I*, 30.    [96] De Villiers (1906), 176–7.

From the beginning, the Dutch tried to be more certain of regular supplies by establishing vegetable gardens and orchards both at Mauritius and St. Helena,[90] and later at the Cape of Good Hope, where by 1661, they were reported to have 1,000 citrus fruit trees.[92] They even tried the expedient of laying out small gardens on board ship, but it did not prove practicable because of waves breaking over the decks in bad weather.[93]

In the absence of fresh fruit on board, the sick were given wine, prunes, and lemon juice. At the end of the century, the standard provision for 100 men for twenty-seven months was one *aam* (150 liters) of lemon juice. This was a small quantity compared with the provision of 132 aams of wine and 20 aams of vinegar.[97] If the lemon juice had been distributed uniformly throughout the whole period, it would have provided about one spoonful per man every five days, or one fifteenth of Lancaster's issue on the first portion of the English expedition in 1601.[58] Almost certainly it was intended for issue to the sick by the surgeon. The daily diet for the sailors at this period started with cooked oatmeal and dried prunes with butter or other fat for breakfast. For lunch they had stockfish and white peas, with butter and mustard, except on two days of the week when they had "gray peas" with salted beef or bacon. Also each man received half a pound of bread and a pot of beer.[98]

The Dutch Company attached great importance to the supply of health-promoting drinking water, and encouraged the use of a distillation apparatus on board. The Directors gathered statistics and concluded that from 1691 to 1696, the death rate in ships in which a still was used was $9\frac{1}{2}$%, compared with $13\frac{1}{4}$% in the others.[99] The ships were also supplied with freshly dried and powdered scurvy grass, and the ship's "watermaker" had orders, whenever scurvy had appeared or was expected, to dip a bag of this for some hours into the water to be distilled. Obviously the expectation was that the active principle in the grass would leach out into the water and then vaporize when it was boiled, and finally recondense in the receiver. This idea may have come from a book published by the Leipzig scientist Andreas Moellenbrok in the 1670s on the antiscorbutic property of scurvy grass. He believed that the property was lost when the plant was dried with heat. To him it also seemed obvious that if the property had disappeared, it must have evaporated with the water; thus he referred to the "volatile salt of scurvy grass" as being the active factor.[100]

At least one ship's surgeon drew attention to warm clothing as being important for health: "Because of the intense cold and inclement weather at Tristan da Cunha . . . the people began to complain of tiredness and stiffness . . . the beginning of scurvy"; and later, "Most of the sickness oc-

[97] Tickner & Medvei (1958), 44. [98] Andel (1927), 88–9. [99] Schoute (1937), 18–23. [100] Lorenz (1953), 320–3.

# Cochlearia
# CURIOSA:

### OR THE
### Curiofities of Scurbygrafs.

Being an exact Scrutiny and careful De-
fcription of the Nature and Medicinal Uer-
tue of Scurbygrafs.

In which is exhibited to publick ufe the moft and
beft Preparations of Medicines. both Galenical and
Chymical ; either for Internal or External ufe , in
which that Plant, or any part thereof is imployed.

Written in Latine by Dr. *Andreas Valentinus*
*Molimbrochius* of *Lipfwick.*

Englifhed by **Tho. Sherley**, M. D. and Phy-
fitian in Ordinary to His prefent Majefty.

*LONDON,*

Printed by *S.* and *B. Griffin*, for *William Cade-*
*man*, at the Popes Head in the *New Exchange,*
and *Middle Exchange* in the *Strand*, 1 6 7 6.

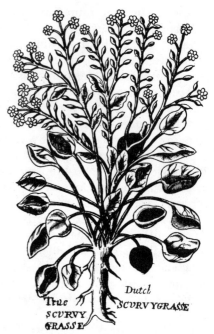

The title page of the English version of Moellenbrok's seventeenth-century book on
the virtues of scurvy grass and his illustration of the plant. (William Andrews Clark
Memorial Library, University of California, Los Angeles.)

cured through lack of clothing . . . [for] instead of giving them woolen
outfits they were given cotton on the thought that they would soon reach
warm climates."[101] In that voyage (1696), the surgeon did not appear to
have lemon juice at his disposal.

The Dutch and the English also shared in attempts to find yet another
route to the Indies – via the North – by traveling either northwest above
Canada or northeast above Russia. We shall return to these heroic attempts
in a later chapter dealing with Arctic experiences over a longer time span.

At this point, it seems fair to conclude, from the records of the early,
distant voyages, that sailors from any one nation of northern or western
Europe were about as subject to scurvy as those from any other, and that
their differences in dress, victualing, and other customs were not therefore
of great significance in relation to the disease. The descriptions of the disease
also coincided, except for the references in some instances to swelling, or
dropsy. In the report of the first Danish expedition to the Indies in the 1620s,
"dropsy" is the only sign associated with their serious sickness and mortality.[102] As mentioned already, it has been suggested that sailors in this condi-

---

[101] Schilder (1976), *I*, 45; de Hullu (1913), 247.     [102] Temple & Anstey (1932), 205, 221–2.

tion were suffering from beriberi rather than scurvy; we will in a later chapter (Chapter 10) consider why one disease rather than another should have occurred in different ships.

Also we must not lose perspective. The quotations selected for this chapter have concentrated on scurvy; however, this was not the only disease risk for sailors and explorers, and it was also not necessarily the most frightening. It became increasingly clear that some of the landing places that were valuable sources of fresh water and foods were also associated with infections, calentures (fevers), and bloody fluxes (dysentery).[103] These could appear suddenly and kill both officers and crew within a few days, with no means of treatment.[104] By contrast, scurvy – with its slow development at a more or less predictable time, and with the known cures such as "refreshing" on land with fresh fruits and herbs – was less frightening.

Thus Hawkins wrote in the account of his 1593 voyage:

It is wisest to shun the sight of them [the Cape Verde Islands], how much more to make abode in them. In two times that I have been in them, either cost us the one half of our people, with fevers and fluxes of sundry kinds; some shaking, some burning, some partaking of both . . . [and] in one of them it cost me six months sicknesse; which I attribute to the distemperature of the air. . . .[105]

In the Lancaster expedition of 1601, the call at Madagascar refreshed the men with oranges and lemons and cured their scurvy, but "here also we lost diverse of our men, which dyed of the flix"; the writer concluded that "it was by reason of the great heate and feeding of[f] the plantaines and lemons, which they did devour immoderately."[106]

Pyrard's expedition had a similar experience in the following year on the opposite coast of the island.

We thought we were arrived at this island most seasonably for our own refreshment and the benefit of the scurvy stricken. . . . But the result was quite otherwise, for they almost all died, and none recovered his health; even those that were whole fell sick of a burning fever, with frenzy, whereof they died at the end of two or three days. The disease was contagious, insomuch that a considerable number of the chiefest among us, and those of gentle birth, to the number of forty-one out of the two ships, died there as well of the scurvy as of the fever; and many that were sick of that disease, whereof he afterwards died. As it was believed that those sick of the fever had contracted it on shore, they were carried aboard, the air there being fresher than on land, while those sick of the scurvy, which is an ailment proceeding from the sea and its fatigues, were carried ashore.[107]

There are many further examples cited by other writers. They include the deaths of both Drake and Hawkins in the 1596 expedition, after they stopped at an island in the West Indies.[108] It is not surprising, therefore, that

[103] Keevil (1958), *II*, 60–6.     [104] Lubbock (1934), *I*, 209.     [105] Hawkins (1847), 45.     [106] Foster (1940), 145.     [107] Gray (1887), 34.     [108] Creighton (1891), 587, 591; Keevil (1957), *I*, 109.

with this experience some captains tried to avoid having their men go ashore unless it seemed essential, and then to have them back on ship before evening.[109] For a voyage made in 1673 and reaching an island off Madagascar, a passenger, Edward Fryer reported that

. . . half the fleet [was] disabled by distempers acquired by salt meats and a long voyage without refreshments. . . . [It is] incredible to relate how strangely they revived . . . by feeding on oranges and fresh limes and the very smell of the earth . . . only minding to fetch them anights that the misty vapours might not hinder the kind operation begun on their tainted mass of blood by the specifick medicines of nature's own preparing.[110]

In his invaluable monograph, Keevil has referred to this passage and has deplored Fryer's theorizing, "which led him to the 'misty vapors' of the night," and considered it an example of the obscurantism that misled practical people.[111] I feel that Fryer was only reporting the Captain's reasonable fear of the acute diseases that his men might contract if they were left on shore at night. The observation was sound enough, even if no one was to know until much later that the "bad quality" of the night air in those situations was that it contained biting insects which transmitted infection.

One is tempted to wonder, in view of the high death rates, how people could be induced to undertake these voyages, but, of course, life was not safe in Europe either. Apart from acute epidemics such as the Great Plague of London in 1665, there were endemic infections which always made the future uncertain to some extent. It was not an age of statistics, giving the relative risks of different ways of life. And, by voyaging to the Indies, there was always the *chance* of getting rich. Commission agents recruiting soldiers for the Dutch East India Company are said to have told them that "out there you hardly need a hammer to knock the diamonds off the rocks." [112]

---

[109] McDonald (1954), 362.   [110] Crooke (1909), 58.   [111] Keevil (1958), *II*, 165.
[112] De Hullu (1913), 248–9.

## Appendix: certain philosophical preparations of food and beverage for sea-men, in their long voyages

An advertisement believed to have been published by Sir Hugh
Platt in London in 1607, with some omissions and modernization
of spelling

And first for Food. A cheap, fresh and lasting victual, called by the names of Macaroni amongst the Italians, and not unlike (save only in format) to the cuscus [couscous] in Barbary, may be upon reasonable warning provided in any sufficient quantity, to serve either for change and variety of meat, or in the want of fresh victual. With this, the Author furnished Sir Francis Drake and Sir John Hawkins, in their last voyage.

2. Any broth or colase [sieved extract], that will stand clear and liquid, and not jelly or grow thick when it is cold, may also be preserved by this fire of Nature from all mouldiness, sourness, or corruption, to any reasonable period of time that shall be desired. A necessary secret for all sick and weak persons at sea, when no fresh meat can be had, to strengthen or comfort them.

3. Now for Beverages: All the water, which to the purpose shall be thought needful to be carried to sea, will be warranted to last sweet, good, and without any intention to putrefaction, for 2, 3, or 4 years together. This is performed by a philosophical fire, being of a sympathetic nature with all plants and animals. In the space of one month, the Author will prepare so many tunnes [casks] thereof, as shall be reasonably required at his hands.

4. By this means also both Wine, Perry, Cider, Beer, Ale and Vinegar may be safely kept at sea, for any long voyage, without fear of growing dead, sour or musty.

5. And, as for Medicine, if any Nobleman, Gentleman, or Merchant shall by his physician be advised to carry any special distilled waters, decoctions or juices of any plant or any other liquid vegetable or animal body whatsoever with him in any long voyage, this Author will so prepare the same only by fortifying it with his own fire of kind, that he may be assured of the lasting and durability thereof, even at his own pleasure.

6. Here I may not omit the preparation of the juice of Lemons with this fire: Because it hath of late been found by that worthy Knight Sir James Lancaster to be an assured remedy in the scurvy. And though their juice will, by natural working and fermenting, in the end so spiritualize itself, as that it will keep and last either simply of it self, or by the help of a sweet olive oil supernatant: yet this Author is not ignorant, that it hath lost much of his first manifest nature, which it has whilst it was contained within its own pulp and fruit: (as is evident in the like example of wine, after it hath wrought long, which differeth exceedingly both in taste and nature from the grape out of which it is expressed) whereas being strengthened with this philosophical fire, it retaineth still both the natural taste, race [distinctive flavor], and verdure [freshness], that it had in the first expression: and so likewise of the Orange.

[Paragraphs 7–12 which deal with various medicines, have been omitted]

Thus much I am bold to offer and publish for the benefit of seafaring men, who for the most part are destitute both of learned Physicians and skillful Apothecaries: and therefore have more need than others to carry their own defensatives [prophylactics] and medicines about them. Which if it shall receive entertainment according to the worth thereof and my just expectation, I may happily be encouraged to pry a little further into Natures Cabinet, and so to disperse some of her most secret jewels, which she hath long time so carefully kept, only for the use of her dearest children: otherwise, finding no speedy or good acceptance of this my proffer (but rather crossed by malice or incredulity) I do here free and enlarge my self from mine own fetters: purposing to content my spirits, with such private and pleasing practices, as may better sort with my place and dignity, and in likelihood prove also more profitable in the end, than if I had thanklessly devoted my self to Bonum Publicum [the public good]. In which course, happy men are sometimes rewarded with good words: but few or none, in these days, with any real recompense.

H. P.

# 2

## The writings of learned men (1540–1700)

As we have already seen, the English sea captain Sir Richard Hawkins said in the 1590s that in his twenty years at sea he could give account of 10,000 men consumed with scurvy, and added that he "wished some learned man would write of it, for it is the plague of the sea." [1]

It was only a minority of the early expeditions that carried a surgeon, and he would naturally have been a lowly member of his profession (or otherwise he could have obtained better employment). He was therefore unlikely to write a treatise on the subject or to find a publisher if he did. Surgeons were also considered inferior to physicians. Even though they had, in practice, broken free from being "barber-surgeons," they still suffered from the old Greek stigma of being mere "mechanicals" rather than members of the academic, intellectual community as physicians were. Their education was often mostly as apprentices to other surgeons, and they were not regarded as "officer class." [2] That they did not, typically, go to a university and receive an academic indoctrination may have been no bad thing if it left them with a fresher mind to see things as they were and make their own observations.

The physicians, of course, were less likely to encounter cases of scurvy. Nevertheless, there had already been some "learned writing" at the time of Richard Hawkins's appeal. In 1541, John Echth, a Dutch physician practicing in Cologne had sent a short treatise to a colleague for his consideration, though it was published only after his death in 1556.[3] It was written in Latin, the international language of educated Europeans, and even the author's name was given as Johannus Echthius. It was intended to be an "epitome" or summary of the subject. He called the disease "scorbutus" and explained that he had Latinized the Danish word *Scorbuck*, which had been taken over

---

[1] Hawkins (1847), 59–60.   [2] Keevil (1957), I; 58, 68–9, 110.   [3] Echthius (1541); Lind (1772), 549.

29

by German-speaking people. (Modern scholars, in turn, have traced the word back through the earlier Scandinavian forms of *skjoerbug* and *skörb-jugg* to the old Icelandic *skyrbjûgr*, which is believed to signify "cut (or ulcerated) swellings."[4] As seen already in Chapter 1, even in English, early forms of the word were scarby and scorby.)

## A disease of the spleen

A medical work of this period makes little sense to the modern reader without some knowledge of the assumptions that must then have seemed so obvious to the community of physicians that they did not need to be spelled out in relation to a specific disease. One assumption was that the world had been in a continual state of decline since the Creation, and that mankind was likewise in a state of steady degeneration. It followed that the ancients were necessarily wiser and better informed than people in later ages, and were consulted as authorities.[5] The main responsibility of the physician was, therefore, to associate his patient's condition with a disease described by an authority, and the earlier the better. This is, of course, the opposite of the modern presumption, which is that of two papers, the later one is more likely to be correct because it has (or should have) been written with additional information to draw on.

The importance of this point becomes apparent in Echth's second sentence: "Scurvy is a disease of the spleen." If this had been a modern work, one would at once assume that the statement had been based on autopsies in which the author had seen that the spleen looked grossly abnormal and/or that microscopic examination showed cellular changes. This is not what Echth had done. He had examined the classical descriptions of different diseases and concluded that "scorbutus" could be identified with a condition described in a number of early writings. His earliest quotation is from Strabo, the Greek geographer and historian born in 63 B.C. In his *Geography* (Book 16.4.23), he described the experiences of a Roman army in Egypt, where a treacherous local leader had misdirected them, hoping that the Romans would be

wiped out by hunger and fatigue and diseases. . . . Gallus, landed his army at Leucê Comê, the men now being sorely tried with "stomakake" and "sceletyrbe," which are native ailments, the former disclosing a kind of paralysis round the mouth and the latter round the legs, both being the result of the native water and herbs. At all events, he was forced to spend both the summer and winter there, waiting for the sick to recover.[6]

Echth also found a rather similar quotation in the *Natural History* (Book 25.6.3) written by Pliny, the Roman naturalist who was born in A.D. 27 and

---

[4] Vassal (1956), 1280 – 1.  [5] O'Hara-May (1977), 18.  [6] Jones (1917) *VII*, 356 – 9.

who died of asphyxiation in A.D. 79, while studying the eruption of Vesuvius that buried Pompeii in its ashes. In the section of his book concerned with the medicinal values of plants, he refers to a unit of Roman army that had been in an encampment in Germany for two years, obtaining all their fresh water from

a single spring in the vicinity of the sea shore . . . [which] was productive of loss of the teeth and total relaxation of the joints of the knees: the names given to these maladies, by medical men, were stomacace and sceloturbe. A remedy for them was discovered, however, in the plant known as the *britannica*, which is good, not only for diseases of the sinews and mouth, but for quinzy also, and injuries inflicted by serpents. This plant has dark oblong leaves and a swarthy root: the name given to the flower of it is vibones, and if it is gathered and eaten before thunder has been heard, it will ensure safety in every respect. The Frisii, a nation then on terms of friendship with us, and within whose territories the Roman army was encamped, pointed out this plant to our soldiers.[7]

The translators explain that *Brittanica* does not mean that it came from Britain, but rather from a local marshy area, which had a similar name. It is not known what the plant was. Certainly the description is not that of scurvy grass.

From these two quotations taken from the writings of general historians, Echth obviously gained confidence that scorbutus was a disease known in classical time. This meant that he could turn to the professional writings of earlier physicians for a detailed diagnosis. Naturally he found them in fair agreement because they were all trying to follow the same tradition. Thus Paulus Aegineta (Paul of Aegina, the Greek island close to Piraeus), who probably wrote early in the seventh century A.D., began the preface to his comprehensive medical work with the statement: "It is not because the more ancient writers had omitted anything relative to the Art [of Medicine] that I have composed this work, but in order to give a compendious course of instruction."[8] Then as Echth saw, in the section of the book dealing with the spleen (which is Book III, Section 49 and *not* 40 as in his reference):

When the melancholic humor is infarcted [trapped and concentrated] in the spleen in the first place inflammation occurs . . . , but afterwards it passes into "scirrhus" [swelling and hardness]. . . . Persons thus affected have fetor of the mouth, their gums are corroded, and ulcers in their legs are difficult to heal. When the liver sympathises, dropsy takes place. . . .[9]

Aegineta, of course, made no claim to be original, and something very similar to the last part of the quotation is to be found in De Medicina (Book II, Section 7.21) written by the Roman physician Celsus in about A.D. 30: "But these in whom that spleens are enlarged, in these the gums are diseased, the mouth foul, or blood bursts out from some part. When none of

---

[7] Bostock & Riley (1856) *V*, 85–6.   [8] Adams (1884), *I*, xvii.   [9] Ibid., 577.

these things happen, of necessity bad ulcers will be produced on the legs, and from these black scars."[10]

The concept of the normal function of the spleen certainly goes back to the Greek physician Galen, who lived from A.D. 130 to 200, finished his education in Alexandria, and practiced in Rome. His writings were accepted as authoritative for the next thirteen centuries, so that he was finally an influence from which the progressive physician struggled to be liberated. But in his own time he was an innovative thinker,[11] and fascinated by the idea that Nature had equipped animals with the best possible bodies; he was determined to show what was the essential function and interrelation of every part.[12]

Writing of the spleen, he ridiculed another Greek physician who had concluded that it was an organ without a function: "I suppose that when Nature had formed the liver on the right side of the animal while still in the uterus, she placed the spleen opposite to it . . . because she wished to make something to occupy that space . . . , as if by extending the stomach slightly in that direction she could have been spared the necessity of creating something useless."[13] As an ingenious speculative physiologist he at once advanced a function:

The spleen is the instrument which eliminates the thick, earthy, atrabilious humor [black bile] formed in the liver. It attracts them . . . by means of a venous vessel like a canal and takes time to elaborate and alter them. . . . Those altered become nutriment for the spleen . . . [and] those that cannot be changed . . . are discharged by another venous channel into the stomach.[13]

The circulation of the blood was not, of course, to be discovered until the early 1600s, so that in 1540 a scholar who had himself done no dissection would see nothing improbable in Galen's conception of one set of veins draining from the liver to the spleen, and another from the spleen to the stomach.

Echth now had all the material for his argument that, in a sufferer from scurvy with the spleen swollen and hard (i.e., with its normal functioning blocked), the "bad" or "putrid" fractions of the blood in the liver, i.e., the black bile, could no longer be cleaned up. These fractions would, therefore, be dispersed throughout the body and rejected in the form of black spots on the skin as well as giving a swarthy complexion. The weakened, unnatural blood also diffused generally, resulting in a lack of energy – physical or mental or both. Lastly the swollen spleen had a direct effect of pressure on the diaphragm, which accounted for the fact that pain with breathing was an early symptom of scurvy.[14]

This is a quite clever reconciliation of the old theory and the sailors' records. Following the custom of his predecessors, Echth felt no need to

[10] Spencer (1935), 125.    [11] Brock (1929), 24.    [12] May (1968), 9–10.    [13] Ibid., 232–3.
[14] Echthius (1541), 181–2.

differentiate in his statements between *facts*, for which he had supporting evidence, and *ideas*, which were merely "possible explanations" or hypotheses. Having given a "theory" of the disease, he went on to give a list of the causes of its appearing among Dutch sailors. These correspond, in fact, to the characteristic hardships complained of by all the seamen of this period – corrupted water, poor quality food (especially meats preserved so as to be virtually indigestible), lack of sleep, hard physical work, and misery.[15] In addition, he listed "warm, ambient air dispersing the subtle parts of the blood, leaving behind thick, fatty residues [clots?] of blood." This is surprising because the sailors had often associated the disease with a sudden transition from hot to cold weather.[16] It is also surprising in view of the melancholic humor which Echth associated with the disease. This needs more explanation.

## The melancholic humor

According to Hippocratic medicine, good health came primarily from a proper balance of all the parts of the body and particularly of the four main fluids (or "humors"): blood, phlegm, yellow bile, and black bile.[17] These, in turn, were thought to be produced by different organs and had distinctive qualities in terms of "hot or cold" and "wet or dry."[18] Then to complete the picture, each humor was associated – particularly when Greek medicine was interpreted by the Arabic school – with a different temperament. Finally we have:

| Fluid (or humor) | Organ of origin | Quality | Temperament associated with excess of humor |
|---|---|---|---|
| Blood | Heart | Hot & wet | Sanguine (courageous, hopeful, amorous) |
| Phelgm | Brain | Cold & wet | Phlegmatic (cold, dull, even-tempered) |
| Yellow bile | Liver | Hot & dry | Choleric (irascible, passionate) |
| Black bile | Spleen | Cold & dry | Melancholic (gloomy, depressed) |

The principle that people with different temperaments fall into "types" and that they are particularly at risk from different diseases is not foreign to us. For example, it is believed that people with a "type A" personality, i.e., competitive and impatient, are particularly subject to heart attacks.[19] Furthermore, it is believed that if people will change their pattern of behavior, they will be less at risk from the disease.[20]

[15] Ibid., 183–4.   [16] Foster (1934), 91–2.   [17] Brock (1929), 9.   [18] Ackerknecht (1982), 53; Temkin (1973), 17.   [19] Friedman & Rosenman (1959), 1286.   [20] Friedman, Thoresen, et al. (1982), 83.

Traces of the old humoral theory itself are still to be found in our language. Thus, "big-hearted" is a synonym for "generous," and "lily-livered" (i.e., with a liver that is pale and therefore deficient in yellow bile) means "lacking the will to fight." Without really believing in the theory, it comes naturally to us to describe an abstract quality such as "generosity" in terms of something physical like "a big heart." It does not seem to us so natural to do the reverse, for example, to feel someone's pulse and say "I can hear your generosity beating." But the Greeks did not seem to feel this difficulty, perhaps because they felt that things were so permeated by qualities that the physical and nonphysical were not really separable.[21] And, to return to our example, it was natural to describe the fluid in a vein leading to the spleen as "the melancholic humor."

One practical effect of the system for Echth was that he could conclude that anyone who exhibited a melancholy temperament was under the influence of that humor, and might therefore develop scurvy even in the absence of any external stresses. As we shall see later, this idea led to scurvy being considered *cachexia universalis* (a universal, chronic disease) by Eugalenus and others. Echth had no specific treatment to propose for the disease, though one presumes that he hoped for a gradual cure after the external causes had been removed by providing good food, good water, rest, and "banishing grief and cares."

From 1560 to 1600, at least nine Dutch or German physicians, including Sennert and Eugalenus, wrote Latin treatises on scorbutus, obviously with much common ground and repetition. Their main points were summarized by James Lind in 1753 in his own *Treatise*,[22] which was reprinted in 1953.[23] Beaudouin Ronsse (Ronsseus) described it in 1564 as a common disease in the damper, boggy parts of Holland, particularly in rainy seasons, and said that it could be cured with scurvy grass and watercress, or infusions of them.[24] He also noted that Dutch sailors had found that they could cure the condition by eating oranges. He thought that this discovery was probably accidental, rather than "guided by reason," and that some Dutch sailors returning from Spain were attracted by the novel richness of oranges, "and by their greedy gluttony unexpectedly drove out the disease and had this happy experience not once only but repeatedly." He concluded that

although this is empirical it seems to have something in common with reason, for inasmuch as in diseased spleens we need, on Galen's authority, reducing drugs without obvious heating qualities, together with moderate astringent action so that the affected part may be strengthened, we shall pronounce oranges not wholly useless in a diseased spleen. For they put an end to and check the excessive flow of blood, and give strength to the affected part.[25]

[21] Siegel (1960), 355.    [22] Lind (1753).    [23] Stewart & Guthrie (1953).    [24] Ibid., 264–5.
[25] Nixon (1937), 197–8.

To the modern reader, this seems extraordinarily arrogant: Surely if oranges worked, they worked and did not need to be pronounced "not useless" by someone without first-hand experience of their effect. The quotation is another illustration of the attitude of mind that ". . . a so-called logical argument, rather than the objective experiment was the way to convince. . . ."[26]

Peter Forest (Forestus) writing at about the same time was rather more modest. Lind said that he "very ingenuously owns that physicians were first made acquainted with those remedies [the juices of different herbs and grasses] by the vulgar; they [the physicians] having only contrived the exhibition [administration] of them in more elegant forms."[27] His medicine, "*Syr. sceletyrb.* Foresti" was prepared by boiling the juices of brook lime and scurvy grass into a syrup with sugar, and is mentioned repeatedly by other doctors well into the next century. From his descriptions, it seems clear that he had treated a great many cases of scurvy in Holland, and he complained that other doctors were confusing it with *lues venerea* (syphilis).

From this time on, one has to note that the sailors' reports may themselves have been colored by their having read the treatises. Thus a translation from Francois Pyrard's report of his expedition to the East Indies in 1602–3 states: ". . . when first overtaken with the disease, the thighs and legs are covered with little pustules and spots like flea-bites, which is the black blood issuing through the pores of the skin."[28] Lind's summary of a treatise published in 1567 by John Wier, a physician in France, includes the description: "smaller spots, resembling blood sprinkled upon the part (or flea bites, but larger) appear on the legs and thighs. . . ."[29]

In England, the first medical references to scurvy appeared in two general manuals of advice for military or sea surgeons. The first, by William Clowes, published in 1596, was said to be for curing all those burned with the flame of gunpowder or wounded with musket shot. However, it did include an account of his successful treatment of two sailors "which fell sick at sea of the scorby," and they had all the usual signs of the disease.[30] His treatment was "performed by the advice and counsel of learned physicians." He began by taking eight ounces of blood from the middle vein of the left arm, and he then gave a strong laxative. As their standard drink, his patients were given new ale which had had scurvy grass, newly picked and bruised in a stone mortar, steeped in it for two days together with cinnamon and ginger. Also, each morning they were given a portion of "almond milk"; this was prepared by beating up almonds with scurvy grass and watercress, bringing the mix to the boil with sugar and rose water. Their meat stews also had scurvy grass and watercress added to them. As a direct treatment of the gums, Clowes gave a gargle made of a variety of ingredients recommended

[26] Renbourn (1960), 142.    [27] Stewart & Guthrie (1953), 273–6.    [28] Gray (1887), 391.
[29] Stewart & Guthrie (1953), 266.    [30] Starnes & Leake (1945), 40–3.

by John Wier; he also put a plaster on their legs. Lastly, he had them inhale a vapor while sitting up in bed, connecting up a flexible tube to a boiling pot containing vinegar with aromatic gums added. This was done "to open their obstructions inwardly . . . and thus by the grace of God and careful diligence they were perfectly cured." He also mentioned that earlier in his career he had been in charge of the children's department in a London hospital and "had 20 or 30 infected with the Scorby at a time."[30]

We have already referred to John Woodall, the Surgeon-General of the British East India Company, in relation to his emphasis on provisioning their ships with juice from oranges, lemons, or limes. He coupled this with a recommendation of two to three spoonfuls of lemon juice, as a medicine against the scurvy – and as a preventive too, if enough could be spared. But what more did he say about the "theory" of the disease? His book, *The Surgions Mate*, first published in 1617, was addressed to young surgeons in the Company's ships, to give them direction "that they may be better able to undertake their charge."[31] Although he wrote that "a learned treatise befits not my pen" and that he would "heartily rejoice to see any good man do [it], knowing my own weakness,"[32] his chapter on scurvy spans twenty-three pages.

He referred to his reading of Echth and other continental treatises, which is apparent in his first sentence: "The scurvy is a disease of the spleen, whereby it is sometimes wholly stopped. . . ."[32] Further on he wrote:

Some judicious writers do affirm this sickness to come by the multitude of melancholic humors gathered in *Vena Porta* by which, it is said, the milt [liver] both draw unto it melancholy humors, and so transporteth it from the milt into the ventricle [heart]. But truly the causes of this disease are so infinite and unsearchable, as they far pass my capacity to search them all out.[33]

Perhaps he meant that he could not suggest why the "accidental" causes of life at sea should result in the "immediate" causes of a damaged spleen and/or liver. He had no doubt that they were damaged: ". . . divers of those which had been opened after death had their livers utterly rotted. Others had their livers swollen to an exceeding greatness, some the spleen extremely swollen."[34] Also, as so many others had done, he remarked on how some could be swollen as with a dropsy and others have their legs withered and apparently dried up.[35]

He attributed the occurrence of the disease on long voyages to the usual factors – the inevitable salt diet, lack of sweet water and wine or beer, and want of fresh clothing. As regards the treatment that was possible at sea, he said: "The use of the juice of lemons is a precious medicine and well tried . . . [so] let it have the chief place. . . ."[36] He went on to advise that where the juice or any kind of citrus fruit was not available, the surgeon

[31] Woodall (1617).     [32] Kirkup (1978), 178.     [33] Ibid., 179.     [34] Ibid., 182.     [35] Ibid., 181.     [36] Ibid., 185.

should use oil of vitriol (sulfuric acid), "as many drops as may make a cup of beer, or water . . . , a little sour." Keevil, writing with hindsight, has castigated him for not emphasizing the unique quality of lemon juice.[37] However, Woodall clearly thought that vitriol was a proven treatment "for of my experience I can affirm that good oil of vitriol is an especially good medicine in the cure of scurvy." [34]

Woodall also referred to the paradox that although scurvy was classified as a "cold" disease and therefore required correction with "hot" medicines, both lemon juice and vitriol were themselves classified as "cold" and were given in cases of burning fevers: ". . . many a medicine hath a seeming show to be cold and yet doth contrary effects . . . all which may easily be proved either hot or cold, by their several strong operations and effects." [38] In other words, he was skeptical of the whole classification of drugs or foods into "hot" and "cold" that had remained influential from the time of Galen.[39]

## A physician's case notes

By a fortunate chance, we can still read some of the case notes of a physician who practiced in the English Midlands in the early 1600s, and who based his diagnosis and treatment of scurvy on the publications of Sennert and Eugalenus. He was John Hall, born in 1575 and a student at Cambridge, graduating with a Bachelor of Arts degree in 1593.[40] He would not have received any medical education in that period, and how he received it subsequently is unknown, but about the year 1600 he began to practice in Stratford-on-Avon. This was, of course, the home town of William Shakespeare, the great dramatist, who still lived there with his wife, Anne Hathaway, when he could get away from his duties in London. They had two daughters, and in 1607 the elder, Susanna, then twenty-four years old, married John. On her father's death in 1616, they moved in to live with his widow. It is perhaps because of his reflected fame as Shakespeare's son-in-law that some years after his death, his notes were purchased from Susanna by another physician, Dr. James Cook, who then transcribed them from an abbreviated Latin. They were finally published as *Selected Observations on English Bodies* in 1657, with a subtitle indicating that these were "cures performed on eminent persons in desperate diseases." [41] John Hall was obviously successful and in demand from leading families in an area stretching over twenty miles from Stratford, which was considerable in view of the time taken to reach patients on horseback.

Altogether, the notes refer to 182 cases, and at least 22 of these patients were diagnosed as having scurvy, or a scorbutic form of another disease –

[37] Keevil (1957–8), *I*, 220.    [38] Starnes & Leake (1945), 194.    [39] Ogden (1938), xvii–xviii, 110–2.    [40] Joseph (1964), 1–16.    [41] Ibid., 31–47.

dropsy, gout, epilepsy, colic, headaches, or wandering pains.[42] The following is an example of a relatively straightforward case (probably in 1622):

Mrs. Mary Talbot, Sister to the Countess of Northampton was troubled with the Scurvy with swelling of the Spleen, erosion of the Gums, livid Spots of the Thighs, Pain of the Loins and Head, with Convulsion and Palsy of the Tongue; her Pulse was small and unequal, her urine was troubled and thick. The Countess asked me whether there were any hopes of Life? I answered, yes, if she would be patient and obedient, although her Scurvy was confirmed.[43]

As usual he began by giving the patient a laxative, and then had her drink nothing but an antiscorbutic infusion. This was prepared by boiling scurvy grass and watercress in new beer for eight hours. In this case, the patient was also given an "electuary" (medicine in the form of a paste) made by pounding up the flowers of scurvy grass. She began walking after about three weeks "and at last was very well."

In 1630, the notes refer to "Wife," which has been taken by editors to mean his own wife Susanna, who would then have been forty-seven years old. She

was troubled with the Scurvy, accompanied with Pain of the Loins, Corruption of the Gums, Stinking Breath, Melancholy, Wind, Cardiac Passion [disorder causing distress], Laziness, difficulty of breathing, fear of the Mother [hysteria], binding of the Belly, and torment there, and all of a long continuance, with restlessness and weakness. The tenth day taking cold, she had again miserable pain in her joints, so that she could not lye in her Bed, insomuch as when any helped her, she cried out miserably.[44]

He gave her an electuary made from a conserve of the tops and leaves of scurvy grass with other plants and other ingredients, with added "oil of sulfur" (sulfuric acid) sufficient to "sharpen it." She was given in infusion to drink that was made with white wine; it had a variety of herbs and even red coral and shavings of ivory infused in it, but the major ingredients were again scurvy grass and watercress. "By these she was cured." [44]

My final excerpt seems particularly removed from previous descriptions of scurvy:

The Lady Brown of Radford, was oppressed with these Scorbutic Symptoms, as with binding of the Belly, Melancholy, Watchfulness, troublesome sleep, Obstruction of the Courses [menstrual periods], continuing for a year, and swelling of the Belly, especially about the Spleen; she felt a continual beating at the mouth of her Stomach, so that it might be felt with the hand. All these happened from the death of her Daughter, dying in Child-bed.[45]

By the use of his treatments she "came to enjoy perfect health." These accounts seem to reflect the influence of Eugalenus, whose treatise, published originally in 1604, went through seven editions and was treated as an

---

[42] Cook (1679).    [43] Ibid., 91.    [44] Ibid., 118.    [45] Ibid., 95.

authoritative account of the disease.[46] He described a long series of cases, which include the characteristics of dysentery, various kinds of fevers, pleurisy, colic, epilepsy, and madness. Scurvy was diagnosed on Euga-lenus's criteria of the urine being either red or "white and turbid," and the pulse being "quick and small but particularly unequal." [47]

It is interesting that Hall never prescribed lemons or lemon juice for scurvy, although it was available. When the Countess of Northampton was ill with a fever, he gave her "the decoction of hartshorn with juice of lemons which she drank liberally." [48] In another case, a newly delivered mother was given a drink of "the juice of lemons and of wood-sorrel . . . by which her stomach was too much cooled. . . . I was sent for and conceived it to be a scorbutic dropsy." [49] Because these were only abbreviated case notes, he did not explicitly state what he believed to be the causes of scurvy. However, he made no mention of previous diet as a possible factor, whereas he did repeatedly refer to its relation to melancholy and some previous tragedy or disappointment such as the death of a child or "slaughter of one in his family."

Shakespeare himself is thought to have been often in his son-in-law's company. In his plays the word "scurvy" is used twenty-nine times, but always as an adjective.[50] The adjective is derived from "scurfy" and was used before the disease was so named (as a modification of "scorby") and, by 1579 at least, it was used with the metaphorical meaning of "sorry, worthless, contemptible." [51]

Lind's review of writings in the seventeenth century includes twenty-seven authors, though Woodall and Hall were not among them. Some unorthodox views, apparently confined to individual writers, were presented, for example, that the disease was hereditary or could be caught from an infected nurse;[52] that it could result from tobacco smoking or "immoderate use of sugar in the present era" [53] (probably less than 20% of our consumption 300 years later!); lastly, that it could be cured with mercury,[54] although others thought it to be harmful.[55] With regard to the controversy as to whether or not mineral acids could be a substitute for lemon juice, Glauber in 1659 urged the value of adding hydrochloric acid to the drinking water on shipboard so as to preserve it and to prevent the corruption of the blood that was the cause of the sailor's scurvy.[56] However, no evidence was presented, so that, presumably, it was a theory considered too obviously rational to need testing.

With such a variety of ideas being put forward by the medical profession, it is difficult to conceive what an *un*orthodox treatment would have consisted of. However, in 1630, in Massachusetts, Nicholas Knopp was fined

---

[46] Stockman (1926), 341.     [47] Stewart & Guthrie (1953), 277–81.     [48] Cook (1679), 137.
[49] Ibid., 163.     [50] Spevack (1973), 1095–6.     [51] Murray (1933), 304.     [52] Stewart & Guthrie (1953), 272.     [53] Ibid., 296.     [54] Ibid., 307.     [55] Ibid., 302.     [56] Glauber (1659), 29.

for "taking upon him to cure the scurvy by a water of no worth nor value, which he sold at a very dear rate, [and was] to be imprisoned till he pay his fine or give security for it, or else to be whipped and shall be liable to any man . . . of whom he hath received money for the said water."[57]

## Acid and alkaline scurvies

We also see the more general adoption of a new concept – that there were at least two forms of the disease, which differed radically in their root cause and consequently in the type of treatment deemed appropriate.[58] In each type there was a "dyscrasia" (abnormal condition) of the blood. But in one kind it was acid or hot, and in another it was alkaline, cold, or "pituitous" (phlegmatic). These terms reflected the ideas of a new school of scientists, the iatrochemists. A more skeptical attitude to the authority of the ancient authorities had been growing since 1500, with new discoveries in astronomy and anatomy.[59] This new attitude came later to medicine than to other sciences, but one pioneer with a nonconformist character was John Van Helmont, who was born in 1577 to an aristocratic family in Brussels. He studied scholastic philosphy at Louvain, but felt it to be worthless, and turned to mysticism.[60] At this point in his life:

Happening to take up the glove of a young girl afflicted with the itch, he caught that disagreeable disease. The physicians whom he consulted, attributed it to the combustion of the bile, and the saline state of the phlegm. They prescribed a course of purgatives which weakened him considerably, without effecting a cure. This circumstance disgusted him with the system of the humorists, and led him to form the resolution of reforming medicine.[61]

He approached this through a concentration on chemistry and spent most of the rest of his life in his private laboratory. He did not believe that disease could be explained by imbalances within the body: "The Elements, Qualities and Temperaments . . . are lying fopperies which have been hitherto stiffly and ignorantly garnished out by the Schools."[62] It was his opinion that "Disease is from an efficient seminal Cause, positive, actual and real, with a Seed, Manner, Species and Order. Defects therefore there are . . . and they are from strange guests received within."[62]

Van Helmont was much impressed by the observation that acids and alkalis were both acrid (irritant) to living tissues, but that they would combine together with effervescence, to give a neutral bland salt. He thought that this type of reaction was important in the process of digestion.[63] He died in 1644, but his ideas were taken a step further in the next generation, by the Franco-Dutch scientist François de le Boe (1614–72) (spelled in several

---

[57] Noble (1904), 11.    [58] Ibid., 293, 297, 300.    [59] Hall (1962), 34–72.    [60] Debus (1977), II, 297–302.    [61] Thomson (1830), I, 179–82.    [62] Pagel (1972), 420.    [63] Debus (1977), II, 368–71.

variations and Latinized to Sylvius).[64] He believed that when the digestive system was not working correctly, ingested foods would "rot" in the body in more or less the same way that they would if left in a warm, moist heap outside it. Some foods such as grains, vegetables, and fruit were acescent, i.e., they turned acid under these conditions, and were thought similarly to result in an "acid acrimony of the blood" when digestion was deficient. This could result in pimples, ulcers, and irritation of the brain, and needed to be corrected by giving ammoniacal preparations and other alkaline drugs.[65] On the other hand, certain animal foods and some vegetables, when left to rot, become "putrid" (i.e., decayed with an offensive smell) and became alkaline. A similar disease condition in the body was obviously extremely serious and characterized by stinking breath and vomit, bilious diarrhea, and gangrene; it needed correction with acid drugs.

The system, simplified here, was fully developed and became orthodox under the influence of Hermann Boerhaave (1668–1738) at Leyden.[66] Acid was also equated to "hot," and alkali to "cold." With the development of these ideas, scurvy was, of course, one of the diseases that physicians were anxious to classify. We can see at once, however, that there was a difficulty: Pimples and ulcers were a sign of "acid acrimony," whereas stinking breath was the result of putrefaction ("alkaline acrimony"); moreover, there had been a continuing belief that the sailors' scurvy was related to their salt meat's being half-putrefied already.

Thomas Willis, the Oxford professor, skirted the problem in 1667 by saying that the disease could arise from both types of blood conditions – i.e., acid (which he called "sulphureo-saline") or alkaline (which he called "salino-sulphureous"). For the first condition he prescribed repeated bleeding and cooling medicines, and for the second, warming medicines.[67] Five years later, Walter Charleton, another Oxford man and a follower of Van Helmont, said that in addition to Willis's categories there was a third form – rancid scurvy. Only the alkaline form of the disease should be treated with scurvy grass because of its "heating" quality.[68]

In 1675, Gideon Harvey, a physician at King Charles's court, wrote that mouth scurvy was due to acid lymph, and leg scurvy to a saponary state (i.e., having an excess of alkaline salts in the blood).[69] This is the opposite of what one would have predicted because the gums and breath were usually described as being putrid. Also, of course, the records indicate that severe cases showed both mouth *and* leg scurvy, so that one would have to suppose that the sufferer was acid at his north end and alkaline at his south! For the first condition Gideon Harvey bled from the left arm, and for the second from above the knee – this despite the acceptance by then of William Harvey's

[64] Ibid., 526–30.    [65] Thomson (1830), *I*, 198; Partington (1961), *II*, 287.    [66] King (1958), 79–83; King (1970), 111–2.    [67] Stewart & Guthrie (1953), 292–3.    [68] Ibid., 297.    [69] Harvey (1675), 17, 176.

discovery of the circulation of the blood.[70] This diversification of the disease was not peculiar to England. Stephen Blancard, a Dutch physician, also divided it into hot (acid) and cold (phlegmatic) forms. Bleeding was not recommended for either; for the first form, drinking tea and coffee were recommended; for the cold form, warm aromatics and spices were needed.[71]

We began the chapter by recalling Hawkins's wish that learned men would turn their attention to "the plague of the sea." One wonders what he would have thought, if he could have come back 100 years later, of the result of their doing so. Sailors were still suffering on long voyages. They had known how to cure themselves in a very short time on returning to land; now the physicians were saying that it was also an endemic disease on land, and had made the subject so complicated that a safe and effective treatment could hardly be chosen without sophisticated diagnosis. This was certainly of benefit to the medical profession – if not to the patient. As a modern French scholar has written: "When theoretical considerations prevailed over empiricism, treatment became more and more complex and less effective."[72]

However, it would be unfair to end on that note. There were some leading physicians who had a restraining influence. Thus Thomas Sydenham (1624–89), sometimes known as the English Hippocrates, reacted against the proliferation of theories, and in the 1660s he wrote that "the two great subterfuges of ignorant physicians were malignity and the scurvy; which they blamed for disorders and symptoms often owing to their ill management . . . [saying that] whatever afterwards obstructs the cure must be the scurvy."[73]

[70] Castiglioni (1958), 515–9.   [71] Stewart & Guthrie (1953), 301–2.   [72] Grmek (1966), 515.   [73] Stewart & Guthrie (1953), 303–4.

# 3

# Scurvy in the British Navy (1700–1772)

By the beginning of the eighteenth century, the intellectuals of the Western World felt themselves to be very modern and liberated from old superstitions. With the work of Isaac Newton, "the unity of nature was made manifest in a grand synthesis revealing the effects of identical physical laws in the heavens and on earth."[1] These successes made it seem as if everything, including the "human machine" would soon be explained by mechanical laws. Medical historians who have examined the period have expressed a wide range of views, characterizing it as "a century of enlightenment and idealism in medicine and allied sciences as well as in politics and philosophy," but also as a time of "much platitudinous philosophizing where formalism dominated literature and even music, and medicine abounded in theories and system-makers."[2]

## Theory versus empiricism

At the beginning of the century, the undisputed master of clinical medicine was Hermann Boerhaave (1668–1738).[3] His teaching at the University of Leyden brought students from many countries, to which they returned as disciples.[4] At the University of Edinburgh, students for at least the period 1735–55 were "taught to think the system of Boerhaave to be very perfect, complete and sufficent."[5] One eulogist has said: "Quite in the spirit of Hippocrates is . . . his attempt to draw from his observations the simplest and clearest possible conclusions. . . . [He is not one who] adapts himself in preconceived systems."[6]

These qualities are certainly not apparent in his treatment of scurvy in 1715. He supposed that the "proximate" (immediate) cause of the disease

---

[1] Hall (1962), 244.　　[2] Veith (1958), vii–viii.　　[3] Tanner (1926), I, 122; King (1958), 59.
[4] Newman, G. (1926), 406–7.　　[5] Thomson (1859), 118.　　[6] Castiglioni (1958), 616.

43

was that the blood serum (the clear fluid remaining after the blood has clotted and the clot settled) was too thin and too acrid in a variety of ways, and that the "other part" (the material in the clot) was too thick and viscid. Thus the serum had to be thickened and its acidity neutralized, whereas at the same time the other part had to be thinned. "There is occasion for the greatest skill in physic to treat this disease with success . . . [for] what is serviceable to one patient must be destructive to another." The acridity may be saline, acid, alkaline, or "oily and rancid"; a successful cure depended on the use of counteracting medicines. Vinegar and Moselle wine were classed with citrus fruit as acid medicines; scurvy grass, ginger, and volatile salts were classified with alkaline ones. He attributed the prevalence of scurvy in Holland to its damp, cold climate and to the fact that in winter, people remained inactive in rooms having tiles or marble floors.[7]

In 1734, a very different evaluation was proposed, again from Holland, by John Bachstrom, a physician whose name does not appear in the standard histories of medicine. He postulated that there was only one cause of scurvy – the absence of fresh (or "recent") vegetable food from the diet for a considerable time.[8] There was no reason to suppose that a cold climate had anything to do with the disease because sailors in the Dutch East Indies fleet developed scurvy in the Tropics. Moreover, in the relatively recent siege of Thorn (Torun, Copernicus's birthplace in Poland), many thousands of the garrison and inhabitants developed the disease, even though it took place in summer. (It lasted from mid-May to October 4, 1703.[9]) The besieging Swedes remained healthy, and those in the town quickly recovered when they had access to fresh greens and vegetables. Nor was there reason to suppose that damp or coastal conditions were required: At the end of a campaign against the Turks, Austrian troops had spent the winter of 1719– 20 in a devastated, inland part of Hungary and there had been a heavy loss of life from scurvy. No drugs were of any help, but with the coming of spring there were fresh green foods available and the men recovered. He gave other examples and urged the value of all kinds of green foods and fresh fruit, and recommended a diet rich in green vegetables as a preventive. He said that mineral acids, and specifically the popular sulfuric acid, were useless. With regard to niter he reserved judgment because it was a natural component of plants.[8]

Bachstrom's treatise seems to the modern reader a straightforward argument and one that deserved at least a serious consideration. But to the contemporary main-line physician it would not have been very impressive because it dealt with a single disease in isolation and did nothing toward establishing a view of the nature of disease in general – an ideal which the medical profession had as its goal, by analogy with the universal laws being

[7] Delacoste (1715), 313–21.    [8] Bachstrom (1734), 348; also summarized in Stewart & Guthrie (1953), 314–7.    [9] Hatton (1968), 193–5.

developed by the physicists at that time. In other words, he was "a mere empirick." [10]

John Wesley, the famous preacher and founder of Methodism, sharply criticized this attitude in his *Primitive Physick*, first published in 1747. His argument, somewhat shortened, is this:

In the beginning Physick was wholly founded on Experiment [meaning experience]. You said to your neighbour, Are you sick? Drink the juice of this herb, and your sickness will be at an end. Has the snake bitten you? Chew and apply that root, and the poison will not hurt you. But in process of time, men of a philosophical turn were not satisfied with this. They began to enquire, how they might account for these things? How such medicines wrought such effects? They examined the human body and all its parts. They explored the several kinds of animal and mineral, as well as vegetable substances. And hence the whole Order of Physick which had obtained to that time, came gradually to be inverted. Men of learning began to set experience aside: to build physick upon hypotheses: to form theories of diseases and their cure, and to substitute these in the place of experiments, until at length Physick became an abstruse Science, quite out of the reach of ordinary men. Profit attended their employ as well as honour; they increased the mysteries of the profession by design, and . . . those who understood only how to restore the sick to health, they branded with the ignominious name of Empiricks.[11]

Wesley's own preferred treatment for scurvy was: "Live on turnips for a month." [12] This was certainly something within the poor man's reach, and the advice could have been founded on the experience of John Guy from the first colonization of Newfoundland in 1601: "This year we had very good turnips grown; they are exceedingly good for the scarby, by trial it hath recovered many of our sick men." [13]

## Scurvy in the British Navy

So far, the British Navy has not appeared in this story. The earlier British explorers and privateers had operated, nominally at least, as private citizens. The role of the Navy, even in the seventeenth century, had been to guard the British coast and shipping approaching it, so that long voyages were not required. Samuel Pepys, the famous diarist, was Secretary to the British Admiralty in the second half of the century, but he was also very much interested in scientific questions and became President of the Royal Society. It is therefore interesting that in all his extensive papers the only reference to scurvy is in a letter received in 1696 listing a large number of needed reforms, one of which was that victualers should not be allowed to supply beef suet in place of raisins and currants "since it's the parent of scurvy." [14] During the next 100 years, as we shall see, the disease was to

[10] King (1958), 32.  [11] Wesley (1751), viii–xii.  [12] Ibid., 105.  [13] Cell (1982), 80.
[14] Tanner (1926), *I*, 122.

become a much more important issue in the affairs of the Admiralty, causing more losses than enemy action.

In January 1740, with war declared against Spain, Commodore George Anson was appointed to capture the Spanish treasure galleon that still went each year from Acapulco (Mexico), carrying silver across the Pacific to the Philippines, and bringing back Chinese silks, spices, etc. He was also ordered to be as annoying as possible to the Spaniards on the west coast of South and Central America.[15] He finally set out in August with seven ships. We do not know of any special victualing prepared for such a long voyage. A typical sailor's ration in the British Navy at that time was one pound of biscuit and one gallon of beer each day (though the beer would last only for a few weeks). The supplements varied with the day of the week but, when averaged out, came to roughly one pound of salt meat (beef or pork), two ounces of cheese, one ounce of butter, seven ounces (by volume) of oatmeal, and 4½ ounces (by volume) of dried peas or beans.[16] In addition there was vinegar and, usually, a ration of spirits when the beer was exhausted. Two ideas may have had some influence on their preparations to deal with the threat of scurvy.[17] One was that lemons could cause enteritis,[18] and that "one must, when ships reach countries abounding in oranges, lemons, pineapples etc, ensure that the crew eat very little of them since they are the commonest cause of fevers and obstruction of the vital organs."[19] Moreover, in 1736, William Cockburn, an influential physician attached to the Fleet, had published a new edition of his *Sea Diseases*, in which he argued that scurvy attacked those who were idle; with greater physical effort, "digestion and nutrition were better performed"; the sailor's traditional victuals were quite adequate, though fresh vegetables were active in curing those already sick.[20] The standard antiscorbutic medicine issued at sea in that period, on the recommendation of the College of Physicians, was "elixir of vitriol," made up of sulfuric acid with added alcohol, sugar, and flavorings.[21]

Anson's voyage makes an extraordinary story, which is readily available to the modern reader.[22] It is famous, on the one hand, for the tenacity and courage of its commander and, on the other, for the extraordinary losses from sickness. Three of the ships were no longer with him in the Pacific. Of the remainder, which started with over 1,000 men, only 145 returned, and the great majority of the rest died of scurvy.[23] Finally, with the survivors concentrated into one ship, they caught up with the treasure galleon and captured it, although it had three times as many men on board, and returned to England in 1744.

The account of their sufferings is appalling but entirely predictable in view of the earlier experiences of others and their own bad luck in encoun-

---

[15] Williams (1967), 34–42.   [16] Lloyd (1981), 10.   [17] Keevil (1958), *II*, 216.   [18] White (1712), 9.   [19] Dulieu (1984), 69.   [20] Cockburn (1736), 12–13.   [21] Lloyd & Coulter (1961), *III*, 294.   [22] Somerville (1937); Wilcox (1969).   [23] Somerville (1934), 303–6.

tering harsh weather that slowed their progress. After a week's stay at Madeira at the end of October, they reached St. Catherine's island off Brazil on December 21.[24] By then many had died of fevers and fluxes. They sent the sick ashore, but, solely from the flagship the *Centurion* with a complement of 520, 26 more died during their four-week stay, and the number remaining sick with fevers increased; this was attributed to the "close air" of the bay.[25] Although they saw all kinds of fruit there, and also onions and potatoes, it was said that they left with only a small store of refreshments.[26] After a further ten days' stop on the Patagonian coast, where there were seals and birds to be had but nothing else,[27] they sailed again and rounded Cape Horn on April 7, and encountered very bad weather.[28]

By this time the crews were seriously weakened. Scurvy had begun to show itself by about March 17, and during April another forty-three sailors died on the *Centurion*. They hoped that as a result of turning northwards into a milder area, "its malignity would abate," yet in May they lost "near double that number"; and when they finally reached land in mid-June, they had lost over 200. In addition, they have referred to

a most extraordinary circumstance – that the scars of old wounds, healed for many years, were forced open again; also many of our people, though confined to their hammocks, ate and drank heartily and were cheerful, yet having resolved to get out of their hammock, died before they could well reach the deck. It was also no uncommon thing for those who were able to walk the deck, to drop down in an instant on any endeavours to act with their utmost vigor.[29]

The same phenomena were reported, with surprise, by other observers of scurvy at sea.[30]

Some of those on the expedition were infirm pensioners sent as substitutes for the active soldiers who should have been supplied. They were among the first to succumb, but it is also clear that they were not the only ones.[31] Pascoe Thomas, the schoolmaster on the *Centurion*, wrote after his return:

I shall endeavour to remove a very great prejudice from which persons who labour under this affliction have most unjustly suffered; which is that none but the indolent are ever sick of this disease. This mistaken opinion has caused many poor sufferers to endure more from their commanding officers than from the distemper itself; being drubbed to do their duty, when incapable of it. Our experience has abundantly testified that the most active, stirring persons are oftenest seized with this disease; and the continuation of their labour only helps to kill them the sooner.[32]

At last, on June 19, the *Centurion* reached the island of Juan Fernandez and found a good anchorage. The flagship then had only seventy-two

---

[24] Walter (1748), 57.     [25] Ibid., 62–4.     [26] Ibid., 120.     [27] Ibid., 87–96; Williams (1967), 165.     [28] Walter (1748), 113–17.     [29] Ibid., 142–5.     [30] Waxell (1952), 200.     [31] Walter (1748), 222–3.     [32] Williams (1967), 87–8.

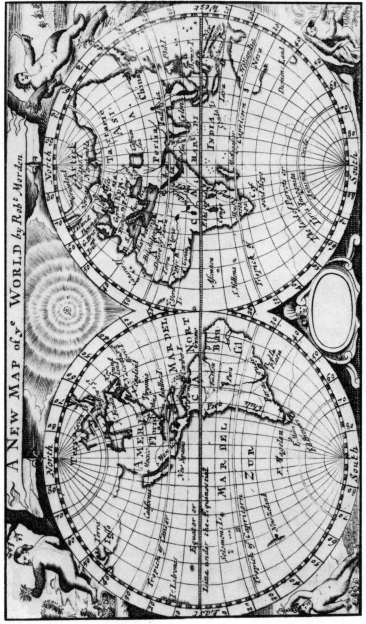

Robert Morden's new map of the world, published in 1693, illustrating the size of the Pacific Ocean. At the time of Anson's expedition in the 1740s, the mid-Pacific Hawaiian Islands were still unknown to Western navigators, and his crews obtained relief from scurvy only after reaching the Ladrone (Mariana) Islands, on the western side of the Pacific. (Bancroft Library, University of California, Berkeley.)

persons capable of appearing on deck.[33] Two weeks later, they were joined by the *Gloucester:* "They had already thrown overboard two thirds of their complement, and of those that remained alive scarcely any were capable of doing duty, except the officers and their servants."[34] The sick were brought ashore, with even the Commodore and his officers helping to carry them to tents.[35] They found there "almost all the vegetables esteemed for the cure of scorbutick disorders," including watercress and turnips. "These vegetables with the fish and flesh we found here, were most salutary for recovering our sick, and of no mean service to us who were well, in destroying the lurking seeds of scurvy and in restoring us to our wonted strength."[36]

In late September, after much refitting of the ships and capturing of some local shipping, they set out toward Mexico, making raids and seizing more prizes on the way. They were unable to catch the treasure galleon at Acapulco, and, after a last call on the coast 100 miles further northwest to get fresh water, they set out at the end of April, 1742, with just one other ship, the *Gloucester*, to sail across the Pacific to intercept it at Manila. Since their departure from Juan Fernandez, there had been no recurrence of scurvy, but now it began to reappear. In addition they were once again dogged by unfavorable winds. The violence of the disease surprised them, because the weather was warm and not stressful, and they had plenty of fresh water from abundant rains and were even catching fish. They also took special pains to keep the ship both clean and well ventilated by having the ports open.[37]

Pascoe Thomas later wrote that during the first epidemic, after rounding Cape Horn,

our surgeon, Henry Ettrick had been very busy in digesting a theory of scurvies; founded on the observations made on a long passage, in a very cold climate. He took abundant pains to prove that the tone of the blood was broke by this cold nipping air, and rendered so thin as to be unfit for circulation; and being thus deprived of a proper force and vigour, stagnation and death must necessarily ensue. From this supposition, he had laid it down, that any food of a glutinous nature, such as salt fish, bread, and several sorts of grains, were alone proper on such voyages. But this passage, in a very hot climate, where the symptoms were not only more dreadful, but the mortality much more quick and fatal, put our scheming doctor to a sad nonplus; he could not account for this, on the same principles with the other. All this obliged him to own that the grand centre was certainly the long continuance at sea and that no cure but the shore would ever take place.[38]

Richard Walter, the Chaplain, suggested that fresh air, so necessary to animal life might be "rendered unfit for its service by the steams arising from the ocean, without its losing its elasticity or any obvious property, unless these steams are corrected by effluvia of another kind which land alone can supply."[39] "The Commodore, having by him some quantity of

---

[33] Ibid., 166.    [34] Walter (1748), 179.    [35] Ibid., 159.    [36] Ibid., 165.    [37] Ibid., 396–7.
[38] Williams (1967), 86–7.    [39] Ibid., 166.

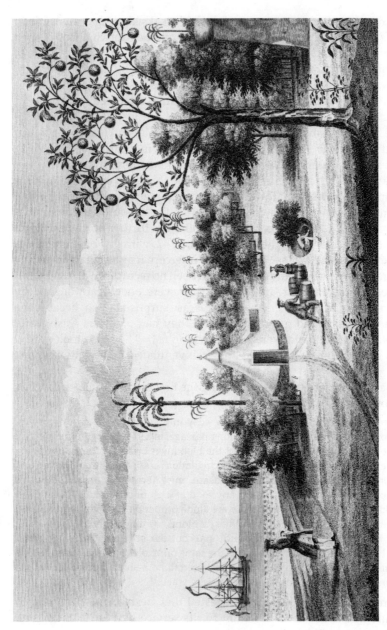

A print showing sailors from Anson's *Centurion* obtaining refreshment on one of the Mariana Islands in 1742, after a serious outbreak of scurvy on their voyage across the Pacific Ocean. (Wellcome Institute Library, London.)

Ward's pills and drops, gave a quantity of them to the surgeon, for such of the sick people as were willing to take them; several did so; though I know of none who believed they were of any service to them." [38]

A lieutenant on the *Centurion* wrote in his journal of this period:

> This distemper . . . expresses itself in such dreadful symptoms as are scarce credible. . . . Nor can all the physicians, with all their *materia medica*, find a remedy for it . . . but I could plainly observe that there is a *Je ne sais quoi* [certain unknown "something"] in the frame of the human system that cannot be renewed . . . without the assistance of certain earthy particles, or in plain English, the land is man's proper element, and vegetables and fruit his only physic. For the space of six weeks we seldom buried less than four or five men a day, . . . [and] I really believe had we stayed ten days longer at sea we should have lost the ship for want of men to navigate her.[39]

The losses were such that even the *Gloucester* had to be abandoned and the survivors transferred into the *Centurion*. Then, finally, all in one ship they reached one of the Ladrone (Mariana) Islands, and on August 28 went ashore. "This island afforded . . . cattle, hogs, lemons and oranges, which was the only treasure which we then wanted." [40] Of course, they did capture the treasure and get home eventually, but the scale of the losses came as a terrible warning for those planning future expeditions.

## *James Lind's experiment*

One naval surgeon who became particularly interested in the problem of scurvy at sea was James Lind, now the most celebrated name in the history of this subject. At least six biographical sketches have been published, all with the same meager information on his early life.[41] He was born in 1716 in Edinburgh, of a well-established merchant family, and left school at the age of fifteen to be apprenticed to a local surgeon. The Medical School of the University of Edinburgh was just getting established at that time, and there is no evidence that he attended lectures there. Normally the apprentice learned his trade by watching his master and gradually being allowed to do more himself.

In 1739, the year in which war broke out between Britain and Spain, Lind, at the age of twenty-three, joined the Royal Navy as a surgeon's mate. He would have had papers certifying the completion of his apprenticeship, but no degree or other qualification. He saw service in the West Indies and off the African coast, as well as in the Mediterranean and home waters. In 1746, he was a full surgeon on H.M.S. *Salisbury*, a fourth-rate man-of-war with a crew of 350.[41] While on cruises in the English Channel in the summer of

---

[40] Ibid., 178.    [41] *D.N.B* (1893) *XI*: 1150–1; Rolleston (1915); Stockman (1926); Roddis (1950); Guthrie & Meiklejohn (1953); Watt (1983).

1746 and again in the following year, serious outbreaks of scurvy occurred, the first involving eighty men.[42] It was during the second outbreak that Lind carried out his famous experiment[43] – probably the first controlled trial in clinical nutrition, or even in any branch of clinical science.[44]

He kept a group of twelve sailors all with scurvy, "as similar as I could have them," in the same quarters; and he saw to it that they all had the same diet: for breakast, gruel with sugar; for dinner, broth (made with fresh mutton) on some days and puddings on other; for supper, barley and raisins, rice, and currants, etc. Then two men were allocated to each of six different daily treatments for a period of fourteen days. The treatments were:

1. One quart (1.1 liters) of "cider" (hard apple cider in American terminology).
2. Twenty-five "gutts" (drops; about 1 ml) of *elixir vitriol*, three times throughout the day; the men also gargled with it.
3. Two spoonfuls (about 18 ml) of vinegar three times throughout the day before meals; the men also gargled and acidulated their food with it.
4. Half a pint of sea water (about 0.3 liters). (The two men on this treatment were the only ones in the group with the tendons of their hams rigid.)
5. Two oranges and one lemon continued for six days only, when the supply was exhausted.
6. An "electuary" (medicinal paste), the size of a nutmeg (about 4 ml), prescribed by another surgeon and made up of garlic, mustard seed, balsam of Peru (resin from the tree *Myroxylon peveirae*), rad. raphan (dried radish root), and gum myrrh. In addition, their drink was barley-water acidulated with tamarinds and, on three or four occasions, *cremor tartar* (potassium hydrogen tartrate) was added as a mild laxative.

Those receiving the oranges and lemons were much improved after six days, and after that they had just a gargle with elixir of vitriol, and were fit for duty or to nurse the others. Those receiving the cider were the next best; at the end of two weeks

the putrefaction of their gums, but especially their lassitude and weakness were somewhat abated. . . . As to the *elixir* or *vitriol*, the mouths of those who had used it by way of gargarism [as a gargle] were in much cleaner and better condition than many of the rest, especially those who used the vinegar; but I perceived otherwise no good effects from its internal use upon the other symptoms. . . . There was no remarkable alteration upon those who took the electuary and tamarind decoction, the sea-water, or vinegar, upon comparing their condition, at the end of the fortnight, with others who had taken nothing but a little lenitive [pain-killing] electuary and *cremor tartar*, at times, in order to keep their belly open; or a gentle pectoral [cough syrup] in the evening, for relief of their breast.

---

[42] Stewart & Guthrie (1953), 83–4.      [43] Ibid., 145–8.      [44] Dudley (1953a), 203; Thomas (1969), 932–3.

His conclusion was "that oranges and lemons were the most effectual remedies for this distemper at sea." [43]

Among the writers on scurvy over the next fifty years, this trial seems to
have made very little impression. It is only in the twentieth century, with the
development of experimental design and analysis as a discipline within
biology, that it has been extolled as an example to be followed.[44] One critic
has protested against such praise, saying that "Lind knew how to carry out a
scientific experiment; it is not so evident that he knew which scientific
experiments should be done." [45] His reason for saying this was that "six
possible cures" were apparently selected arbitrarily from those currently
favored, and that this reduced the experiment to the level of "controlled
empiricism" rather than a critical test of a hypothesis; if all six treatments
had given the same result, either positive or negative, the experiment would
not have succeeded.[45] The argument has already been made that Lind may
have had good reasons for his choice of treatments, but may have thought
that his readers would have been interested only in *what* was done, rather
than *why* it was done.[46] Newton, himself, can be quoted as saying: "*First*
search carefully for the properties of things, establishing them by experiment, and *then*, more warily, assert any explanatory hypothesis." [47]

Certainly, it should be a mark of respect, rather than the reverse, to treat
Lind's work as being worthy of detailed analysis. What Lind did should
clearly be classified, in modern terminology, as a controlled clinical trial. But
can we criticize him for an empirical "selection" of treatments? They probably represented the *full* range of practice of different surgeons in the Navy at
that time, and had all been recommended in print. There were many other
suggestions for treatment on land with various kinds of vegetables or vegetable extracts, but none of them was available on ships.

It seems clear that Lind regarded the treatment with oranges and lemons
as his positive controls: "Their experienced virtues have stood the test of
near 200 years." [48] If he had really wanted to study their value, he should, of
course, have fed them separately because the results, as they stand, do not
prove that *either* oranges *or* lemons separately were active, only that one, or
the combination of them both was. Also, Lind did keep some men as "negative controls" – those treated just with a "lenitive electuary" (pain-killing
paste), laxative, and cough syrup, even though he did not list them as
experimental subjects in the "design" of his experiment.[49] It is interesting
that the two subjects in worst condition both received the seawater treatment. Was this chance, or had Lind perhaps been a believer in it and
expected that they would give a dramatic response from "worst" to "best"?
He does refer in his *Treatise* to ". . . numberless instances of giving salt
water in very bad scurvies . . . with great benefit." [50]

[45] Hughes (1975), 343–4.    [46] Wyatt (1976), 433.    [47] Turnbull (1959), 169.    [48] Stewart &
Guthrie (1953), 154.    [49] Ibid., 148.    [50] Ibid., 160–1, n2.

The true significance of the experiment at that time was that it demonstrated the *in*activity of sulfuric acid, vinegar, etc., which were the officially recommended treatments. Forty years earlier, Martin Lister had said that, from his experience of twelve cases, the acidity of lemons did not seem to be the full measure of the antiscorbutic value and that there "reside (in them) a special exotic principle."[51] But he had not carried out a controlled trial, nor, obviously, had his remark been persuasive. Today, of course, it would seem merely laughable, if in trying to tell students in one or two sentences why James Lind was a great man, we were to say that it was because he proved the sulfuric acid did *not* cure scurvy; so instead they have been told something more positive, but not really true, for example: "The connection (of scurvy) with dietary deficiency was not established until James Lind demonstrated the curative effects of lemon juice."[52]

## Lind's treatise

In 1748, Lind left the Navy, returned to Edinburgh, and was granted the Doctor of Medicine degree and a license to practice as a physician, and in 1750 was elected a Fellow of Edinburgh's Royal College of Physicians.[53] At this time he set out to write a short paper on scurvy for the Society of Naval Surgeons, but it expanded into a 400-page book, which was published in Edinburgh in 1753 as *A Treatise of the Scurvy. Containing an inquiry into the Nature, Causes and Cure of that Disease. Together with a Critical and Chronological View of what has been published on the subject.*[54] It is of interest that it was written in English rather than Latin.

The treatise begins with a "critical history" of the subject, and has, as Part III (a kind of appendix to the book), a synopsis of each of the earlier publications on scurvy that Lind had been able to discover. This is impressive and scholarly work, and, wherever I have been able to compare his summary with the original, it appears objective and accurate. He made a thorough review of the claims of Echth and the other sixteenth-century writers that scurvy was known to Hippocrates and his successors (Pliny, Avicenna, etc.), and he argued that *stomakake* and *sceletyrbe* would not have been scurvy because there was no mention of the spots that are so characteristic of the disease. In conclusion, he stated that

it may appear a matter of no great importance, to be rightly informed whether this disease was known to the ancients or not, if a misplaced esteem for their works had not been productive of ill consequences . . . in the cure of this disease. Many, believing the spleen the seat of it, have adapted their medicinal intentions to the relief of that bowel. . . . But as people are apt to run from one extreme to another, such has been here the case. Many not finding the disease in any description of the

[51] Lorenz (1953), 311.     [52] Castiglioni (1958), 469–70.     [53] Rolleston (1915), 182.
[54] Stewart & Guthrie (1953), title page.

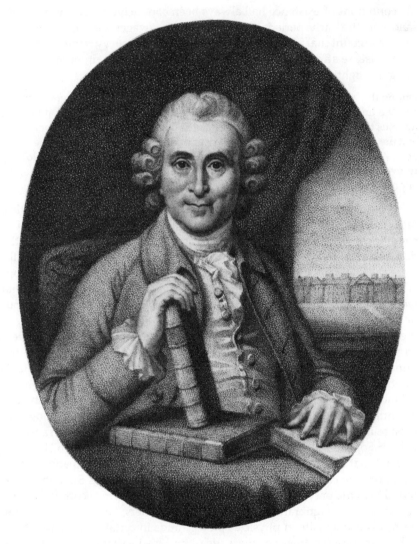

Portrait of the Scottish physician, James Lind (1716–94), holding his famous *Treatise of the Scurvy*. (Wellcome Institute Library, London.)

ancients, have supposed it a new calamity, making its appearance in the world, like the *lues venerea* [syphilis], at a certain period of time; an opinion equally, if not more censurable than the former.[55]

Lind suggested that the ancients were not familiar with the disease because they had no reliable information about the northern countries where

[55] Ibid., 255–6.

the conditions of existence had always been conducive to scurvy,[56] nor did sailors in the early periods go for extended voyages far from land. The earliest account that in his opinion represented true scurvy is the description of the disease affecting the French Army that spent the winter of 1249–50 in Egypt, fighting the Saracens.[57]

During the whole of Lent we ate no fish except eels. . . . It was this wretched diet and the unhealthiness of the country, where not a drop of rain falls, that brought upon us the "camp fever" which caused the flesh on our legs to dry up completely and the skin to become covered with black and earth-coloured spots, just like an old boot. When we caught the disease, the flesh on our gums began to rot away. Nobody recovered from it, and it was always fatal. Bleeding at the nose was a sure sign of the approach of death.[58]

Turning to the seventeenth-century writers, Lind was particularly critical of Eugalenus, who was largely responsible for describing as "scorbutic," conditions which were quite different from the characteristic pattern of the disease as it appeared at sea.[59] Eugalenus believed that scurvy and syphilis were the *only* new diseases. In consequence, many conditions more properly described as nervous, or allied to rheumatism or rickets (diseases that were also not described in ancient writings), had to be classified as "scorbutic." He further believed that patients could die of the disease before any of the classical symptoms appeared and that the true and infallible signs were "a small, quick and unequal pulse, together with a peculiar state of the urine." [60] We have already seen the effect of this teaching in Dr. Hall's casebooks in the 1630s.

Lind apologized for his long treatment of Eugalenus: "his vanity and presumption are indeed intolerable," [61] but "succeeding authors follow him most religiously and minutely"; at times, "they even exceed him in absurdities." [62] For the well-known Oxford professor, Thomas Willis (1621–75), it seemed that any case, "which cannot properly be referred to any disease, may justly be called scorbutic." [63] For Lind, as for Thomas Sydenham, referred to in the previous chapter, falling back on the term "scorbutic" was a convenience for ignorant and indolent practitioners, "as if an unmeaning term was as requisite in physic as pious frauds in certain religions." [64]

His skeptical treatment of these ideas, and his insistence on evidence to support theories, provided a refreshing blast of common sense. He was equally critical of the eighteenth-century divisions of scurvy, among others, into "hot or cold," "acidic or lixivial [alkaline]," "sea or land," and "hereditary or adventitious." [65] To take an example, he pointed out that writers were in general agreement that any "alcalescent" disease would be characteristically hot and putrid and accompanied by loss of appetite, belchings,

[56] Magnus (1972), 316, 570.     [57] Stewart & Guthrie (1953), 255n.     [58] Hague (1955), 97. The original in old French is reproduced in Hirsch (1885), *II*, 511n.     [59] Stewart & Guthrie (1953), 14–29.     [60] Ibid., 31.     [61] Ibid., 28.     [62] Ibid., 30.     [63] Ibid., 32–6.     [64] Ibid., 61.
[65] Ibid., 38–63.

and the body's being hot to the touch. Yet the typical scurvy case showed none of these things, even though "hot scurvy" was said to be the most common type. Also, it was quite inconsistent with this theory that scurvy should be so consistently curable with plants like the mustards and cresses, which were themselves classed as "hot and alkaline." [66] He argued particularly that the first descriptions of land scurvy by physicians were the same in all points as those of the disease seen at sea.[67] Extraordinary ideas are thus perpetuated, in part, because "there are few now who . . . read these authors; and by that means their merit is little examined into, and is admitted upon the credit of others." [68]

He also made a comment relating to the official recommendation of elixir of vitriol and vinegar as antiscorbutics:

. . . caution is at all times necessary in our reasoning on the effects of medicines, even in the way of analogy. . . . For some might naturally conclude, that oranges and lemons are but so many acids, for which, vinegar, vitriol, etc. would prove excellent substitutes. But, upon bringing this to the test of experience, we find the contrary. Few ships have ever been in want of vinegar, and, for many years were supplied with vitriol. Yet the Channel fleet often had a thousand men miserably over-run with this disease. . . . Although acids agree in certain properties; yet they differ widely in others, and especially in their effects upon the human body. Of theory in physic the same may perhaps be said, as has been observed by some of zeal in religion, that it is indeed absolutely necessary yet, by carrying it too far, it may be doubted whether it has done more good or hurt in the world.[69]

After reading Lind's brilliant review of other people's ideas, which was so much ahead of its time, one turns eagerly to his own theory of the disease. But this is extremely difficult – even painful – to read, let alone summarize, and few have attempted it. None did so at the symposium in Edinburgh in 1953, celebrating the bicentennial of the *Treatise*.[70] A French naval surgeon, in his review of the *Treatise* in 1867, wrote: "It is astonishing that Lind, that rigorous and severe spirit, who in matters of therapeutics will recognize no authority but experience, should have accepted too readily, as the basis of his arguments, ideas that are far removed from any kind of scientific precision." [71] Also, because he had separate chapters entitled "Cause," "Prevention," "Cure," and "Theory," some of the same ground is covered several times in rather different terms.

## The "blocked perspiration" theory

Lind's theory was based on the concept that a cold, wet climate (and also an unhappy psychological state and inactivity) could result in either a constriction or a clogging of the pores in the skin and a consequent reduction in

---

[66] Ibid., 49–50.    [67] Ibid., 53–4, 57.    [68] Ibid., 59.    [69] Ibid., 152–3.    [70] Dudley et al. (1953).    [71] Rey (1867), 58.

"insensible perspiration." The idea that the skin was a major route of excretion of undesirable "vapors and humors" from the body dates back to Galen's time, but was very much developed by Sanctorious in the early 1600s.[72] The idea that obstruction, caused by cold and damp, could result in a variety of "putrid" diseases became increasingly popular in the mid-eighteenth century and was also put forward as the cause of fevers and cholera in military units.[73] Another Edinburgh physician wrote in 1759: "There is no discovery next to that of circulation of the blood, that has so much affected our reasoning in Medicine as that of insensible perspiration. The origin of most diseases and the operation of most medicines are accounted for from it." [73]

To return to Lind, he began his argument by pointing out that with the uninterrupted circulation of the body's fluids, the friction and mutual interaction with the solid tissues resulted in sweet and healthful components being "abraded and degenerated" into "various degrees of acrimony and corruption." Just as food had to be ingested to replace these components, so had the end products to be excreted.[74] This seems a reasonable statement for someone to make in a period dominated by the success of physical (i.e., mechanical) theories in explaining different natural phenomena. He went on to say that minerals and acid salts we mostly excreted in the urine, but that a greater part of the total excretion was through the skin.[75] He was impressed (we would say overly impressed) by the quantitative experiments that were supposed to have proved this beyond doubt. They involved a subject weighing his food and drink and also his excreta over a period, and also himself at the beginning and end. If the intake weighed more than the urine and feces, together with any gain in body weight, it was said that the excess was lost by perspiration. If the subject had not visibly sweated, then this loss was entirely "insensible perspiration." [72] It was probably the quantitative aspect that particularly appealed to Lind, but of course, there was no measure of the carbon dioxide gas and water vapor lost in the air expired from the lungs.

He then went on to argue that, if the insensible perspiration were blocked, the quantity of urine and fecal material could certainly be increased, but "the most subtile and putrescent of the animal humors . . . (could) not conveniently pass another way . . . [and] when retained long in the body were capable of acquiring the most poisonous and noxious qualities . . . and [could] then give rise to various diseases according to the habit or constitution of the person." [76] He agreed with Sanctorius, who had stated that the consequence of moist air could be retention of the matter of transpiration, which induced a cachexy (chronic disease) of a scorbutic character.[77] Addington had put forward essentially the same theory in his

[72] Renbourn (1960), 138–9.    [73] Ibid., 145; Pringle (1750).    [74] Stewart & Guthrie (1953), 201.    [75] Ibid., 202.    [76] Ibid., 203.    [77] Ibid., 207.

*"Essay on the Sea Scurvy,"* published in 1753, just before the *Treatise*. He, too, said that "the extraordinary moisture of the sea-air lessens perspiration," and reasoned that "the resulting plenitude of humours disposes the fluids to corrupt . . . as it is the nature of all animal fluids by such confinement . . . to degenerate into a state of putrescence." [78] He concluded that this plenitude should be removed by repeated bleeding and by purging with seawater (using it as a laxative), and wrote that "the antiseptic quality of the sea-water is improved if it is acidulated with spirits of salts [hydrochloric acid]." [79]

Lind suggested yet a second mechanism for the action of moisture:

It weakens the spring and elasticity of the air, and makes it unfit for the many salutary purposes obtained by respiration. . . . There can be no good digestion without pure air. . . . it assists the lung in converting crude chyle [lymph] into blood. Hence during a moist constitution of the air, improper food, or such as affords too viscous and tenacious chyle, can never rightly be converted to this vital juice.[80]

The reader is anxious, by this point, to see how the theory can be related to the curative effects of lemon juice and green vegetables. Lind wrote that one important property of vegetables was they they were "acescent" (i.e., if not immediately acid, they became so if left to ferment). This property balanced the chyle resulting from a purely meat diet, which had an alcalescent and putrefying character.[81] However, on this argument, mineral acids and vinegar should be just as antiscorbutic as lemon juice. Indeed, he stated that "acids of any kind are useful . . . but wanting some other properties much more necessary than acidity." [82] This *special,* "other property" he described as "a saponaceous, attenuating and resolving virtue [emulsion-forming]." He believed that the salts in vegetables combined with oil in the chyle to form soap. In turn, the soap helped to break up the gross particles in the chyle so that even an imperfectly functioning lung could complete their "concoction" into true blood, or into such fine residual particles that they could be excreted through even partly blocked pores in the skin. He felt that the particular resolving quality of summer fruits was shown by the fact that eating them in excess caused the body's humors to "melt down," resulting in the diarrheas so common in summer.[83]

Lind's ideas that air in ships had a "weaker spring and elasticity" were close to those of Richard Mead (1673–1754), the fashionable London physician who had published his *Discourse on Scurvy* in 1749. "The air is, even more than any other agent, concerned in bringing on the mischief." [84]

Whatever therefore alters this gravity and elasticity, makes the air unfit for the purposes, for which it was designed. In the first place, moisture weakens its spring; next, a combination of foul particles, such as are contained in the breath of many

---

[78] Addington (1753), 9.   [79] Ibid., 19.   [80] Stewart & Guthrie (1953), 208.   [81] Ibid., 221.   [82] Ibid., 222.   [83] Ibid., 223.   [84] Mead, (1762), 439.

persons crowded together, and some perhaps diseased; then, the filthiness of water stagnating in the bottom of the ship . . . insinuate themselves into the blood, and, in the nature of a ferment, corrupt its whole mass.[85]

From this concept, Mead encouraged the adoption of ventilators in ships to remove stagnent air.[86] However, Lind felt that this would not solve the problem. Foul air was also to be found in crowded prisons, but scurvy did not usually result from it. Also, at sea, ship's carpenters had to spend most time down below in noxious vapors, yet were no more liable to scurvy than their mates.[87] Lastly, scurvy had still occurred after ships had been fitted with ventilators.[88] "The *principal and main pre-disposing cause* is a manifest and obvious quality of the air, namely its *moisture.*"[89] "I will venture to affirm, that, without any one exception, *'Scorbutus locis aridis ignotus est'* [scurvy is unknown in dry places]. . . . Stugart [sic], in Germany, was formerly noted for being a place where the scurvy raged much; but, upon drying up a large lake in the neighbourhood of the town, the disease has since quite disappeared."[90]

Cold, moist open winters greatly inforce the disease; but by the return of warm, dry weather, these scorbutic complaints are much mitigated. Where the indisposition is but beginning, and even when the gums have been pretty much affected, there are numerous instances of a perfect recovery, without having the benefit of fresh vegetables; provided the patient is able to use due exercise.[91]

He suggested that a ventilation apparatus adapted to force in air warmed and dried by the galley fire might prove more advantageous:[92]

The exhalations of aromatics, though, they do not dry up moisture, yet prevent the pernicious effects of it upon the human body, by diffusing through the air a subtile acid, of an antiseptic and astringent quality, opposite to the putrid and relaxing tendency of moisture. . . . So I would recommend . . . , in damp seasons, putting a red-hot loggerhead in a bucket of tar, which should be moved about, so that all the ship may be filled with this wholesome antiseptic vapour.[93]

Other precautions were "to go well clothed and with dry linen" and "to eat a bit of raw onion or garlic" before being exposed to rain or spray – this was to promote perspiration.[93] "The lazy and indolent, and those of a sedentary life are most subject to scurvy; those that are of a cheerful and contented disposition, are less liable to it, than others."[94] This, of course, is a repetition of the view of Cockburn, already quoted, who believed that physical activity assisted in digestion. "In the inactive, digestion is weak, yielding a gross chyle which is not easily converted into blood, and transpiration is diminished."[20] For Cockburn, the consequence of the excessive volume of circulating fluid was a rise in pressure that forced out the spots of extravasated

[85] Ibid., 440.    [86] Zuckerman (1976–7).    [87] Stewart & Guthrie (1953), 76–7.    [88] Ibid., 79.    [89] Ibid., 85.    [90] Ibid., 98n.    [91] Ibid., 134.    [92] Ibid., 171.    [93] Ibid., 172–3. [94] Ibid., 105.

blood seen on the back and legs of scorbutics. He had been a pioneer in attempts to explain biological effects in terms of Newtonian mechanics.[95]

## The role of diet

Turning to matters of diet, Lind wrote that salt was not in itself either helpful or harmful; however, salted meat might be "rendered improper to afford that soft, mild nourishment, which is required to repair the body."[96] However, it could be "corrected by bread, vinegar or vegetables."[97] "Flour well leavened and baked into fresh bread is an excellent anti-scorbutic";[98] and ". . . it is adapted by its acescency to correct a flesh diet."[99] These statements are almost identical to Addington's recommendation of flour and rice in the same year.[100] Elsewhere, Lind wrote that "diet and moisture . . . are each but half-causes, neither of them singly being able to produce it: but both of them concurring, constitute all that is requisite and sufficient to form the scurvy."[101] And again, "such hard dry food as a ship's provisions, or the sea-diet, is extremely wholesome; and no better nourishment could be well contrived for people, using proper exercise in a dry pure air."[102] However, for those at sea, fresh vegetables and greens "correct the quality of such hard and dry food as they are obliged to make use of."[103]

Chick has written that "to Bachstrom and Lind must go the recognition of scurvy as a nutritional deficiency disease."[104] However, Lind made it quite clear that he did *not* accept Bachstrom's "supposition that . . . the constitution of the human body, is such that health and life cannot be preserved long, without the use of green herbage, vegetables, and fruits; and that a long abstinence from these, is alone the cause of the disease."[105]

If this were truly the case, we must have had the scurvy very accurately described by the ancients; whose manner of besieging towns was generally by a blockade. . . . Now, as they held out sometimes years, without a supply of vegetables; we should, no doubt, have heard of many dying of the scurvy, long before the magazines of dry provisions were exhausted. . . . likewise . . . there are persons every where, who, from choice, eat few or no green vegetables; and some countries are deprived of the use of them for five or six months of the year; as in the highlands of Scotland where, however, the scurvy is not a usual malady.[105]

In his last point Lind disregarded other vegetables such as turnips, carrots, onions, and potatoes, which were more available in winter months.

Later, he returned to his own experience:

I have been three months on a cruise, during which time none of the seamen tasted vegetables or greens of any sort; and for a great part of that time, their beef and pork

[95] Brown (1968), 241–9.   [96] Stewart & Guthrie (1953), 72.   [97] Ibid., 95.   [98] Ibid., 167.
[99] Ibid., 94.   [100] Addington (1753), 31.   [101] Stewart & Guthrie (1953), 99n.   [102] Ibid., 92.   [103] Ibid., 91.   [104] Chick (1953), 212.   [105] Stewart & Guthrie (1953), 73–4.

were boiled in the sea-water, yet without one scorbutical complaint. But, in two cruises where I had an opportunity of making observations, it began to rage upon being less than six weeks at sea; and after having left Plymouth, where plenty of greens were to be had; by which, one would have thought, the sailors had sufficiently prepared their bodies against the attack of this malady. Now both these cruises were in the months of April, May, and June; when we had . . . a continuance of cold, rainy weather . . . : whereas in our other cruises, we had generally very fine weather. . . . Nor could I assign any other reason for the frequency of this disease, and our exemption from it at other times, but the influence of the weather; the circumstances of the men, ship, and provisions, being in all other respects alike.[106]

To the modern reader, with the benefit of hindsight, the weak point in the argument is the assumption that sailors had been eating "plenty of greens" in the winter period, January through March, prior to the voyages in which the disease occurred.

Turning to the cure of people with the disease, Lind first divided the disease into "adventitious" and "constitutional" forms of scurvy. Sailors, in general, were placed into the first class, for whom "the cure is very simple, *viz.* a pure dry air, with the use of green herbage or wholesome vegetables, almost of any sort; . . . the first step to be taken towards its removal, when contracted either at sea or land, is change of air.[107] Thus, "numberless people have recovered without the assistance of many medicines." [108] In fact, according to Lind, none of the medicines available to a surgeon in his sea chest was of real value, except for easing local inflammations or ulcers.[109]

"Constitutional" scurvy was the designation given to the condition of people with

the peculiar tendency and disposition of their humours to the scorbutic corruption, from much slighter causes, . . . such people should also have recourse to other medicinal helps. . . . The physical intentions must be, to keep the outlets and emunctories of the body open and clear, for the gentle evacuation of the scorbutic acrimony, (*viz.* the belly [bowels], urinary passages, and excretory ducts off the skin): while, the remaining mass of humours is rendered mild, soft, and balsamic, by proper antiscorbutic food and medicine.[110]

(To digress for a moment, Voltaire, the great French writer and philosopher, complained in his correspondence in 1752–3 that the loss of most of his teeth was due to an inborn scorbutic humor, resulting in his blood being "saumuré" [pickled in brine], so that his organs had lost their elasticity and softness; and that this was a different condition from adventitious sea scurvy and would not respond to the same remedies.[111] This is surprisingly similar to Lind's comments on adventitious and constitutional scurvy, though neither could have read the other.)

---

[106] Ibid., 83–4.    [107] Ibid., 178.    [108] Ibid., 179.    [109] Ibid., 141–2, 196.    [110] Ibid., 180–1.
[111] Besterman (1956), XX, 276; XXIII, 297.

Lind then tackled the problem of what antiscorbutics could be carried on long voyages, because fresh vegetables and citrus fruit would spoil so easily. The Admiralty had proposed dried spinach, which could be moistened and boiled in the sailor's food, but he thought that Cockburn had probably been correct in his assessment that this would not "restore the natural juices of the plant lost by evaporation, and, as he imagined, altered by a fermentation which they underwent in drying." This seemed to be confirmed by the failure of dried herbs to help the Austrian Army wintering in Hungary.[112]

He therefore proposed "a method of preserving the virtues (of oranges and lemons) entire for years in a convenient and small bulk. It is done in the following easy manner." [113] The squeezed juice was allowed first to stand for a period so that impurities settled. It was then poured into open, glazed earthenware bowls, which were stood in almost boiling water for several hours ("at least 12–14 hours" in the third edition),[114] until the juice had evaporated down to a syrup that was only about 12% of the original volume. "Thus the acid, and virtues of twelve dozen of lemons or oranges, may be put into a quart-bottle, and preserved for several years." [115] Lind also recommended sailors to lay in a store of onions, green vegetables stored dry in layers of salt, cabbages "pickled in the Dutch style" (sauerkraut), and fermented drinks such as cider and spruce beer.[116]

After the *Treatise* was published, Lind remained in Edinburgh for a further five years. Then, in 1758 he was appointed by Anson, now First Lord of the Admiralty, to be Physician to Haslar Hospital near Portsmouth. This was a prestigious appointment to the largest and newest of the naval hospitals, soon to be further expanded to house 2,000 patients. He retained the position until his retirement in 1783, at the age of sixty-seven.[53] Scurvy continued to be a serious problem for the Navy, even in the fleet stationed in the English Channel but remaining at sea for months at a time in order to maintain a close blockade of the French ports. Lind recorded that at Haslar alone, he often had 300–400 cases at one time.[117] He therefore had unique opportunities for studying the disease and comparing different treatments; thus it is of interest to see what changes there might have been in his thinking by the time he revised the *Treatise* for its third and final edition that appeared in 1772.

## A variety of other ideas

But first, we should consider some other events that occurred during the period between 1753 and 1772. In 1755, Charles Bisset, another Edinburgh graduate, who had served at sea and in Jamaica, published his own treatise.[118] He believed that the principal causes of sea scurvy, as he had seen it

---

[112] Stewart & Guthrie (1953), 140n.    [113] Ibid., 155.    [114] Lind (1772), 161.    [115] Stewart & Guthrie (1953), 156.    [116] Ibid., 160–3.    [117] Lind (1772), iii.    [118] Bisset (1755), Chap. XVII.

in the West Indies Fleet, were the heat and salted food; vegetable foods and fruits were a cure, but so was wine and a punch made from rum and sugar; Lind was wrong to condemn the use of spirits. He particularly recommended rice as an antiscorbutic.

In 1757, John Travis, a surgeon practicing at the English seaport of Scarborough, presented the hypothesis that the scurvy so prevalent in the British Navy was caused by copper poisoning.[119] He argued that men on merchant ships, which generally had iron boilers for cooking their food, where much less affected that those on naval ships, which always had copper boilers, even though the provisions on the latter were usually of higher quality. He believed that the motion of a large quantity of food in a briskly boiling copper pot caused the metal surface to react with salt to form verdigris (a copper salt, actually copper acetate), which dissolved in the grease that was usually present.

The acrimonious mineral corpuscles are sheathed by the oil so that when the food is eaten they do not cause vomiting or gripping, and are then absorbed into the tissues – tearing the extremities of the capillary arteries, irritating, and wounding the nerves. Though the quantity taken at once be so small as not to do any sensible mischief, yet being daily repeated, it gradually, and insidiously, brings on a train of the most dreadful complaints.[120]

For the present-day reader, this paper is very suggestive, and we shall return to it later. At the time, it was ignored, perhaps because the theory seemed inconsistent with the curative properties of fruits and vegetables.

In 1768, Nathaniel Hulme published his *Proposal for Preventing the Scurvy in the British Navy*.[121] He disagreed with Lind's theory that moist air could cause scurvy, and instead believed that it could be entirely explained by the basic indigestibility of the sailors' food. Because oranges and lemons were curative, they should also be used as preventives at one-third of the curative level – and idea already proposed by Huxham in 1747.[122] Hulme also gave instances of problems occurring due to spoilage of the lemon juice, and he recommended procedures for preserving it in good condition.[121]

The most influential papers published in the period were those of David MacBride.[123] They will be considered more fully in the following chapter. For the moment, we need only to know that they were based on ideas put forward earlier by John Pringle. In lectures to the Royal Society in 1750, Pringle had reported the results of tests as to which substances either slowed or speeded up the putrefaction of meat soaking in warm water. He found that adding bread resulted in no immediate effect, but that later the fermentation of the bread checked the putrefaction with release of much air.[124] This he considered an ideal effect because "neither vegetable nor animal substances can become aliment [provide nourishment] without undergoing

---

[119] Travis (1762).     [120] Ibid., 13–14.     [121] Hulme (1768), 21–5.     [122] Huxham (1747), 467.     [123] MacBride (1764, 1767).     [124] Pringle (1750), 555.

some putrefaction." [125] However, excessive putrefaction led to "putrid diseases," of which scurvy was one. In 1753, Pringle went further, suggesting that the increased use of sugar might be a reason for the decline of scurvy in Britain because, again, it encouraged fermentation at first, and then the acid that was produced checked it.[126] David MacBride (1726–78) was ten years younger than Lind, but had served for a short period in the Navy as a surgeon's mate before the Peace of 1748. He then attended some lectures in Edinburgh and London before returning to practice in Dublin.[127] He had the idea that malted barley might prove to be the perfect material for use on board ships as an antiscorbutic, because it could be stored indefinitely, and then "sweet wort" could be made from it when required; this would then ferment rapidly in the body of the person drinking it, just as it did during the brewing of beer.

What follows is an eighteenth-century description of the preparation of malt: Whole barley grains are steeped in water for about three days. The grains are then heaped on a floor to drain; they begin to germinate in this period and develop roots. At this point they are spread out for a further two days to begin to dry and stop further development. The husk then separates and is winnowed away; the residue, i.e., the malt, is dried slowly on sieves in hot air above a fire. When fully dry, it is ground to a powder. The characteristics of the malt depend on the severity of the heat that it receives during drying; the best malt is no darker than amber-colored.[128] For the brewing of beer, the malt would be incubated with warm water and hop leaves, and then the extract fermented with yeast. For use as an antiscorbutic on ships, the malt was stored on board in a dry state, and, when needed, "3 measures of boiling water were poured on one of the ground malt, left to stand for 4 hours, when the liquor was strained off and each of the patients served an allowance." [129] The usual dose appears to have been in the range of two to four pints per day.[130]

The Sick and Hurt Board, the organization responsible for having new remedies tested for use of the Navy, gave instructions in 1762 for a trial of sweet wort at the Royal Naval Hospital, Plymouth, by giving it to a group of scorbutic sailors in place of vegetables and fresh meat. After one man died, the remaining sailors refused to continue with the experiment.[131] Lind put 130 scorbutic patients on a course of wort for two weeks at Haslar. He said that they found it a pleasant drink, and that it was a nourishing liquor, but he said nothing about its curing their condition.[132] In 1763, orders were given for it to be tested at sea, where vegetables and fresh meat would not be available, but this was not carried out, perhaps because hostilities ceased in that year and thus there were fewer ships at sea.[131] MacBride himself said

[125] Ibid., 553.    [126] Pringle (1753), 347.    [127] *D.N.B.* (1893) *XII*, 424–5.    [128] *Encyclopaedia Brittanica* (1797), *III*, 543–7.    [129] MacBride (1767), 33.    [130] Badenoch (1776), 63, 69. [131] Smith (1918), 814.    [132] Lind (1772), 539n.

that the failure "may easily be accounted for, from that aversion to innova-
tion and experiment which is so prevalent among the bulk of mankind, but
expecially among seamen." [133] Finally, he persuaded his own brother, who
was a ship's captain, to have the wort evaluated, and his brother's surgeon
gave a strongly favorable report.[134] The wort was then tested, with the
encouragement of Pringle, on a naval circumnavigation, as we shall see
later.

## Trials on long voyages

Two expeditions were organized by the Navy in the period under consideration, and they had returned in time for the results to be known to Lind when
he was preparing his third edition. A small expedition, under John Byron,
sailed in June of 1764 and returned after only twenty-two months.[135] The
Admiralty had given Byron special permission to purchase all the vegetables
he needed at ports of call, but despite this, scurvy broke out when they were
crossing the Pacific.[136] At the first island where they were able to go ashore,
"the scurvy grass proved of infinite service." [137] They also took with them,
on the next leg of the voyage, a store of coconuts, and recorded: "It is
astonishing the effect these nuts alone had on those afflicted. . . . Many in
the most violent pain imaginable, . . . and thought to be in the last stage of
that disorder, were in a few days by eating those nuts (tho' at sea) so far
relieved as to do their duty, and even to go aloft as well as they had done
before." [138] Scurvy broke out again a few weeks later, but they recuperated
for two months at Tinian and laid in 2,000 coconuts for the voyage home.[139]
Although Byron's men suffered severely, none of them actually died from
scurvy. Watt has suggested that the outcome demonstrates the benefits of
Byron's having adopted some of Lind's proposals, in having his men
dressed warmly in cold weather, and in taking on vegetables wherever
possible.[140] The results were, of course, very similar to those obtained by
Francis Drake 200 years earlier.

With Byron's safe return, the Admiralty ordered another expedition of
two ships under Captain Wallis, to be fitted out immediately for further
exploration of the South Pacific.[141] They sailed in August of 1766, with
special supplies consisting of three materials recommended as antiscorbutics.[142] The first was dried malt for the preparation of wort. The second,
called "portable soup," was made by first preparing a soup from the offals
of cattle, flavored with salt and vegetables, and then evaporating it down to
form hard, gluelike cakes.[143] The third was "salep" (also spelled "saloop,"
"saloup," "salop," and "salope"), a powder made from dried orchid roots; it

---

[133] MacBride (1767), 5.   [134] Ibid., 32.   [135] Gallagher (1964), xxv, lxii.   [136] Ibid., 92–4.
[137] Ibid., 101.   [138] Ibid., 116.   [139] Ibid., 122.   [140] Watt (1979), 64.   [141] Wallis (1965), *I*,
19.   [142] Ibid., *II*, 448–9.   [143] Lloyd & Coulter (1961), *III*, 87–9.

was popular for thickening jellies and broths, and, weight for weight, had greater thickening power than any other of the starchy materials available.

Lind was thought by Wallis to have recommended a combination of the last two as antiscorbutics.[144] This may have been a misunderstanding, though he did write:

An ounce of powdered salep, and another of portable soup, dissolved in two quarts of boiling water, become a rich thick jelly, capable of receiving any flavour from the addition of spices. This is sufficient sustenance for one man a day; two pounds of each would serve him a month; and being a mixture of both animal and vegetable food, it is more wholesome that either used alone.[145]

The modern reader may feel that there has been some misreading of the text here, because the quantities per day are very small and we can estimate that they would have provided no more than 250 kilocalories, or less than 10% of a man's needs. But the idea that animal heat and energy were produced solely from the energy of the combustion of food was a much later one. Provided that the soup was mucilaginous or jellylike, it was considered to be raw material for conversion into blood. Even Count Rumford, who came later and had a special interest in both heat and latent heat, used very dilute soups when he designed economical diets for the poor. He apparently believed that water itself was a food, provided that it was thickened:

Our knowledge in regard to the *Science of nutrition* is still very imperfect, but I believe, that we are upon the eve of some very important discoveries. . . . It is now known that Water is not a simple element, but a compound, and capable of being decomposed. . . . one single spoonful of salope, put into a pint of boiling water, forms the thickest and most nourishing soup that can be taken; . . . The barley in my soup, seems to act much the same part as the salope in this famous restorative; when it is properly managed, it thickens a vast quantity of water; and, as I suppose, prepares it for decomposition.[146]

We know that Wallis's own ship, the *Dolphin*, with a complement of 150, was provided with 3,000 pounds of portable soup, the equivalent of 320 ounces (i.e., servings) per man. We do not know how much saloop was provided. The other material supplied as an antiscorbutic was sauerkraut (i.e., pickled cabbage).[142] There is no mention of lemon juice. By the time they were well down the east coast of South America in late December, scurvy was becoming serious. They treated it successfully with green vegetables boiled up in the portable soup, and with berries similar to cranberries.[147]

In April, while trying to beat out of the Straits of Magellan against the prevailing wind, the two ships were separated and did not see each other again. The *Dolphin*, which was the better sailer, reached home first in 1768.

[144] Wallis (1965), *II*, 448.    [145] Lind (1788), 352.    [146] Thompson (1800), 194, 199.
[147] Hawkesworth (1773), *I*, 384–5.

They had discovered the island of Tahiti on June 16, but before that were again afflicted with scurvy, despite Wallis's distribution of generous quantities of all the supplies already mentioned, as well as of wine, vinegar, and mustard.[148] They refreshed themselves at Tahiti for five weeks, than had a relatively quick voyage to the East Indies, where each sailor was provided with 500 limes, with extra limes kept on deck so that the sailors could squeeze the juice into their water at will.[149] From there they came home in the usual way, with contagious agues (malarial conditions) and fevers contracted at Batavia as their main problem.[150]

The second ship, the *Swallow*, under Carteret, was much slower and was also leaking. It took many months to cross the Pacific with one short stop at an inhospitable island, and the crew suffered serious scurvy including deaths.[151] Carteret wrote a report assessing the usefulness of the materials with which he had been supplied.[152] In short, he said that the portable soup made green vegetables (when available) much more palatable, also that both wort and salop provided a nourishing diet for scorbutic men, who presumably had difficulty in chewing solid food with sore gums, but that these provisions did not in themselves prevent scurvy. The malt, however, was inconvenient because it took up a great deal of room, became infested with insects, and resulted in a waste of water.[153] It is thought that only the *Dolphin* included pickled cabbage in its stores.[154]

Captain Cook's famous voyages will be considered in the next chapter. Although he returned from his first circumnavigation just before Lind's final revision, it seems unlikely that the reports of it would have been available to Lind when he was writing, and he makes no reference to them.

It is difficult to know what was the generally accepted opinion in 1770 as to the cause of scurvy. Buchan's *Domestic Medicine*, published in 1769, followed Lind quite closely in its review of the principal causes: "by cold moist air; by the long use of any kind of food that is hard of digestion, . . . the want of proper exercise. . . ."[155] The first edition of the *Encyclopaedia Brittanica* was published in Edinburgh in 1771, and most of the article on scurvy is an epitome of Lind's *Treatise*, but it ends with three rather contradictory paragraphs that refer to the contrasting treatments required for the "hot" (or alkaline) form of the disease and the "muriatic" form produced by an excess of salt.[156]

Rouppe, a surgeon with long experience in the Dutch Navy, published a treatise on sailor's disease in 1764, which was translated into English eight years later. He repeatedly referred to Lind and followed him on almost every point. In particular, he stressed the importance of insensible perspiration and the need for exercise and fresh air. He had obviously seen many

---

[148] Ibid., 422.    [149] Ibid., 500.    [150] Ibid., 511.    [151] Wallis (1965), *II*, 377.    [152] Ibid., 444–7.    [153] Ibid., 447.    [154] Ibid., 449.    [155] Buchan (1769), 470–1.    [156] *Encyclopaedia Brittanica* (1771), *III*, 106–10.

cases of severe scurvy but nevertheless believed that Dutch sailors had less of it than the British, because they ate less flesh and more pickled cabbage; roots were also as valuable as fruits or herbs.[157] In both France and Spain, there had been early writings urging the importance of providing citrus fruit as antiscorbutics, but their navies did not receive them as a regular issue, and they continued to suffer severely from scurvy on many occasions.[158]

## Lind's last writings

Now we can return to Lind's own revision of his *Treatise* that appeared in 1772, and we are immediately confronted in his Introduction (titled "Advertisement") with a mood of deep pessimism. He wrote:

> I can carry my researches no further. . . . A work, indeed, more perfect, and remedies more absolutely certain might have been expected . . . ; but, though a few partial facts and observations may, for a little, flatter with hopes of greater success, yet more enlarged experience must ever evince the fallacy of all positive assertions in the healing art.[159]

This seems surprising, but the text sets out the grounds for his disappointments.

First, his investigations at Haslar had failed to confirm his previous belief that sufferers from scurvy were in a state of putrefaction. Blood drawn from them tasted bland and did not corrupt sooner than blood drawn from a healthy subject, nor did the tissues of those who had died from the disease corrupt more quickly.[160] If scurvy was not, after all, a putrid condition this, of course, undercut Pringle and MacBride's theory, just as much as it did Lind's.

Second, there had been no confirmation of the value of his recommended procedure for concentrating lemon juice to a "rob." His friend, Dr. Ives, had judged it to be actually less potent than ordinary stored lemon juice, which was in turn less potent than the fresh fruit; though he did confirm Lind's finding of the uselessness of sulfuric acid.[161] The Admiralty's Sick and Hurt Board had said in 1767 that they thought that the rob would not be efficacious in preventing scurvy and that it would, in any case, be impracticable to supply the Navy in general because of the quantities required.[162] They had arranged for a small batch of twenty-two pints of rob to be prepared at Haslar for testing on a long voyage, but no results were available by 1772. The revised *Treatise* still claimed that the concentrated rob contained all the virtues of the original fruit, but Lind did add a warning that the evaporation should not be carried out in a glazed vessel.[114] The reason was that the

---

[157] Rouppe (1772), 111, 118, 132.  [158] Guerra (1950), 22; Dufrenoy, Dufrenoy, & Rousseau (1954), 995.  [159] Lind (1772), vi.  [160] Ibid., 511–14.  [161] Ibid., 543.  [162] Letter dated 1 July 1767 and filed as ADM/FD/IO at the Naval Museum Library, Greenwich.

acidity of the juice had been found to dissolve lead from the glaze, thus making the product poisonous.[163]

Third, it had recently become more obvious that scurvy could attack armies in a variety of situations on land as seriously as it did sailors at sea. Lind alluded to the great losses from this disease in an Austrian garrison that had been besieged for three months in 1758, and also to the losses in British troops fighting in North America in 1756 and 1759.[164] An outbreak had also occurred during a warm summer in 1761, which could not be associated with the men eating salt meat.[165] Another outbreak occurred very close to home, at Winchester Castle, among French prisoners of war, some of whom had never served at sea.[166] These observations were not in keeping with his theory that the disease was initiated by cold, moist air.

Yet another disappointment for Lind was that, despite that facilities and the large number of cases available at Haslar, he had been quite unable to repeat the kind of experiment, with clear-cut results, that he had organized as a young man at sea on his first attempt.

At different times, I selected a number of patients in Haslar hospital, and administered antiscorbutic remedies . . . the juice of scurvy-grass, the Peruvian bark in large quantities, infusions of berries, stomachic bitters, . . . etc. . . . Patients selected for the trial were confined in wards by themselves; they were strictly watched, and debarred from eating any green vegetables, fruits, or roots whatever, though many of them had not tasted any thing of that sort for several months; they were not even permitted to taste the hospital broth. Their breakfast was balm tea with bread and butter, for dinner they had light pudding, and for supper, water gruel with bread and butter. Upon a daily comparison of the state of those patients, I was surprised to find them all recovering pretty much alike, and though they abstained altogether from vegetables, yet they in general grew better. This . . . convinced me, that the disease would often, from various circumstances, take a favourable turn, which cannot be ascribed to any diet, medicine, or regimen whatever.[167]

In another series of trials, Lind compared the values of different sorts of salads and of different fruits such

as plums, apples, currants, etc. But I could not observe a superior antiscorbutic virtue in any of those, as the patients who ate them did not recover sooner than those who had daily given them the hospital broth, with boiled beef and green. On the other hand, this disease sometimes proves very obstinate, . . . as to prove a lasting affliction to them during a great part of their lives.[168]

Lastly:

there are frequent occurrences in this disease, which I think very difficult to account for; thus . . . some are afflicted with the scurvy, while their constant food consists of vegetables, well baked bread, fresh soups, and other articles of light and easy

---

[163] Lind (1754), 228–9.  [164] Lind (1772), 268–71.  [165] Ibid., 517n.  [166] Ibid., 272.
[167] Ibid., 537–8.  [168] Ibid., 539.

digestion, as was the case of many in Haslar hospital, in the year 1759; while the same diet proves a certain means of relief to others from this disease. Another remarkable, and not an unfrequent occurrence, is, . . . that five or six hundred men, in a long voyage, while living the whole time on salted and hard meats, often continue in perfect health, but soon after they come into a harbour and begin to eat ripe fruits and green vegetables, many of them will be seized with an obstinate scurvy. Several hundred such seamen have been admitted into Haslar hospital . . . ; and notwithstanding the most proper remedies, joined with the utmost care that could be taken of them, the scurvy continued in several of them for five or six weeks.[169]

Against this background it is no wonder that Lind should have concluded that "enlarged experience must ever evince the fallacy of all positive assertions in the healing art."[158] He accepted this, although it was well established that

a moist or cold air, damp lodgings, together with the want of fresh green vegetables, and too long and strict confinement . . . are the general causes which produce a universal and heavy calamity; yet a slighter degree of the disease, or its attack upon a few individuals, will often take place where those general causes do not subsist.[170]

Of the triad of causes, he now put confinement in first place, rather than cold, moist air.[171] The lack of opportunity for exercise might work, he thought, through its weakening effect on the powers of digestion.[172] With regard to his original theory that scurvy was caused by a stoppage of perspiration, he still thought it probable,[173] but he had already said in his Introduction that he retained "some doubtful theoretical doctrines . . . as being agreeable to the present theories of physic," but advised that "the theory of this, as well as of many other diseases, is in general merely conjectural."[174]

Modern reviewers have, as already mentioned, generally preferred not to consider Lind's theory and even to assume instead that he *really* regarded the disease as a straightforward dietary deficiency. Thus, Lloyd and Coulter have said that Poissonière, his French contemporary, *misunderstood* Lind when he quoted him as believing that cold and damp air were causes of the disease.[175] They also have suggested that because of Cockburn's influential position, Lind could not be as rude about the former's theory as he would have wished.[176] Yet the theory was based on bad air, laziness, and indigestible food – all points to be found in his own *Treatise*.

As Lind himself had predicted, he did not carry out any further revision of the *Treatise* after 1772. However, there is an interesting paragraph in the 1779 edition of his "Essay on the Most Effectual Means of Preserving the Health of Seamen." After saying that "syrup of lemons ought always to be put in the surgeon's medicine chest," and describing how orange juice, an

---

[169] Ibid., 540.    [170] Ibid., 516–17.    [171] Ibid., 519, 544.    [172] Ibid., 516.    [173] Ibid., 515.
[174] Ibid., iv.    [175] Lloyd & Coulter (1961), *II*, 303.    [176] Ibid., *III*, 299.

excellent alternative, could be preserved under a layer of olive oil, he went on to say:

For want of these fruits, or their juices, I would suggest another vegetable acid for the use of the navy, which is Cream of Tartar [potassium hydrogen tartrate]. . . . The eighth part of an ounce of this will be sufficient for each man a day, and for half a pint of spirits, mixed with a pint and half of water. . . . If the officers, and others in the ship, who make use of lemons or oranges, would reserve the peels to be put into the spirits served to the men, it would greatly improve the flavour of the punch, and make it little inferior to what is made with lemon-juice. It has hitherto been the aim of those, who have made marine diseases their study, to find out a proper agreeable acid, which sailors might be induced to use, as the best preservative against many of their diseases. Vinegar, spirit of salt, elixir of vitriol, and many others, have been severally recommended, and have been experienced, under proper circumstances, to have produced good effects: Cream of Tartar has the advantage not only of being much more palatable than any of these acids, and, according to . . . my own experience beneficial . . . but is also the cheapest. . . . An allowance of the eighth part of an ounce a day, will not cost the government one shilling yearly, for each man in the West Indies.[177]

He did not say specifically that he was referring here to the prevention of *scurvy*, but one would have expected that if he did *not* believe cream of tartar to have been a substitute for orange juice for that particular purpose he would have been careful to make himself absolutely clear on the point.

Lind retired in 1783 and died eleven years later at the age of seventy-eight. It has been pointed out that he received no honors or public recognition of any kind from the Admiralty or from any of the learned bodies in London, and that he died in comparative obscurity.[178] In recent years, a number of writers, mostly connected with Edinburgh University or with nautical medicine, have sought actively to raise his status in the history of medicine both for his work on scurvy and his advice on hygiene (not considered here) for preventing the spread of infection in the Navy.[179] One eulogist has gone so far as to say that "one of the greatest names in the whole history of medicine is that of James Lind," and: "The discovery of the cause and prevention of scurvy is one of the great chapters in all human history; this discovery was largely the work of James Lind."[180]

Others have attributed Lind's relative obscurity to his lack of the social connections possessed by some other physicians and to their jealousy when they were passed over for the senior appointment at Haslar.[181] I find it difficult to believe that this factor could have continued to operate over a period of more than twenty years. Some of his supporters are perhaps claiming things for him that go beyond the record. Thus Chick has written: "Lind devoted his energies to securing a regular issue of lemon juice in the

---

[177] Lloyd (1965), 43.     [178] Stockman (1926), 336; Watt (1983), 2.     [179] Roddis (1950), 152–5.
[180] Ibid., 2–3.     [181] Meiklejohn (1954), 305, 308; Watt (1979), 64.

Royal Navy."[182] Indeed, this is what one might have expected, but another sympathetic biographer, in a more detailed study, has said: "Lind died 41 years after his book was published without seeing his recommendations carried into any practical effect or any diminution in the terrible ravages of scurvy. It is difficult at this distance of time o say why he did not show more energy in this matter."[183]

Certainly we have no record of Lind ever having set out specific recommendations for the victualing of ships. It was Nathaniel Hulme, rather than Lind, who published *A Proposal for Preventing the Scurvy in the British Navy* in 1768, and argued that to supply every ship with enough citrus juice to provide 1½ ounces per man per day, together with two ounces of sugar, was both practicable and economical. Sources of supply, prices, and means of controlling quality were all discussed, together with the admonition that it must be the responsibility of the Government, rather than of individual sailors, to do this.[184] There was nothing comparable to this in Lind's *Treatise;* advice was given only to individual sailors, who were recommended to carry onions, have some "rob" prepared for them in foreign ports, and so on. Moreover, in his final work in 1779, he seemed to be saying that cream of tartar was an adequate substitute. The dietary advice on scurvy prevention was coupled with hygienic measures for drying the ship and fumigating it with burning tar.[185] He also included examples of people failing to get scurvy when it might have been expected, so that there was no clear final message to those in authority.

Stockman, who had obviously pondered this subject, concluded that Lind's character could be summed up in his remark: "The province has been mine to deliver precepts: the power is in others to execute."[186] We should not take this to mean just that he was not in a position where he could make recommendations; he clearly was. Rather, Lind has told us, and his writings confirm it, that he was by nature a scholar and research worker, concerned with the complexities of the diseases he was studying and not feeling himself suited to take on the very different job of lobbying for administrative actions. A senior naval surgeon in this century, and another admirer of Lind, referred to his "apparent hatred of publicity and self-advertisement" and went on: "This contempt of public opinion, social status, and honours is not so uncommon among real scientists. It is a kind of pride . . . which is to be deplored in so far as it holds up the development of social science and social health."[187]

We should honor Lind for what he was and for his truly pioneering controlled clinical trial. Some well-intentioned claims for things he did not do have led to hypercritical assessments of Lind's work. Thus Mettler's *History of Medicine* states: "Lind . . . could never have cured any real cases

[182] Chick (1953), 213.    [183] Stockman (1926), 340.    [184] Hulme (1768), 53–9, 78–83.
[185] Stewart & Guthrie (1953), 158–73.    [186] Stockman (1926), 340.    [187] Dudley (1953a), 204–5.

of scurvy with the boiled and evaporated syrup that he recommended so highly. It is difficult to believe that Lind was an absolute fraud, and we can only conclude that he over-embroidered his account in order to achieve greater elegance."[188] In fact, Lind never claimed that "rob" prepared by his recipe had cured scurvy, and we have seen that he included in his third edition Dr. Ives's evaluation of it as "inferior to stored fruit juice."[161] On the other hand, he still retained the claim in the description of the procedure, that "it preserves their virtues entire for years."[189] He must have assumed that as long as the juice did not actually come to a boil and the flavor was not lost, the activity would be retained; we shall see later that this was unjustified.

This last point is the weakest in Lind's record, especially in view of his claim that "the means of preventing and curing . . . are found upon attested facts and observations without suffering the illusions of theory to influence and prevent the judgement."[190] It has led to the most recent criticism that "by recommending . . . the 'rob' . . . and other remedies of low or negligible antiscorbutic value he complicated, if he did not delay, the successful management of scurvy in British and Western European shipping."[191] This seems overly critical if we remember that the other treatments in use during the period included bleeding, purging with salt water, and dosing with mercurials. Certainly, not every one of Lind's recommendations is seen now, with our benefit of hindsight, as being antiscorbutic, but if his recommendations, *taken as a whole*, had been adopted, there can be no doubt of their favorable effect. Let us respect the man in the context of his period and by what he *did*, rather than by what, from our viewpoint, we think he *might* have done.

---

[188] Mettler and Mettler (1947), 410.    [189] Lind (1772), 160.    [190] Stewart & Guthrie (1953), 7.
[191] Norris (1983), 334.

# 4

## Captain Cook and pneumatic chemistry (1770–1815)

We have seen in Chapter 3 how the rapid rise in general scientific knowledge from 1700 to 1770 was accompanied by an actual worsening of the problem of scurvy at sea. The European naval powers were engaged in wars that required the maintenance of large fleets in foreign stations and also, in the case of Britain, the continuous blockade of the European coast, with ships having to remain at sea for long periods, even though they were at no great distance from their home ports.

The magnitude of the problem, in turn, stimulated considerable interest in medical circles, with numerous proposals as to the cause of the disease and its prevention. Most writers, as we have seen, felt that although eating fresh fruit and vegetables would cure scurvy, it was not just the inadequacy of the diet that precipitated the disease at sea; they therefore looked for some positive cause. In the eighteenth century the properties of gases were a new and exciting field of research. First to be explored was the physical property of elasticity; then, in the period to be covered in this chapter, came the discoveries of "pneumatic chemistry," through which it was found that air was a mixture of gases with different properties, one of which, "fixed air" (or carbon dioxide, in modern terminology), could dissolve in water and be "condensed" into solid chemicals.[1]

Two quite different theories associating scurvy with the quality of the air breathed by sailors had already been put forward. The first was that inadequate ventilation below decks resulted in a buildup of a toxic component and that the problem could be cured by forced ventilation. The second (held by Lind) was that the moistness of the air was a sufficient cause through its effect of inhibiting natural perspiration.

By 1770 it had appeared that improved ventilation of ships really had little relation to scurvy. The increasing number of reports of scurvy out-

[1] Leicester (1974), 128–37.

75

breaks among armies on land also undermined the belief that it was caused by moist air. The practical question for the Admiralty, therefore, reduced to the kind of supplies they could issue to ships, that would (a) be effective antiscorbutics, (b) be stable for at least one year and preferably two, (c) not be unduly bulky or require the use of a lot of fresh water, and (d) be regularly available in large quantities and at a reasonable cost.

## Cook's first expedition

We have already seen that some naval expeditions had been given different preparations to try out, and that the conclusions had been rather equivocal. At the beginning of the period to be covered by the present chapter, a further expedition was at sea under Captain James Cook, and the Admiralty hoped that their instructions for careful testing would lead to a resolution of some of the questions.

Cook is, of course, the second name (along with that of Lind) popularly associated with the elimination of scurvy as an inevitable risk on long voyages. He is also a hero both for his successful voyages of exploration and for having made his way from very humble beginnings.[2] The son of a Scottish farm laborer, he left school at the age of thirteen, and at eighteen went to sea as an apprentice in a ship carrying coal in the British coasting trade.[3] This was hard training, and he graduated after five years to the rank of "Mate." Then, after nine years at sea, he transferred in 1755 to the Royal Navy, starting as an "Able Seaman," but quickly being promoted to Warrant Officer.[4] Again, after showing extraordinary skill as a surveyor and chartmarker, he was commissioned in 1768 as a First Lieutenant and given command of a small ship, the *Endeavour*.[5] His orders were to carry a scientific expedition to the South Pacific to observe and time an astronomical event – the predicted transit of Venus across the Sun's disc in June 1769 – and then to continue the exploration of the area.[6]

Obviously, Cook would have known of the outbreaks of scurvy on other voyages in the Pacific, and he had already seen a severe outbreak of the disease when serving in 1757 off the coast of Canada.[7] In addition, he received instructions to test and report on the value of the same variety of antiscorbutic remedies that had been supplied earlier for Wallis and Carteret's expedition, i.e., sauerkraut, portable soup, saloup, malt, and "rob of oranges and lemons."[8] He was given a particularly large supply of malt, was provided with copies of MacBride's *Experimental Essays*, and was told that there was "great reason to believe that malt made into wort may be of great benefit to seamen in scorbutic and other putrid diseases."[9]

---

[2] Cook's life has been the subject of many books. In connection with scurvy a biography of moderate length by a naval surgeon (Muir, 1939) is of particular interest.    [3] Beaglehole (1974), 3–8.    [4] Ibid., 11–25.    [5] Ibid., 67–98, 128.    [6] Ibid., 147–9.    [7] Muir (1939), 24.    [8] Beaglehole (1955), *I*, 610–13.    [9] Ibid., 622.

The outcome of the expedition was that during the entire three-year voyage, no one died of scurvy or was seriously ill with it. By a coincidence, at one point when he was exploring the coast of New Zealand, a French expedition was, unknown to him, in the same area and with many already dead from scurvy and with most of the rest too weak to go ashore.[10] Forty-one of the ninety-four men starting out with Cook did die, but mainly from dysentery contracted at Batavia on the return journey.[11] One of those dying was the ship's surgeon, and it was left to his mate to make the medical reports on the voyage. Here we are directly concerned only with scurvy, but Sir James Watt has made an analysis of all the diseases encountered on Cook's voyages.[12]

The conditions were very different from those in the ordinary Fleet. The crew were all picked men, and the ship was victualed on a lavish scale for the period. Also, unlike some of the earlier Pacific explorers, they never had to be away from land for more than seventeen weeks at a time.[13] Cook took every opportunity of gathering green leafy material or yams and coconuts at each landing place and then ensuring that they were eaten by his men. As the editor of his *Journals* says:"It was not that Cook was unique or original in his approach to the problem of diet at sea . . . but his . . . determination to replenish and vary his supplies was reduced to a sort of passionate system."[14] Interestingly, he makes no reference to searching out citrus fruits. He also makes no mention of Lind, and it is thought that he had never seen his *Treatise*.

In a famous passage from his journal he describes how the men, at first, would not eat the sauerkraut provided; he then

had some of it dressed every day for the (officers') cabin table and left it to the option of the men either to take as much as they pleased or none at all; but . . . before a week I found it necessary to put every one on board to an allowance, for . . . whatever you give seamen out of the common way, although it be ever so much for their good yet . . . you will hear nothing but murmurings against the man that first invented it; but the moment they see their superiors set a value upon it, it becomes the finest stuff in the world and the inventor an honest fellow.[15]

(In this and subsequent notes of Cook's voyages the spelling has been standardized.)

Of course, with such a combination of measures against the scurvy, it was really impossible to sort out which was active and which was not. Thus in reporting on the value of the sauerkraut, he said:

The sour krout together with the many other antiscorbutics my Lords Commissioners of the Admiralty were pleased to order to be put on board did so effectually

[10] Dunmore (1981), 124, 212, 245.   [11] Lloyd & Coulter (1961), *III*, 311–12.   [12] Watt (1979), 69–72; 75–81.   [13] Lloyd & Coulter (1961), *III*, 304.   [14] Beaglehole (1955), *I*, clxvii. [15] Ibid., 74.

preserve the people from a scorbutic taint that not one dangerous case happened in that disorder during the whole voyage, and it is our opinion that sour krout had a great share in it . . . ; it has the good quality not to lose any part of its efficacy by keeping; we used the last of it in September last after having been above two years on board and it was then as good as at the first.[16]

Cook was, presumably, making the dangerous assumption that so long as the sauerkraut retained its original appearance and taste, it also retained its original antiscorbic value. Moreover, it seems illogical, when so many treatments had been used, that he could even venture to put a value on one of them. The same point holds for the following comments by Perry, the surgeon's mate:

Sour Krout, Mustard, Vinegar, Wheat, Inspissated Oranges and Lemon Juices, Saloup, Portable Soup, Sugar, Molasses, Vegetables (at all times when they could possibly be got), were some in constant, others in occasional use: these were of such infinite service to the people in preserving them from a scorbutic taint, that the use of the Malt was, with respect to necessity, almost entirely precluded. Again, cold bathing was encouraged and enforced by example, the allowance of salt beef and pork was abridged from nearly the beginning of the voyage and the sailors' usual custom of mixing the salt beef fat with their flour etc strictly forbad: . . . throughout the voyage raisins were served with the flour instead of pickled suet. What opportunities have occurred of using [Mr. MacBride's medicine] have constantly been embraced; . . . [Describes four cases of scurvy that occurred in March and April of 1769] From [April 12, 1769] while at sea the wort became a part of our diet, so that, excepting five cases, . . . not a man more suffered any inconvenience from this distemper. In the cases I have mentioned, a trial was made of the robs and attended with success. It is impossible for me to say what was most conducive to our preservation from scurvy, so many being the preventives used, but from what I have seen the wort perform, from its mode of operation, from Mr. MacBride's reasoning I shall not hesitate a moment to declare my opinion, viz. that the malt is the best medicine I know, the inspissated orange and lemon juices not even excepted.[17]

The naturalist in the *Endeavour* was Joseph Banks, later to succeed Pringle as President of the Royal Society. It was unfortunate that his journal of the voyage was not published for another century, because his experience did not fit what Perry had said.[18] In April 1769, when they had just reached Tahiti, and seven months after leaving home, he wrote:

As I am now on the brink of going ashore after a long passage, thank God, in as good health as man can be, I shall fill a little paper in describing the means which I have taken to prevent the scurvy in particular. The ship was supplied by the Admiralty with sour-crout, of which I eat constantly, till our salted cabbage was opened, which I preferred: as a pleasant substitute, wort was served out almost constantly, and of this I drank a pint or more every evening, but all this did not check the distemper so entirely as to prevent my feeling some small effect of it. About a fortnight ago my gums swelled, and some small pimples rose on the inside of my mouth, which

16 Ibid., 633.     17 Ibid., 632–3.     18 Lloyd (1961), 126.

threatened to become ulcers; I then flew to the lemon juice, which had been put up for me according to Dr. Hulme's method . . . [described in his letter, which is inserted here in Banks's journal]. Every kind of liquor which I used was made sour with lemon juice No. 3, so that I took nearly six ounces a day of it; the effect of this was surprising, in less than a week my gums became as firm as ever, and at this time I am troubled with nothing but a few pimples on my face, which have not deterred me from leaving off the juice entirely.[19]

Hulme's letter explained that he was sending a concentrated rob of lemon juice, also a cask of seven gallons of orange juice with one gallon of brandy added and, lastly, cask no. 3 containing five quarts of lemon juice with one quart of brandy.[20] Banks noted that both the rob and the juices appeared to be in good condition, but that he chose to use up cask no. 3 because it had been leaking.

This experience seemed to indicate a clear superiority of lemon juice to wort. Nevertheless, a year later, Banks paid an unexpected tribute to the sagacity of MacBride in his *Journal*:

Our malt having turned out so indifferent that the surgeon made little use of it, a method was thought of some weeks ago to bring it into use, which was, to make as strong a wort with it as possible, and in this boil the wheat, which is served to the people for breakfast. . . . I myself . . . , either received, or thought I received, great benefit from the use of this mess. It totally banished that troublesome costiveness [constipation] which I believe most people are subject to when at sea. Whether or not this is a more beneficial method of administering wort as a preventative than the common, must be left to the faculty, especially that excellent surgeon Mr. Mac-Bride, whose ingenious treatise on the sea-scurvy can never by sufficiently commended. For my own part I should be inclined to believe that the salubrious qualities of the wort which arise from fermentation might in some degree at least be communicated to the wheat when thoroughly saturated with its particles, which would consequently acquire a virtue similar to that of fresh vegetables, the greatest resisters of sea-scurvy known.[21]

This is an unexpected statement because Banks's only direct experience was of the laxative properties of wort, and a year earlier, as we have just seen, he had started to develop scurvy while taking wort, and had cured himself by taking lemon juice. The only explanation seems to be the intellectual attraction of MacBride's theory, which we shall return to shortly.

## Cook's apparent success with malt

Cook arrived in the Admiralty for the success of the expedition and, in less than three months, was ordered to prepare another. This time he was to take two ships towards the South Pole and to look for the hypothetical Southern Continent. At one point an invitation to be Astronomer to the expedition

---

[19] Banks (1896), 71–2.   [20] Ibid., 69.   [21] Ibid., 258–9.

was sent to "Dr. James Lind." [22] This has caused some confusion among historians.[23] However, the invitation was not to "our" Lind but to a namesake, also with an Edinburgh Doctor of Medicine degree, but twenty years younger and an amateur astronomer. He did not, in fact, go with Cook but later traveled with Banks in Iceland and became a Fellow of the Royal Society.[24]

Cook again received exceptional help with the issue of the supplies that he wanted. For a total complement of 200 men, he took nearly 100 pounds of sauerkraut per head, twenty-five pounds of salted cabbage, and fifteen pounds portable soup, together with smaller quantities of malt, saloup, and mustard, all of which were classified as antiscorbutics.[25] Something new was a total consignment of thirty gallons of carrot marmalade. This had been highly recommended as an antiscorbutic by a Baron Storch of Berlin, and the Victualling Board had had it prepared by evaporating carrot juice to the thickness of treacle.[26] He was also supplied with Joseph Priestley's instructions and equipment for making "water impregnated with fixed air" (soda water).[27] Cook, as always, was willing to increase the variety of the supplements available to his men. He also asked for a further supply of "rob of oranges and lemons which we found of great use in preventing the scurvy from laying hold of our men, . . . a quantity in proportion to what the Endeavour had." [28] That, as we saw in Chapter 3, was just a few gallons in total, so that again, it could have been intended only as part of the surgeons' supplies.

The ships finally set off in July 1772 and reached the Cape of Good Hope in good health after a three-month voyage, with a call at Madeira for "refreshment" that included the purchase of onions. While they were at the Cape, two Dutch East Indiamen arrived from Holland; they had lost 150 men from scurvy in a four-month voyage. From there Cook traveled south, and by mid-December was in latitude 50° S and sailing among icebergs. On December 20, it was noted that three men had been seriously affected by scurvy, and that two had been cured by rob but one had not. Cook ordered that everyone beginning to have symptoms should receive wort; Mr. Wales, the Astronomer, recorded: "Unhappily I am one of them." [29]

They went even further south, below 60°, for a further two months and then headed north toward New Zealand. Before reaching land, the two ships were separated in heavy fog. Cook in the *Resolution* anchored in a bay in the southwest corner of the country, on March 26, after 117 days at sea. He felt that it was very creditable, under these conditions, to have only one man ill from scurvy and two or three others on the sick list with slight complaints. Even the one serious case was "occasioned chiefly by a bad habit of body, and a complication of other disorders. . . . We are not to

[22] Beaglehole (1961), *II*, 902–3.　　[23] Lewis (1972), 41.　　[24] *D.N.B* (1893), *XI*, 1151–2; Guthrie & Meiklejohn (1953), 398.　　[25] Beaglehole (1961), *II*, 13.　　[26] Ibid., 15, 910. [27] Ibid., 917; Gibbs (1965), 59.　　[28] Beaglehole (1961), *II*, 917.　　[29] Ibid., 64.

attribute the general good state of health in the crew wholly to the sweet wort and marmalade, this last was given to only one man; we must allow portable broth and sour krout to have had some share in it; this last article can never be enough recommended." [30]

The two ships met again on May 17 at another prearranged rendezvous on the New Zealand coast. Captain Furneaux, in the *Adventure*, had reached the rendezvous some weeks earlier, and then erected tents on shore because of "several on board much afflicted with the scurvy." [31] The difference in the health record on the two ships persisted. At the end of July, when they had been at sea again for another six weeks, the *Adventure's* cook, described as indolent and dirty, died of scurvy, and others were seriously ill with it, whereas on the *Resolution* there were only mild symptoms. [32] Cook ordered the usual dietary supplements for both ships and speculated that

the crew of the Adventure being more scorbutic . . . than we were . . . [might be owing to] their eating few or no vegetables when they reached New Zealand, partly for want of knowing the right sorts. . . . To introduce any new food among seamen requires both the authority and example of a Commander. . . . Many of my people at first disliked celery, scurvy grass, etc being boiled in the pease and wheat . . . but this obstinate prejudice, by little and little, wore off. [33]

Cook also organized the brewing of spruce beer which may have been of some value. [34]

He learned that the *Adventure* had been using wort and noted: "It would be proper to examine the Surgeon's journal to know when and in what quantity the wort was given to these scorbutic people, for if it was properly applied, we have a proof that it alone will neither cure nor prevent the sea-scurvy." [35] Two weeks later, Furneaux told Cook that his men were improved "due to giving them cyder, wort and some of the things that had been proposed." [36] However, when they reached Tahiti after a further two weeks, "many were so weak they were unable to get on deck without assistance," whereas none in the *Resolution* had "the least touch of scurvy." [37] They soon recovered with the fruits and coconuts to be had on the island.

For the remainder of the voyage, suffice it to say that Cook brought the *Resolution* home in July 1776 with only one man lost from sickness, and that not due to scurvy. Again, after a three-year voyage he had returned with an astonishing health record, and his opinions were attended to with the greatest respect. As usual, he reported to the Admiralty on the value of the different antiscorbutic supplies. [38] He also submitted a very similar report to

[30] Ibid., 111.   [31] Ibid., 737.   [32] Ibid., 185n, 186n; Burney (1975), 58, 59n.   [33] Beaglehole (1961), *II*, 187–8; see also Hoare (1982), *II*, 297.   [34] Kodieck & Young (1969), 55–6. [35] Beaglehole (1961), *II*, 188n; Kodicek & Young (1969), 54, give the final part of this quotation without the qualifiying "if."   [36] Beaglehole (1961), *II*, 191.   [37] Ibid., 205.   [38] Ibid., 954–5.

Pringle, the President of the Royal Society, who had it published in their *Transactions*.[39] This is what he wrote, with a slight condensation at some points:

Many expressed surprise at the good state of health which the crew of the Resolution experienced during her late voyage. Much was owing to the attention given by the Admiralty, in causing articles to be put on board, judged to tend most to preserve the health of seamen. I shall confine myself to such as were found the most useful.

We had a large quantity of malt, of which was made sweet-wort, and given to those who had manifest symptoms of the scurvy, and to such also as were judged to be most liable to that disorder from one pint to three quarts in the twenty-four hours. This is without doubt one of the best antiscorbutic sea-medicines yet found out; and if given in time will, with proper attention to other things, I am persuaded, prevent the scurvy from making any great progress for a considerable time: but I am not altogether of opinion, that it will cure it in an advanced state at sea.

Sour krout, of which we had also a large provision, is not only a wholesome vegetable food, but, in my judgement, highly antiscorbutic, and spoils not by keeping. A pound of it was served to each man, when at sea, twice a week, or oftener when it was thought necessary. Portable soup or broth, was another essential article, of which we had likewise a liberal supply. An ounce of this to each man, or such other proportion as was thought necessary, was boiled with their pease three days in the week; and when we were in place where fresh vegetables could be procured it was boiled with them. It was the means of making the people eat a greater quantity of greens than they would have done otherwise.

Further, we were provided with rob of lemons and oranges; which the surgeon found useful in several cases. Also we were furnished with sugar in the room of oil. Sugar, I imagine, is a very good antiscorbutic; whereas oil, has the contrary effect. Proper care was taken of the ship's coppers. The fat, which boiled out of the salt beef and pork, I never suffered to be given to the people . . . being of opinion that it promotes the scurvy.

But the introduction of the most salutary articles, either as provision or medicines, will generally prove unsuccessful, unless supported by certain rules of living. . . . The crew were at three watches [four hours on and eight hours off] except upon some extraordinary occasions. By this means they were not so much exposed to the weather as if they had been at watch-and-watch: and they had generally dry clothes to shift themselves when they happened to get wet. Care was also taken to expose them as little as possible. Proper methods were employed to keep their persons, hammocks, bedding clothes, etc constantly clean and dry. . . . To this and cleanliness, as well in the ship as amongst the people, too great attention cannot be paid; the least neglect occasions a putrid, offensive smell below, which nothing but fires will remove.

I never failed to take in water wherever it was to be procured, even when we did not seem to want it; because I look upon fresh water from the shore to be much more wholesome than that which has been kept some time on board. . . . I am convinced, that with plenty of fresh water, and a close attention to cleanliness, a ship's company will seldom be much afflicted with scurvy, though they should not be provided with any of the antiscorbutics before mentioned. We came to few places

[39] Cook (1776), 402–6.

[which] . . . did not afford some sort of refreshment. It was my first care to procure what could be met with, and to oblige our people to make use thereof. . . .

These, sir, were the methods, under the care of Providence, by which the Resolution performed a voyage of three years and eighteen days, through all the climates from 52° North to 71° South, with the loss of one man only by disease, a complicated and lingering illness, without any mixture of scurvy.

Pringle added, as a postscript to this paper, an extract from a reply by Cook to some points made by Pringle himself: "I entirely agree with you, that the dearness of the rob of lemons and of oranges will hinder them from being furnished in large quantities, but I do not think this so necessary for though they may assist other things, I have no great opinion of them alone. Nor have I a higher opinion of vinegar." [39]

Perhaps, inevitably, Cook somewhat adjusted the tone of his report so as to be as pleasant as possible to Pringle, the progenitor of the theory behind the use of wort. His original report to the Admiralty had some additional points: "We were happy in having few or no opportunities in giving full and fair trial, to either the marmalade of carrots or water impregnated with fixed air, my opinion is not very favourable to either and that [of ] the surgeons worse. . . ." Then, he said that wort "will, with proper attention to other things prevent the scurvy from making any progress, but I am afraid it will seldom be found to cure it," and added: "We have been a long time without any, without feeling the want of it, which might be owing to other Articles." [38]

Pringle announced the award of the Copley Medal of the Royal Society to Cook for his success in keeping his expeditions free from scurvy. Cook could not receive it in person because he had already left on yet another voyage, in which he was to be killed by natives on a beach in Hawaii. It seems that illness had changed his normally even-tempered nature, and he became involved in an altercation.[40]

Obviously, Cook had shown that it was possible to conduct long voyages without scurvy having to appear as a serious threat. He is rightfully considered a "hero," and in consequence all sorts of claims are made for him. A surprising one is that "Lord Anson and Captain Cook were the first navigators who employed lemon juice on their crew for the treatment of sea-scurvy." [41] Another recent paper in a scientific journal stated that: "On his three round-the-world voyages, Captain Cook ordered daily lemon juice for the crew and none of his sailors got scurvy." [42] This is obviously pure myth. The final assessments in the most recent studies of naval medicine of the period are that Cook "confused the scurvy problem," [43] and that "contrary to general belief, . . . Cook's voyages delayed rather than hastened the introduction of the true cure of scurvy." [44]

It seems, at first, illogical that his successes could be considered "confusing." The essential point, of course, is that he took such a range of measures

[40] Watt (1979), 80; Beaglehole (1974), 667–72.     [41] Parkes (1830), 265n.     [42] Pratt (1984), 118.     [43] Watt (1982), 41.     [44] Lloyd & Coulter (1961), *III*, 318; Lloyd (1961), 124, 129.

that he, himself, could not be sure which were the really effective ones. Then, influential people at home were already convinced of the value of wort and used Cook's endorsement of it to promote the idea that it would be sufficient of itself to prevent scurvy at sea.[45] Certainly the statistics for disease in the Navy show no improvement in the following decade. In 1780, the Channel Fleet returned to Portsmouth after a ten-week cruise with 2,400 men ill from scurvy, of whom nearly 1,500 were taken to Haslar Hospital.[46]

We have been concentrating on Cook's experience from 1768 to 1776, but other papers continued to appear at the same time. In 1773, John Clark published the results of six cases of scurvy which were treated with wort at sea and showed no improvement.[47] On the other hand, in 1776, James Badenoch published notes of several cases in which scorbutic patients had at least been kept in stable condition by dosing with two quarts of wort per day.[48] He also described one "perfect cure" in three weeks during which time the patient received nearly nine gallons of wort and one quart of lemon juice; he added that "it may perhaps be suggested by some, that the lemon-juice had a considerable share in this cure; but the contrary is well known to every practitioner who hath tried that remedy in the cure of the scurvy at sea, the utmost to be expected from it being only to mitigate or to prevent the increase of that disease."[49]

## Fermentation versus putrefaction

Also in 1776, David MacBride published further ideas on the mechanisms by which putrefaction could be prevented.[50] Today, with 200 years of hindsight, his ideas about the cause and cure of scurvy seem totally wrong, though one modern writer has referred to "the happy chance by which MacBride stumbled upon a method . . . which was responsible for the success of Cook's voyages."[51] This is certainly incorrect. At the other extreme, he has been treated as something of a "villain" by biographers of Lind, and charged with arrogance in using Lind's ideas without acknowledgement and with cynically adopting Pringle's ideas on putrefaction only to enhance his own reputation.[52] This seems equally out of proportion. He did have an original idea, and we must go back a few years further into the history of research on gases, in order to place that idea in perspective and to understand why the use of fermentable materials in the treatment of disease seemed such an exciting advance in the 1760s and 1770s.[53]

Stephen Hales, with the encouragement of Newton in his old age, had returned in the 1720s to the problem of gases or "air," which apparently

[45] Watt (1979), 76.    [46] Lloyd (1965), 202–3.    [47] Clark (1773), 283–99.    [48] Badenoch (1776), 63–7.    [49] Ibid., 68–72.    [50] MacBride (1776).    [51] Oliver (1973), 206.    [52] Watt (1979), 67.    [53] Scott (1970), 46–9.

consisted of particles that repelled each other at a distance so as to occupy a large volume in the gaseous state, and yet would stay in a compressed form in a substance like marble (calcium carbonate) until released by heat or the action of an acid.[54] He urged the importance of the study of air, which obviously played such an important part "in a continual round of the production and dissolution of animal and vegetable bodies."[55]

This line of thought was then taken up at the medical schools in Glasgow and Edinburgh under the influence of Professor William Cullen, a strong believer in the importance of chemistry as a basis for further medical advances.[56] His student, Joseph Black, showed that constant, weighable amounts of "fixed air" were expellable from calcareous earths heated to form caustic alkalies, and that the same quantity could then be reabsorbed. This "fixed air" was "not air in its ordinary form, but one particular species only."[57] He also said that both food and living animal tissues contained fixed air "which serves many great uses."[58]

These and other discoveries stimulated a new field of "pneumatic chemistry," which seemed suddenly to add a new dimension to the possibilities of understanding the interactions of humans with their environment. It takes an effort of imagination for us to understand this. Perhaps there was something analogous to the explosion of interest in DNA and Molecular Biology in the 1960s, at which time there was the feeling that for research in any division of biology to be current, it must make use of these new concepts.

David MacBride, the young physician practicing in Dublin, was told of Black's work by a friend of Black who had returned to Dublin from Glasgow, and MacBride was the first person to refer to it in print, in his own *Experimental Essays* published in 1764.[59] He had also been impressed by the idea that dissolution of animal bodies was characterized by an evolution of air, which he thought of as an escape of previously trapped air. He thought that it must follow logically that it was this "held" or "fixed" air that was responsible for the cohesiveness of living, healthy tissue.[59] Then he took Pringle's work, published in 1750, indicating that fermentation inhibited putrefaction, one step further by suggesting that the fermentation worked *because* the special "fixed air," which it produced, was at the very site in which there was risk of putrefaction. He must have thought, though it is not explicit in his writing, that the pressure of the external "air" somehow prevented the air already "fixed" in the material from escaping; and that the treatment or prevention of putrefactive disease, through the subjects consuming a food that fermented rapidly in the digestive tract, would be effective because the air released would penetrate into the recesses of the alimentary tract and other tissues.

[54] Hales (1727), 312–13.   [55] Ibid., 314.   [56] Donovan (1975), 39–41.   [57] Ibid., 201–12.   [58] Ibid., 191–92; Scott (1970), 47.   [59] Guerlac (1957), 453–4; MacBride (1776), 117–18.

MacBride now carried out other experiments. He believed that, as judged by their smell, he had either prevented or delayed putrefaction in small pieces of meat, both by preventing the escape of air (by coating the meat with melted suet) and by having them surrounded by "fixed air," either by hanging them in the neck of a flask in which fixed air was being evolved from a fermentation, or by immersing them in a fermented liquor such as wine.[60]

As a former naval surgeon, he had an obvious interest in scurvy and accepted the current views that it was one of the putrefactive diseases, and also that it could be cured with fresh fruit or vegetables. As one might have expected, he thought that these acted by being more rapidly fermented in the digestive tract than hardened vegetable material like ship's biscuit. He then took it as axiomatic that it was impracticable to supply such fresh foods on long voyages, so that some alternative was required, and he suggested that malt was a promising one.[61]

These ideas attracted considerable interest. Joseph Priestley found that he could make soda water by shaking water with "fixed air," and suggested that it, too, be tested at sea. We have seen already that Cook took the equipment for its preparation on his second voyage. It has been said that Priestley received the Copley Medal in 1773 for his discovery of the method of making soda water and its presumed medical importance.[62] Certainly Pringle, now the President of the Society, who gave the discourse at the presentation of the Copley Medal, praised him for using this discovery in the public interest, but it is clear that the Medal was given for the whole of his extensive work on gases.[63]

A number of physicians examined the effect of fixed air on patients with supposedly "putrid" diseases. One reported that his tuberculous patients "inspired the steams of an effervescing mixture of chalk and vinegar through the spout of a coffee pot."[64] He did not claim any cures, but thought that the fever was lessened. Others were more skeptical, and, already in 1771, William Alexander, an Edinburgh physician, had reported that he had been unable in his own tests to keep meat from putrefying to the extent described by MacBride. He suggested that the loss of air was "rather a circumstance attending putrefaction than the cause of it."[65] As another modern writer has pointed out, the main criterion of putrefaction in the experiments was smell, and the sense of smell is quickly deadened when going from sample to sample.[66]

Pringle, in his discourse on the occasion of the presentation of Cook's Copley Medal in 1776, again praised MacBride's theory and assumed that the value of "fixed air" was now a fact: "Before the power of the fixed air in subduing putrefaction was known, the efficacy of fruits, greens and fer-

---

[60] MacBride (1776), 45, 72–3, 146.    [61] MacBride (1767), 3–4.    [62] McKie (1961), 2.
[63] Ibid., 7; Priestley (1772).    [64] Percival (1774), 303–14.    [65] Scott (1970), 50.    [66] Ibid., 51n.

mented liquors [in curing scurvy] was attributed to the acid in their composition. . . ." [67] He suggested that the "rob of lemons" was of little value because "by evaporating upon a fire . . . their aqueous parts had lost not a little of their aerial, on which so much of their antiseptic virtue depended." [68]

In 1778, Hulme, who had earlier urged the use of lemon juice in the Navy, now recommended "salt of tartar" (potassium carbonate) mixed with weak spirit of vitriol as an effervescing drink and therefore a good source of fixed air.[69] Watt has characterized this change as showing that he "lacked the moral fibre to sustain a correct but unpopular theory." [70] In the following year, Matthew Dobson reported further successes with fixed air in the treatment of putrid diseases. A young lady with all the signs of scurvy "drank water saturated with Fixed Air, took the effervescing draughts [salts of tartar acidified with lemon juice] and was allowed to eat ripe fruit at pleasure: she was perfectly recovered in the course of three weeks."[71] The young lady was fortunate, we would think, in the choice of acidifying agent.

However, by this time it was beginning to be accepted that combustion, fermentation, and respiration all yielded the same "fixed air" product.[72] No one in the 1780s formally withdrew the earlier claims for the virtues of "fixed air," but it obviously became ridiculous to think that something which the body was continually producing and excreting in the breath would also be a valuable medicine. As a naval surgeon put it in 1792: "The very process necessary for its production abundantly refutes the idea that this is . . . the cure of scurvy." [72] Whether or not malt could be expected to show antiscorbutic activity by any other mechanism will be discussed in Chapter 10.

At the siege of Gibralter in 1780, there was a serious outbreak of scurvy. "Extract of malt was used without success," but when a cargo of lemons was purchased, "the salutary effects were almost instantaneous; in a few days men who had been considered irrecoverable, left their beds." [73] In 1782, Professor Milman criticized the idea that scurvy was a disease of putrefaction (as Lind had done already in his third edition), and, therefore, also the relevance of Pringle's type of experiments on antiseptics.[74] He himself attributed scurvy to weakness resulting from sailors having to consume such an indigestible diet of salted meat and hard biscuit; he believed that the sufferers needed a stimulant such as brandy.[75]

Sir John Pringle had resigned the Presidency of the Royal Society in 1778 (at age sixty-five) because of infirmity, and lived only another four years.[76] He appears, when judged solely in terms of the history of scurvy, and with our modern hindsight, to be another "villain." Certainly, he did seem to use

---

[67] Pringle (1776), 19.  [68] Ibid., 21.  [69] Hulme (1778).  [70] Watt (1979), 85.  [71] Dobson (1779), 61.  [72] Trotter (1792), 189.  [73] Drinkwater (1786), 114–15.  [74] Milman (1782), 202–3, 210.  [75] Ibid., 91.  [76] Singer (1949–50), 179–80.

his position as President to publicize the "fermentation" theory for the treatment of scurvy, which fitted and supported his own published ideas that disease was generally the result of putrefaction; also, by selective quotation, he seriously distorted the record of Cook's experience. In other respects, he has a quite different reputation. His interest in "putrefaction" grew out of his experience as Physician to the Army in Flanders in the 1740s. And his unquestioned reforms, aimed at increasing the ordinary soldier's comfort and hygiene, have led to his being described as the father of military medicine. He also had the reputation of being extremely liberal in trying to break down the religious intolerance shown by professional bodies in London, of assisting young people in need of help, and of patching up quarrels, including that between James Boswell (Dr. Johnson's biographer) and his father.[77] Benjamin Franklin described him as a good friend, and they spent at least one summer vacation together, traveling in France.[78]

## The oxygen theory

The loss of belief in carbon dioxide as a treatment of "putrid disease" did not mean the end of "pneumatic chemistry" as a source of ideas for both the cause and the cure of diseases and of scurvy in particular.[79] The same period saw the discovery of oxygen and its essential role in animal life,[80] and soon there was a new school arguing that it was a lack of oxygen in the tissues that was responsible for the scorbutic condition. The pioneer in this school was Thomas Trotter, still another Scot who had studied medicine in Edinburgh, and had then gone to sea as a surgeon's mate at the age of nineteen, in 1779. He saw severe dysentery and scurvy and was himself a sufferer in his first ship when it struggled home in a partly disabled condition from the West Indies.[81] In 1783, with the end of the fighting, he was paid off and could find employment only in a merchant ship taking slaves from West Africa to the Caribbean. Scurvy broke out among them, which Trotter attributed partly to the foul air in the hold where they were confined. He had noticed that the slaves seemed to prefer unripe, acid-tasting guavas to those that were ripe and sweet, and he surmised that this might represent an instinctive preference for those with the greater antiscorbutic value. From a controlled experiment with nine victims of the disease, he concluded that the three receiving unripe guavas recovered as well as the three receiving limes, whereas those receiving the ripe fruit showed little change.[82]

He was disgusted by the conditions of the trade and left at the end of the voyage. After a short period of private practice, he returned to Edinburgh to study for his M.D. degree.[81] There he was dissatisfied with the teaching on

[77] Ibid., 138–46, 153–62.     [78] Clark (1983), 207–9.     [79] Stansfield (1984), 145–69.
[80] Partington (1962), *III*, 471–9     [81] Cockburn (1845), 430–1; Rolleston (1919), 414–16; Porter (1963), 155–64.     [82] Trotter (1792), 136–8.

scurvy and produced his own *Observations on the Scurvy with a Review of the Theories Lately Advanced on that Disease*, in 1786, when he was still only twenty-six. He was, as was to be expected, particularly skeptical of its being defined as a disease of cold regions, and needing stimulants for its treatment.[83] He also denounced the still popular idea regarding the existence of both acid and alkaline scurvies. However, the thesis for which he obtained his medical degree in 1788 had drunkenness as it subject.[81]

In 1789 he was reappointed as a naval surgeon, and in 1792 he published the second edition of his book, which first introduced his new theory. His argument brought together two observations. One was that the spots and also the blood in scurvy had a black or livid color, and the other was that experiments had shown that oxygen was "the principle in nature which restored the florid color to the vital fluid." This suggested a lack of oxygen in scorbutic tissues.[84] Second, the fruits and berries with a reputation for being strongly antiscorbutic were all acid. And though "each acid has its own radical, what communicates acidity to the whole is vital air . . . [and] no room is left to suspect its certainty. Since vital air, or what is more properly called *oxygene,* is a component principle of the acid fruits, we have reason to conclude that this is the quality which they restore to the human body in scurvy."[85] Until the realization that hydrochloric acid consisted only of ionized hydrogen and chlorine atoms, it had indeed seemed a firmly established fact in chemistry that all acids contained oxygen.

"It will no doubt be asked . . . how comes it that every acid is not equally effectual in the cure of scurvy, since they all possess this common principle?"[86] To answer his own question, Trotter quoted from a French paper, published in 1787, giving the degrees of "elective attraction or affinity" of different acids, and which showed oxalic, gallic, citric, and malic acids at the bottom of the table (i.e., well below nitric, carbonic, and sulfuric acids); he concluded that these were the ones that decomposed more easily to give up their oxygen.[87] He also believed that they were the active principles in unripe apples, green gooseberries, citrus fruit, etc. He realized that it was difficult to explain the inactivity of the acetic acid in vinegar, but suggested that this "most highly oxidised organic acid" was also the most stable. The stability of nitric and sulfuric acids was confirmed by their being recovered unchanged in the urine.[88] He ended by admitting that "many facts and experiments are, no doubt, wanting to give his theory stability," but he felt that it "has to recommend it, that it holds out no new method of cure, supported by partial observation; but tends to confirm the old, and lead the way to a more certain practice than has hitherto been done."[89]

In the following year, Dr. Beddoes published a treatise in which he said that many persons could testify that he, too, "had long supposed scurvy to

---

[83] Trotter (1786), 9.   [84] Trotter (1792), 140–1.   [85] Ibid., 139–40.   [86] Ibid., 143.
[87] Ibid., 144–5.   [88] Ibid., 146–7.   [89] Ibid., xxvii.

be owing to a gradual abstraction of oxygen from the whole system, and that acid fruits and vegetables acted by their contribution of oxygen to the system."[90] However, he believed that Trotter had misunderstood the French ranking of different acids, and that this did not represent the tenacity with which they retained their oxygen. There was reason to think that tartaric acid would prove the most useful of the materials that could be "cheaply procured and long preserved."[91] He also thought that fresh (or frozen) meat, in addition to fresh vegetables, could be a source of oxygen because the Laplanders and Eskimos ate no vegetables but nevertheless remained free from scurvy.[92] He also made the point that although oxygen could normally be obtained in sufficient quantities through the lungs, the reason why sailors suffered the disease so commonly was the lack of oxygen in the confined atmosphere below decks.[93]

In 1795, David Paterson went further. In his experience, as a naval surgeon for over fifteen years, limes and lemons were very powerful antiscorbutics, but vinegar by itself had little effect, even though sufferers seemed instinctively to take large quantities of it, and this did them no harm.[94] He had hypothesized that if the vinegar could only be charged with oxygen, it might prove highly beneficial.[95] He chose to try niter (potassium nitrate) as his source of oxygen, and this, he said, had proved highly successful. He dissolved four ounces in one quart of ship's vinegar and gave one to two ounces two to four times per day.[96] Altogether, he treated 100 cases at sea with this remedy when no fruit or citrus juice was available, and all but four recovered before reaching land.[97] On one occasion, when a few limes were available, he compared their activity with that of his nitrous vinegar, and the patients recovered better with the latter.[98] The only other advantage that all the patients received was to be brought up each day into a situation where they received plenty of fresh air; their usual sea diet was unchanged.

In his booklet, Paterson reproduced a letter from another naval surgeon, Fairfoul. He had been treating ten cases of scurvy at sea from April 25 to mid-May with the usual treatments: essence of malt, sulfuric acid, and fresh meat, but the disease was gaining. He then started to use 1½ ounces of nitrous vinegar three times per day. By June 5, two were fit for duty; by June 12, on reaching port, three more were off the sick list.[99]

Paterson also carried out an experiment that seemed to confirm the great oxygenating power of nitrous vinegar; when it was added to a specimen of drawn, dark blood from a scorbutic patient, the color changed to a beautiful red, even more florid than arterial blood.[100] He, too, believed that scurvy arose from breathing contaminated air, rendered so, probably, by its high content of nitrogen and hydrogen.[101] He calculated that in an eight-hour

[90] Beddoes (1793), 45.    [91] Ibid., 84–6, 91, 94.    [92] Ibid., 58–60.    [93] Ibid., 52–3; 57–8.
[94] Paterson (1795), 9.    [95] Ibid., 11.    [96] Ibid., 12.    [97] Ibid., 23.    [98] Ibid., 24.    [99] Ibid.,
81–3.    [100] Ibid., 41.    [101] Ibid., 50.

period, 580 men sleeping between decks, together with candles and infusions of foul air from the bilges, consumed 556,800 gallons of air, and that this was an overwhelming argument for the need for more attention being paid to ventilation.[102] Paterson's booklet was apparently distributed by the Admiralty in 1797.[103] However, the value of nitrous vinegar was not confirmed by other surgeons,[104] though we shall see the report of a later advocate in the following chapter.

In 1800, Trotter reported that he had "succeeded in the cure of scurvy by the citric acid, in the concrete form, as prepared . . . after the manner of Scheele." [105] This Swedish chemist had reported his procedure for obtaining a crystalline organic acid, which he called "citric acid," from lemon juice in 1784.[106] Articles for the next thirty years or more continued to refer to the use of "the citric acid" in treating scurvy. Sometimes authors did mean the crystalline chemical, but more usually citrus juice, whose activity they assumed to come from its content of the citric acid. This was elaborated in one paper referring to "the speedy and complete cure of scurvy by the citric acids (the scientific term in chemistry for the juice of the fruits of the genus *Citrus* . . .)." [107] In some cases we still cannot know for certain in which sense the term was used. Crystalline citric acid would certainly have been a much more convenient store than lemon juice on long voyages, and Lloyd has referred critically to the Admiralty's decision not to follow Trotter's recommendation of changing to the crystals.[103] But in actuality their conservatism was fortunate in this instance because, as we shall see later, his claim for the crystals could not be confirmed.

## The return to lemon juice

We now resume our discussion of what had actually been happening in the British Navy since the serious outbreak of scurvy in the Channel Fleet in 1780. In the first six months of the following year, there were nearly 3,000 cases of scurvy in the West Indies Fleet under Admiral Rodney.[108] It was fortunate for him that the conditions in the French Fleet opposing them were even worse. The British admiral had brought with him, as his personal physician, Gilbert Blane, then thirty-one years old and yet one more graduate of the Edinburgh and Glasgow Medical Schools, already with his M.D. degree and something of a reputation as a physician in London society. Rodney treated Blane as a personal friend and appointed him Physician to the Fleet. This was an irregular appointment but productive of good results. Rolleston has judged that his subsequent work makes his one of the two great names (i.e., along with James Lind) of the Royal Navy's Medical Service.[109]

[102] Ibid., 60–1.   [103] Lloyd (1961), 131.   [104] Trotter (1804), 402n.   [105] Trotter (1800), 154; Trotter (1804), 391–8.   [106] Scheele (1966), 361–3.   [107] Blane (1819), 24.   [108] Lloyd (1965), 142.   [109] Rolleston (1916), 72–3.

In particular, Blane attached importance to the collection of factual, statistical data in a systematic way.

I have followed what I conceive to be the only true method of cultivating any practical art, that is, to collect and compare a great number of facts. A few individual cases are not to be relied on as a foundation of general reasoning, the deductions from them being inconclusive and fallacious, and they are liable to be turned and glossed, according as the mind of the observer may be biased by a favorite prepossession or hypothesis. It has been my study . . . to take the average of numberless particular facts and to analyse and collate them . . . into the form of Tables, as the most certain and compendious way for finding their general result.[110]

After only ten months with the Fleet, Blane returned to London with Rodney, and submitted a strongly worded "memorial" (written representation of facts) directly to the Admiralty. Presumably his social standing gave him the self-assurance to act directly in this way. In his document he pointed out that in a twelve-month period, the deaths in a fleet of 12,000 men had amounted to nearly 1,600, of whom only 60 were killed by the enemy.[111] As was usual in the West Indies, infections were the first cause of death, and he made recommendations for increasing cleanliness on board. Cases of scurvy, which was not contagious, should be treated on ship rather than transferred to hospitals, "where a number of cases of it terminate fatally from flux and fever." [112]

Secondly, scurvy, one of the principal diseases with which seamen are afflicted, may be infallibly prevented, or cured, by vegetables and fruit, particularly oranges, lemons, or limes. These might be supplied by employing one or more small vessels to collect them at different islands: policy, as well as humanity, concur in recommending it. Every fifty oranges or lemons might be considered as a hand to the fleet, inasmuch as the health, and perhaps the life, of a man would thereby be saved.[113]

After three months in London, Blane again sailed to the West Indies with Admiral Rodney and served there for two more years, until the American War of Independence was concluded, and his sea service ended.

Certainly the Lords of the Admiralty made no great change in their practices as a result of Blane's memorial. Lloyd and Coulter have described the conditions in the Fleet during the last years of the War, with continuing heavy losses from disease, but also the successful use of lemons and limes as antiscorbutics by some individual surgeons.[114] In 1785, the Admiralty received a letter from a surgeon in the service of the East India Company who said that in six long India voyages, he had seen scurvy "through all its progressions" and had adopted a method of cure which had proved certain. This was to add two quarts of good French brandy to five gallons of juice

---

[110] Lloyd (1965), 138.      [111] Ibid., 167.      [112] Ibid., 170.      [113] Ibid., 168–9.      [114] Lloyd & Coulter (1961), 3, 125–37.

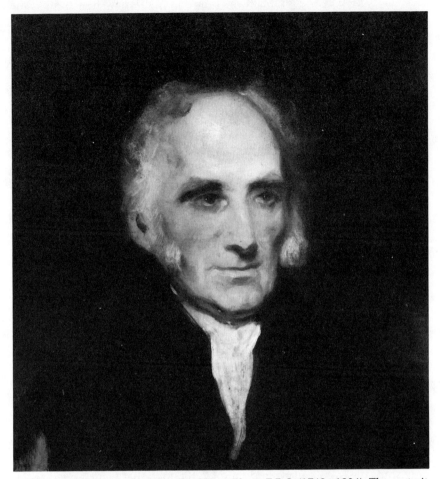

Portrait of the Scottish physician, Sir Gilbert Blane, F.R.S. (1749–1834). The portrait must have been painted late in his life when it had become acceptable for a gentleman to be seen without a wig. (Royal College of Physicians, London.)

carefully expressed from sound lemons or limes, and then carefully casked. In the early stages of the disease, a tablespoonful should be given five or six times a day, or in later stages, a tablespoon every hour. The cure was generally effected in six to eight days, and he felt it to be his duty to communicate it to their Lordships.[115] The Admiralty, in turn passed the letter to the Office for Sick and Hurt Seamen, asking them to report on their opinion. Their report was submitted on March 28, 1786, and the core of it reads as follows:

[115] Sick and Hurt Board (1786).

The remedy proposed by Mr. Matthews is not new. Trials have been made of the efficacy of the acid of lemons in the prevention and cure of scurvy on board several different ships which made voyages round the globe at different times, the surgeons of which all agree in saying the rob of lemons and oranges were of no service, either in the prevention, or cure of that disease, which we mentioned in our letter of the 18th December 1781. Therein we explain our idea of the scurvy and point out what appears to be the only means of prevention. Although the rob, with which the trials were made may be inferior to the juice, we do not think the latter so far preferable as to render any further trial necessary. The method already pursued with the preparation of substances, such as the portable broth, wort, sour krout etc. are much more efficacious both in the cure and prevention of the scurvy.[115]

These two letters are in the library of the National Maritime Museum, London. The report of December 1781 that is referred to was presumably a reply to Blane's memorial of October in that year. It does not seem to be in the Museum's collection of manuscripts, but its contents seem clear enough from the later letter. In short, the administrators at the Admiralty were counseled by their professional advisers *not* to adopt Blane's suggestion, and they can hardly be blamed for following that advice. The other extraordinary thing, from our position of being able to review the earlier literature, is that a sea surgeon in 1784 should have thought the suggestion of using citrus juice preserved with brandy to be an original one!

From the published papers of naval surgeons in that period, there is also no clear recommendation that oranges and lemons were of *special* importance. Gillespie, in 1785, certainly advocated the use of lemons or limes rather than malt and sauerkraut.[116] Thomson, in 1790, though including lemons in his list of useful antiscorbutics, gave precedence to having bread freshly baked at sea, beer made with hops, and the issue of brown sugar instead of butter and cheese.[117] Even Blane had written in 1785 in high praise of molasses: "The first trial of molasses was in the *Foudroyant,* and it answered so well that, in a cruise under Admiral Geary in 1780, this was the only ship free from scurvy, and out of 2,400 men that were landed at the hospital with this disease, there were none from this ship."[118]

In 1793, when scurvy appeared in the Mediterranean Fleet under Lord Hood, the ships affected could not be sent to port for refreshment because of the imminence of battle. The chief physician wrote later:

I proposed to his lordship the sending a vessel into port for the express purpose of obtaining lemons for the use of the fleet . . . and the good effects of its use were so evident that an order was soon obtained that no ship under his lordship's command should leave port without being previously furnished with an ample supply of lemons; and to this circumstance becoming generally known, may the use of lemon juice, the effectual means of subduing scurvy be traced.[119]

---

[116] Gillespie (1785), 375.　　[117] Thomson (1790).　　[118] Lloyd (1965), 161.　　[119] Laughton (1911), 132–3.

This is yet one more extraordinary claim to have discovered the value of lemons, and especially extraordinary, because Hood himself had written in 1781, while in the West Indies: "I have got lemons and limes for my poor fellows from every place I could, which has prevented the scurvy from taking that root which I am sorry to say it has in other ships." [120]

What had Gilbert Blane been doing in this decade? On returning to London in 1783, he was appointed Physician to St. Thomas's Hospital. He also built up an obviously successful private practice and was soon Physician to the Household of the Prince of Wales and to the royal Duke of Clarence. In addition, he published two editions of his *Observations on the Diseases of Seamen.*[121] As mentioned already, he referred in his book to the antiscorbutic value of other foods such as sauerkraut, sugar, and molasses, but he also emphasized: "Of all the articles, either of medicine or diet, for the cure of the scurvy, lemons and oranges are of much the greatest efficacy. They are real specifics in that disease, if anything deserves that name." [122]

In the autumn of 1793, he advised his friend, Admiral Gardner, who had been appointed to sail out and command the fleet in the East Indies, to ask the Admiralty for a supply of lemon juice, and the Sick and Hurt Board approved the idea.

An experiment was made of supplying her [the *Suffolk*] with a quantity of lemon juice sufficient to serve out two-thirds of a liquid ounce every day, to every man on board. This was mixed with their grog, along with two ounces of sugar. She was twenty-three weeks and one day on the passage [to India], without having any communication with the land, and arrived in Madras road, on the 11th of September, without losing a man, with only fifteen men on the sick list, all slight cases, and none of them affected with the scurvy. This disease appeared in a few men in the course of the voyage, but soon disappeared on an increased dose of lemon juice being administered.[123]

In 1795, Blane himself was appointed to be a Commissioner of the Board of the Sick and Wounded Sailors. The name of the Board changed slightly from time to time, but its responsibilities continued to include the provision of adequate medical supplies. The success of the "experiment" on the *Suffolk* must have added weight to the recommendation made by the Board, soon after Blane had joined it, that lemon juice be authorized as a regular issue in the Navy.[121] The Lords of the Admiralty agreed to a daily allowance of three-quarters of an ounce, and there was a dramatic decline in the incidence of scurvy from 1796 on. Although it appears that individual admirals still had to request an issue of lemon juice before it was supplied, Fleet physicians, such as Trotter, actively encouraged its adoption. Over the period from 1795 to 1814, the Admiralty records show a total issue of 1.6 *million* gallons of lemon juice![124]

[120] Barnes & Owen (1938), 160.     [121] Rolleston (1916), 73–5.     [122] Lloyd (1965), 159.
[123] Ibid., 178.     [124] Lloyd & Coulter (1961), 320–4.

Lord Nelson, true to his reputation for taking a special interest in the needs and comfort of his men, obtained permission to order an additional 20,000 gallons of lemon juice locally for his fleet in the Mediterranean, in addition to the regular issue of 30,000 gallons.[124] The correspondence from the British agent in Sicily is preserved at the Wellcome Institute in London. Ironically, the agent had to say that he would have a problem in fulfilling the contract because of the unusually poor crop that year. In the previous year, he had written, in reply to an enquiry from Nelson's Fleet Physician as to the best way of shipping lemons:

Great quantities are sent every year to Hamburg, Petersburg and other Ports in the North; they are usually wrapped in double paper and put into light boxes which contain about 400 each. . . . Another method of packing lemons has lately been adopted for the Russian market which has succeeded very well, viz, to put them in barrels, or casks which are afterwards filled with sea water and bung tight.[125]

By contrast, a U. S. naval ship sailing home from the Mediterranean in 1803 carried only a few lemons, and the surgeon tried to deal with an outbreak of scurvy with Peruvian bark (rich in quinine), sulfuric acid, and vinegar.[126]

There seems no doubt that the issue of lemon juice, perhaps combined with other improvements in victualing, resulted in the elimination of scurvy from the British Navy as a major problem and, by increasing the time which ships could remain at sea, greatly increased its efficiency during the Napoleonic Wars. We know that some outbreaks still occurred as a result of breakdowns in victualing arrangements, but they were the exception and quickly treated.[127] The statistics collected by Blane for *total* annual sickness (i.e., from all causes) also show a great decline – from 24% of the total manpower for the years 1780–95, to under 11% for the years 1798–1806.[128] The years 1796–7 are omitted because of the disruption caused by the mutinies in that period.

And so the problem of scurvy in the British Navy was solved just in time to maintain the resistance to Napoleon through the continental blockade, whereas the French Services were less fortunate.[129] It is a humbling moral to the story that, after all the attempts to apply new scientific concepts and hypotheses, the final solution came from rejection of theory and a return to the practical experience of previous centuries. Blane was one who had the necessary humility and could say: "Lemons and oranges . . . are the real specifics . . . [as] first ascertained and set in a clear light by Dr. Lind. Upon what principle their superior efficacy depends . . . I am at a loss to determine."[130]

Surgeon Vice-Admiral Sir Sheldon Dudley, who himself had great responsibilities for maintaining the health of the British Navy during World

[125] Letters & Documents (1780–1805), 11: Letters by J. Broadbent, 13 June 1804 and 13 January 1805.  [126] Estes (1982), 250–1.  [127] Lloyd (1965), 240, 244, 306.  [128] Ibid., 200.  [129] Mahé (1880), 51–4, 61; Acerra (1981), 75.  [130] Lloyd (1965), 159–60.

War II, has made some interesting comments on the contribution of Sir Gilbert Blane (as he was to become in 1812).

Lind himself had not the patience, the aggressive spirit or the powers of persuasion to overcome the resistance of his executive masters; few doctors have, or if they have, they soon give up in disgust and despair. This is where the great Sir Gilbert Blane was useful as Lind's mouthpiece; he could employ his gifts of oratory and eloquence in persuading admirals and administrative naval officials to listen to reason and become hygiene-conscious. Blane may be likened to Huxley in the Darwin–Huxley partnership. . . . Perhaps Blane did dearly love the society of lords and of senior officers. . . . But, considering the times, there is no need to condemn him as a snob. Thank God he was, if it meant that he had the power of using cajolery and flattery to get his own way with the powers-that-be. . . . Without Blane's popularity with Admiral Rodney and the rulers of the King's Navy, the country might have had to wait even more than forty years to see Lind's recommendations for preserving the health of seamen put into force.[131]

[131] Dudley (1953b), 378–9.

# 5

## Land scurvy, potatoes, and potassium
## (1810 – 1905)

From 1810 to 1840, there was little medical interest in scurvy. Cases still occurred at sea, but they were usually to be explained by exceptional circumstances or failure to carry out the recognized precautions.[1] Authors were agreed that the disease was now virtually unknown in a big city such as London; the only controversy was over whether the conditions had really changed so much for the better, as was argued by Blane,[2] or whether what had earlier been described as evidence of the "scorbutic humor" was really a quite different disease.[3]

In 1830, Dr. Elliotson was giving a course of lectures at St. Thomas's Hospital in London. At one lecture he was able to demonstrate a case of scurvy, and he began, "Gentlemen, this case is important because of its rarity."[4] The patient was a young sailor who had reached London after a seventeen-week voyage from Buenos Aires on a merchant ship supplied with salt meat and bread but no lemon juice or medicine of any kind. He had all the usual signs of scurvy including loose teeth. Nowadays, said Dr. Elliotson, such a case was so outside normal experience that it might be misdiagnosed – for example as a cancer of the gums. After an excellent historical survey of the disease, he concluded:

The remedy for this state is fresh food, vegetable and animal food, and particularly lemon juice. . . . Scurvy is a purely *chemical* disease . . . [in that] each part of the system is ready to perform all its functions, but one of the external things necessary for its doing so is taken away. . . . [As] in the case of suffocation, the body is not at all in fault, but it suffers from a want of fresh air. This is very different from some other diseases. . . . in the case of diabetes, it is not that the body is overloaded with an excessive supply of sugar . . . but that the functions of the body which form urine are diseased . . . [and] sugar appears in it. . . . Scurvy is exactly like

---

[1] Hirsch (1885) *II*, 531; Mahé (1880), 54–9.  [2] Blane (1813), 96.  [3] Hall (1820), 205–6 .
[4] Elliotson (1831), 649–51.

. . . impending suffocation – the body would be in good health if not deprived of its proper external supply.[5]

This interpretation of the disease, together with Dr. George Budd's lectures in 1842 on "Disorders Resulting from Defective Nutriment," [6] which presented a similar analysis, will be considered more fully in the final chapter.

## Problems in prisons

In reality, scurvy had not been quite as rare in London as Elliotson had implied. In 1823, there had been something of a parliamentary scandal over its outbreak in the new National Penitentiary (prison) at Millbank, the site now occupied by the Tate Gallery in London.[7] This building had been designed as part of the "new scientific, utilitarian approach to the problem of crime in society." The idea had been to provide hygienic conditions of housing and diet – "since the prisoners' sentence had not included disease and death" – but to impose psychological punishment through isolation and hard, physical labor.[8] In 1822, the diet was criticized as "luxurious" because it was superior to that available to the honest poor. Reluctantly, therefore, the committee-in-charge reduced the rations in July of that year. The daily allowances of approximately 3½ ounces of meat and one pound of potatoes were eliminated. The men still received 1½ pounds of bread, two pints of soup (made with some vegetables and a very little meat), and one pint of gruel.[9] By February 1825, disease had become rife and out of control.[10] It was diagnosed, by two physicians called in to investigate the problem, as being a combination of infectious dysentery and sea scurvy. The scurvy was the prevailing disease, and was seen in over half of the 860 inmates, though in none of the 24 who worked in the kitchen; nor were any of the 106 officers and servants affected. The inspecting physicians recommended an issue of three oranges daily to each inmate and a restitution of their meat allowance.[11] The scurvy quickly cleared up, but the infectious dysentery became epidemic, and no class in the building was immune from it for a further year.

Over the next twenty years, many more unintentional experiments were carried out as governors of prisons and pauper institutes wrestled with the problem of feeding their inmates without providing "luxury." The results were analyzed by Baly in 1843. His interest in this was stimulated by the recurrence of scurvy at the Millbank penitentiary among one particular class, the military prisoners, and typically after four to six months of imprisonment.[12] The main difference in their conditions, as compared with the

---

[5] Ibid., 653.     [6] Budd (1842).     [7] McConville (1981), 144.     [8] Ibid., 146.     [9] Baly (1843), 700.     [10] Latham (1825), 5.     [11] Ibid., 11.     [12] Baly (1843), 699.

civilian prisoners, was that they did not receive the latter's weekly issue of five pounds of potatoes and one pound of onions. Dr. Baly arranged first for the military prisoners to receive pea soup with added vegetables, in place of the two pints per week of rice soup that they had previously received. However, this did not stop the occurrence of further cases. He therefore arranged for the further addition of three pounds of potatoes per week "and not a single case of scurvy has since occurred." [9]

Spurred on by these results, Baly went on to analyze the reports of the Inspectors of Prisons over the previous decade. Scurvy had been a problem in twenty county jails, and at every one, potatoes were either wholly absent from the standard ration or "given occasionally on Sunday when the prison garden would furnish them." Where diets had been subsequently changed to include a regular ration of potatoes, no more was heard of the disease.[13] There was no relation between the occurrence of the disease and how much meat was provided, and nowhere were fruit or green vegetables supplied. The antiscorbutic value of cooked potatoes seemed clear, and because potatoes were so much less expensive than other succulent vegetables, Baly urged that they should, and could, be included at a rate of three to six pounds per week, even where the food of inmates was regulated by principles of strict economy.[13]

By coincidence, Baly's study was published just after the appearance of two letters from ship's surgeons advocating the use of potatoes to prevent scurvy at sea. The first reported continued health on long voyages when no lime juice was supplied but when the crew ate raw potatoes "sliced with a little vinegar." [14] The second surgeon reported that potatoes were regularly relied on for their antiscorbutic quality by the crews of whaling ships spending many months at sea off Australia, that they would keep for four months if kept dark and dry in large hampers, and that they could be cooked without losing their value.[15] In the latter's experience, they were a more reliable antiscorbutic than lime juice. Even these were not the first references to the use of potatoes at sea. In the 1780s, Blane had recommended them when eaten raw, but along with other materials that were later regarded as worthless; and in the 1820s, two French surgeons had recommended the use of decoctions of potatoes, or else the tubers very lightly cooked.[16]

The potato had, of course, been introduced to the Old World by explorers bringing tubers back from Central and South America in the late sixteenth century.[17] There it had been a staple food for the Inca and Aztec civilizations. In Europe the potato plant was regarded with great suspicion, partly because its flowers resembled those of the poisonous nightshade, partly because the "scabby" skin of the tubers was associated with leprosy and, for

[13] Ibid., 701–2.    [14] Dalton (1842).    [15] Berncastle (1842).    [16] Lloyd (1965), 161; Pereira (1843), 378.    [17] Salaman (1949), 142–8.

some groups, because it was not a food mentioned in the Bible.[18] However, it began to be generally cultivated and eaten throughout Europe in the eighteenth century. In many parts of Scotland, where scurvy had previously been endemic, it had disappeared by 1800, i.e., in the same period during which potatoes became a regular item of the diet.[19] There was a similar association in Norway, where the disease had been a great problem.[20]

In Ireland, for complicated reasons, the potato had become the typical peasant's staple food as early as 1700. For someone supporting a family on a small area of land, the first advantage was that its yield was so much greater than that of grain, even after allowing for the fact that the potato was nearly 80% water, whereas mature grains were only some 10–12% water.[21] However, because of the high moisture content of the potato tubers, it was more difficult to store them after harvest than it was to store dry grain. In practice, they could not be kept for more than about ten months unless they had been sliced and dried, and this was not generally practiced by peasants in northern Europe.[22]

## The Great Potato Famine, 1845–8

The weather in the summer of 1845 through much of Britain, Ireland, northern France, and Belgium was most unusual. Until the beginning of July, it had been particularly good, but then for six weeks it became uniformly cold, wet, and foggy.[23] On August 23, the *Gardener's Chronicle*, published in London, announced: "A fatal malady has broken out amongst the potato crop. . . . In Belgium the fields are said to have been completely desolated."[24] In the following weeks it became clear that every variety of the plant was being attacked – from Poland to Ireland. Not only were the leaves turning black, and covered with a fungus, but the tubers, when dug up, were discolored and rapidly turned putrid. The minute fungus on the leaves belonged to the genus *Botrytis* and appeared similar to that associated with a disease of silkworms in France. There was controversy as to whether the fungus actually caused the trouble, or merely grew on the already damaged tissue. Whatever the truth of the matter, there was no way to prevent the disease or to keep the tubers in good condition. Worse, with this "blight," many crops dug up in apparently good condition would rot after a few weeks of storage.[25]

In 1845, about half the potato crop was lost.[23] Prayers were focused on the hope that the following year would see a better crop. Again the plants seemed at first to be healthy, and then at the end of July, turned into "one wide waste of putrefying vegetation."[26] In Ireland, as in Britain generally,

---

[18] Ibid., 112, 116, 119.   [19] Ibid., 356.   [20] Nicolaysen (1980), 304.   [21] Kahane (1978), 111–12.   [22] A. Smith (1880), 171.   [23] Salaman (1949), 291–2.   [24] Large (1940), 13.   [25] Ibid., 15–21, 27.   [26] Ibid., 36.

the 1846 crop was almost completely lost. The consequence was a most appalling famine, relieved only to a small extent by Government and voluntary organizations which arranged the import and distribution of maize
meal.[27] With so many people in weakened condition, typhus and relapsing
fever broke out in epidemic form and killed many more.[28] Many people who
were forced to change their staple from potatoes to maize meal, and who
had no source of any other vegetables, let alone fruit, developed signs of
scurvy.[29] But this seems almost trivial in the context of a famine that was
responsible for the loss of something like a million lives.[30] Dr. Curran who
was the author of a scholarly article on the Irish scurvy epidemic, that
appeared in August 1847, was himself dead of typhus at the age of twenty-
eight, before the end of September.[31]

In England and Scotland, there was hardship but no actual famine because grain was still the main staple. However, a Scottish physician wrote in
1847:

it is familiar to everyone that the failure of the potato crop for two successive seasons
did, with the stunted growth of our pastures  . . .  lead to a rise of 30 – 40 percent on
all kinds of provisions during the last Winter. . . . The Winter was protracted and
severe. . . . one effect was to render fresh succulent vegetables unattainable by
nearly every class; another was to raise the price of milk and other dairy produce
beyond the reach of the poor.[32]

With hindsight and the lesson of Baly's review of previous experience in
prisons with diets low in vegetables and milk, the consequences seem inevitable, though they came as a surprise at the time.

By June 1847, a flurry of papers were appearing in the British medical
press referring to the appearance of scurvy.[33] An editorial in the *Lancet*
concluded that no part of the country appeared to be exempt.[34] Typically,
the physicians admitted that they had at first failed to diagnose the condition correctly, because it was something not previously encountered; some
cases were at first classified as *purpura*.[35] It was also generally agreed that
rice and corn were not complete substitutes for potatoes, and that the condition could be both cured and prevented by adding succulent vegetables back
to the diet, either as potatoes (where there were any to be had) or as green
vegetables.

It is particularly interesting to read the reactions of the physicians in
Edinburgh and Glasgow to the appearance of scurvy in their midst, because
Scotland had been the home base of so many ideas and writing about the
disease some fifty to one hundred years earlier. It was agreed that, indeed,
they were beginning to see "a distinct disease presenting the precise fea-
tures  . . .  of the scorbutus of our navies."[35] Although the first outbreak

---

[27] Woodham-Smith (1962), 73–6, 134–6.    [28] Ibid., 188–90.    [29] Curran (1847), 109.
[30] Aykroyd (1974), 30.    [31] Anonymous (1847), 500–11.    [32] Ritchie (1847), 77.    [33] Laycock (1847), 575; Lonsdale (1847), 97; Shapter (1847), 281; Sibbald (1847), 413; Stiff (1847),
392.    [34] Editorial (1847), 312–13.    [35] Ritchie (1847), 40; Barrett (1849), 149.

had occurred in an institution, the General Prison at Perth,[36] in the winter of 1845–6, it was later present in the general population also. By the end of May 1847, doctors at the infirmary in Glasgow had seen 122 cases of scurvy,[37] and in Edinburgh 143 cases had been admitted to the infirmary, where no case had been seen for the previous thirty years.[38] In Edinburgh, three-quarters of those admitted were laborers (or "navvies" working on the construction of railway lines in the area. Dr. Christison, President of the Royal College of Surgeons in Edinburgh and a Professor in the University, wrote: "Who could have expected such a disease as scurvy among the labourers on our railways, men mostly in the prime of life, engaged in an athletic occupation, working in the open fields and breezy moors, earning ample wages. . . . "[39] However, further investigation showed that they were not really so well off. The laborers were compelled to buy all their provisions at the contractor's store on credit against their monthly wage paid in arrears, and the food available there was practically limited to bread, salt pork, and cheese (all of poor quality), coffee, tea, and sugar.[40] One patient's daily diet had consisted of 900 grams (g) of bread, 65 g butter, 65 g sugar, and 150 g salt pork, which Dr. Christison calculated to have contributed 750 g total "anhydrous nutritive matter": "130 g were nitrogenous, but of this only 35 g were animal in nature."[40]

## The protein theory

To understand Christison's analysis of the diet in this way and his subsequent theory for the cause of scurvy, we must go back to the developments in the science of nutrition (often referred to as "Animal Chemistry" in this period) that had been taking place since 1800. These included the discovery of new elements and the development of quantitative analysis of materials for their content of each chemical element. The study of nutrition and metabolism could therefore begin to be put on a quantitative basis.

First there was the discovery that the atmosphere contained a third gas in addition to carbon dioxide and oxygen. Animals could not breathe in it, and it was called in France "azote" (meaning "not life-supporting"). In English, it was called "nitrogen" because, when sparked with oxygen and water vapor, it would react to form nitric acid. It was then discovered that all living tissues – vegetable as well as animal – contained a certain amount of nitrogen in organic combination: Moreover, animal tissues generally contained a significantly higher proportion of nitrogen. From this knowledge the idea arose that vegetable foods relatively rich in nitrogen were more nutritious than others as a food for animals because they were closer to the composition of animal tissues, and that the function of food was to replace the wear and tear of tissues in adults, and to provide for growth in young animals.

[36] Christison (1847a), 877.     [37] Ritchie (1847), 40.     [38] Christison (1847b), 5–6.     [39] Ibid., 8.
[40] Ibid., 9.

Experiments indicated that atmospheric nitrogen could not be utilized by animals for incorporation into their tissues.[41] In the 1830s, the French worker, Boussingault, carried out practical experiments in feeding young cattle on different materials, and he confirmed that their value for growth correlated well with their nitrogen content as determined by analysis.[42] He made it clear in his text that, of course, animals must need other components also, such as lime (or calcium) for their growing bones. However, he suggested that, as a practical approximation it would be useful for farmers to compare the prices of different animal feeds in terms of the nitrogen that they contributed.[43]

With further developments in food analysis, the nonnitrogenous organic material was divided into an oily fraction (the fats), starches, and sugars – in addition to vegetable fiber, which was considered indigestible, at least for humans. The principal nitrogenous components of animal tissues were divided, according to their solubility under different conditions, into serum "albumin," blood "fibrin," and "muscle fiber." They were thought to be only relatively slight modifications of each other, and, as a group, they were later called "proteins"; milk was also found to contain material, named "casein," of the same general class.[44] Vegetable foods contained variable quantities of components similar in properties to animal albumin and casein, but grains, in particular, had most of their nitrogen in a different form, named "gluten" because of its gluey character.[45]

Justus von Liebig, the German chemist, gave lectures which were published in English in 1842 as *Animal Chemistry*, a book that had a great influence for the next fifty years. In retrospect, it seems unfortunate that his ideas were often accepted, even by their author, as dogma rather than as a series of imaginative hypotheses to form the basis for further experiment. He outlined three main principles that are relevant to the present study:

1. The proteins (as we would call them) are readily converted to each other in animal digestion because of their common fundamental character.
2. The energy needed for muscular contraction is derived from the breakdown of the muscle proteins themselves.[46]
3. The only function of the nonnitrogenous starches and sugars in foods is to protect the tissues from the destructive effects of oxygen, by themselves reacting with oxygen and, at the same time, giving out heat that keeps animals at their optimal working temperature.[47]

From this scheme the idea arose that only nitrogenous foods had true nutritional value and that other organic compounds merely acted as "respiratory" materials, i.e., as the source of animal heat. In addition, the need for inorganic salts was appreciated, but it was thought that, in practice, they were unlikely to be in short supply. We can now, of course, see the errors in

---

[41] Munro (1964), 1–9.   [42] Boussingault (1845), 525–6, 553–4.   [43] Ibid., 553–4.   [44] Liebig (1842), 40–4, 52.   [45] Ibid., 45–9.   [46] Ibid., 220–3, 245.   [47] Ibid., 52–3, 69.

Liebig's reasoning. But his air of certainty supported by an array of quantitative analyses meant that for many years other investigators started with his system as the foundation, i.e., their paradigm (to use a twentieth-century term),[48] and tried to explain any discrepant findings by a relatively minor modification or elaboration of the same scheme. The *Lancet* in 1842–43 published a series of ten papers reviewing Liebig's work and finally extending it to an analysis of British diets.[49] However, the author of another *Treatise on Food and Diet* did add a warning that Liebig's concept overemphasized nitrogen, and ignored the need for succulent vegetables and for variety in the human diet.[50]

We return now to Dr. Christison's analysis of the problem of scurvy that had appeared first in Perth General Prison in 1845–6 and then in the population of Edinburgh. His report on the epidemic at the prison began with statements about its good ventilation and absence of any surrounding marshland.[51] Dampness was still considered to be scorbutic by some, particularly in France.[52] He also referred to the plentiful supply of good water.[51] At his inspection of the 330 prisoners at the end of October 1846, he had found about 40 definite cases of scurvy and 10 more doubtful or incipient cases. The disease had first been noticed towards the end of June, and those who had been longest in prison were the most affected; there seemed no doubt that they were seeing all the signs of true *scorbutus*, or sea scurvy.[53]

Turning to diet, Dr. Christison noted that the prisoners had shown a good health record from the opening of the prison in 1842 until 1845. In that period, the longer-term prisoners had received the Scottish standard ration which supplied oatmeal porridge and milk for breakfast and supper, and bread and broth (containing meat and vegetables) for the midday dinner, with a list of approved substitutions that added variety to the diet. In March 1845, treacle-water (syrup diluted with water) was substituted for milk at breakfast, and in May for supper also. In addition, potatoes had occasionally been served instead of oatmeal at supper, but in 1846, this was stopped because of their scarcity. The original standard ration, with approximately 700 ml milk, supplied altogether 720 g nutritive dry matter (protein + fat + starch + sugar); 170 g were nitrogenous (55 g of which were from animal sources). The omission of occasional potatoes would have had no significant effect on these values, but the change from milk to treacle-water meant that the modified diet had 690 g nutritive dry matter, of which 135 g were nitrogenous but only 15 g were from animal sources.[54]

Christison's conclusion was that "the main cause of scurvy in that year had been the substitution of treacle for milk"; the faulty diet, though still liberal in quantity, had then become essentially "saccharofarinaceous" (sugary–starchy). The prisoners were therefore given "skimmed milk

<hr />

[48] Kuhn (1970), 43–51.     [49] Ancell (1843), 670.     [50] Pereira (1843), 46–8, 77–88.
[51] Christison (1847a), 874–5.     [52] Scoutten (1847), 505–6.     [53] Christison (1847a), 877.
[54] Ibid., 876.

again, morning and evening and, in severe cases, half a pound of meat at dinner," and the disease was arrested without prescribing the use of lemon juice or extra vegetables.[55]

He accepted that the total amount of nitrogenous constituents (135 g) in the "treacle diet" was higher than that found in some other diets that maintained health. However, he suggested that Liebig was wrong in considering "gluten" to be equivalent in nutritive value to muscle fiber and casein, and in the treacle diet all but 23 g of the nitrogenous material was in the form of gluten. With such an unbalanced diet, individuals would be subject to scurvy whenever stressed by "co-operating causes hitherto unascertained." In his opinion, succulent vegetables had cured scurvy in other outbreaks because of their content of "vegetable albumen," which was not found in grains.[56]

Dr. Christison's investigation of the scurvy cases in Edinburgh led him to the same conclusion; the railway laborers and poor people with the disease had been eating too little of what would later be called "first-class protein," and their response to his treatment convinced him that milk was the antiscorbutic of choice under the circumstances. Equally, he admitted that scurvy could also occur in people "when their food abounded in too much animal nutriment," and then it would need different treatment.[57]

Dr. Anderson of Glasgow replied to Dr. Christison three months later. He argued that scurvy could not typically be caused by a lack of nitrogenous compounds in the diet because it had responded so uniformly to the use of lemon juice. Four ounces (115 g) of lemon juice was an effective daily dose, but this contained less than 2.5 g of dry matter, virtually none of which was nitrogenous.[58] He went on to point out that this small amount of dry material could not itself be sufficient to provide the substance of the healthy blood needed for the cure of scurvy, and he suggested that it acted "by, in some way, promoting the assimilation of the nutritive part of the food." He suggested that where milk had shown antiscorbutic activity, it could have been due, not to its casein, but to its lactose (milk sugar); thus whereas Nature had provided the casein in milk for growth of tissues, and butter for "caloric" (heat or energy), perhaps the function of the milk sugar was to supply lactic acid as a result of fermentation in the gut. This then made up for the want of vegetable acids in the infant diet. The crucial test for this idea, he said, would be to give whey to scorbutic cases.[59] This by-product of cheese making still contains the lactose of milk but not the casein. He suggested that lactic acid and also "nitre + vinegar" "probably exert in the process of assimilation an agency more-or-less like that of citric acid, although not so uniformly powerful." [58]

Another critic of Christison's views as to the cause and cure of scurvy was Dr. Lonsdale. In the northwest of England, he had been seeing cases of

---

[55] Ibid., 885.     [56] Ibid., 888–90.     [57] Christison (1847b), 20.     [58] Anderson (1847), 177–8.
[59] Ibid., 179.

scurvy among three groups with quite different backgrounds: handloom weavers in the city of Carlisle, railway excavators working in the country, and farm laborers. The first two classes had typically been getting little milk, but the third had received it regularly in generous quantities. The only change in diet common to all three groups was the omission of potatoes or other succulent vegetables from their diet over the last six months.[60] In the one town that seemed to have escaped the disease, there had been a particularly good supply of local turnips. Lastly, there had been a local scarcity of milk in the winter of 1842–3, but no cases of scurvy.[61]

## The potassium theory

Dr. Curran of Dublin had also seen Christison's papers when preparing his own article that appeared in August of 1847. He was doubtful of the general value of cow's milk in curing scurvy because many of his patients had come from a poorhouse where they had continued to receive one pint of milk per day.[62] On the other hand, he marshaled evidence that most of the recorded outbreaks of scurvy had occurred in spring, and suggested that it was "due to some peculiarity of diet or climate found only, or chiefly during the (preceding) winter season." [63] He himself believed that "an 'epidemic constitution' exists in the air in certain seasons, giving a *tendency* to the development of scurvy, but that other predisposing causes are necessary to its actual outbreak." [63] The principal and predisposing cause he took to be the want of fresh succulent vegetables. The one really consistent feature of the previous diets of his patients was that their diets had contained no green vegetables or potatoes.[64] In terms of the chemical composition of scorbutic diets, Dr. Christison had concluded that their specific deficiency was in "albumin + casein"; however, "by overlooking *the salts* contained in foods, he has committed an error which totally destroys all the value of his reasoning." [64] He referred the reader to another paper read earlier that year in Dublin for the evidence that the salts in roots, stems, and leaves of vegetables complemented those found in a "grain + meat" diet.

Dr. Aldridge, the author referred to, had spoken to an agricultural group in April. His main point was that the nutritional requirements of humans (or of farm animals for that matter) could be calculated by measuring their daily losses in breath, feces, and urine, and he gave typical values for nitrogen and for six individual elements. If the diet did not replace the losses, then the body tissues would waste away. Specifically he showed, from published analyses, that the ratios of calcium to nitrogen, and of "soda + potash" to nitrogen, were higher in potatoes and other roots than they were in bread and peas.[65] He went on to say that "the cure of sea-scurvy consists in eating

---

[60] Lonsdale (1847), 100–3.     [61] Ibid., 104.     [62] Curran (1847), 100–1.     [63] Ibid., 103–5.
[64] Ibid., 109.     [65] Aldridge (1847), 137–9.

the herbaceous parts of plants abounding in sulphur, lime and alkalies; and the circumstances under which this disease occurs show it to be dependent upon a deficiency in these necessary elements of food."[66]

Dr. Anderson of Glasgow replied to Curran in the paper already referred to. He pointed out that dried vegetables had, on many occasions, been found to be of much lower antiscorbutic activity than vegetables in the fresh, succulent state; yet there should be no change in the salts as a result of drying.[67] Second, turning Curran's own phrase, he said: "Dr. Curran has committed an error which totally destroyed the value of all his reasonings"; this was that he had ignored analyses showing that there was no diminution in the level of salts in the blood of scorbutics.[67]

That was not the end of the belief that scurvy resulted from a deficiency of mineral salts. In January 1848, Dr. Garrod, a junior member of the staff at University College, London argued somewhat as follows:

1. There is general agreement that scurvy arises from some deficiency in the diet rather than from the presence of a toxic material. This must be *either* an *organic* material (a carbon compound) or an *inorganic* one (i.e., a simple salt).
2. It used to be thought that citric acid (an organic compound) was the active factor in lemon juice, but it has now been found not to be antiscorbutic. Nor can albuminous matter be the active factor when a small amount of fruit cures the disease.
3. Although the total level of saline matter in scorbutic blood is approximately normal, that of potash (potassium) in particular is reduced.
4. Scorbutic diets are all low in their content of potash, and the antiscorbutic remedies are rich in it.
5. In his (Garrod's) experience, treating scorbutics with 12–20 grains (0.8–1.3 grams) of simple potassium salts such as the bitartrate, acetate, and carbonate resulted in as rapid a recovery as treatment with milk and vegetables. Also, the literature had reported cures with niter (potassium nitrate) or potassium oxalate, though the importance of the potassium, rather than the acid had not been recognized at the time.[68]

The potassium theory could be critized on the same grounds as Aldridge's more general "sulfur and alkalies" theory, i.e., that vegetables lost their antiscorbutic qualities when they were dried just as lemon juice did when it fermented; yet the mineral elements were still present. In October 1848, an exhaustive review of the lessons to be drawn from the scurvy epidemic firmly rejected the "mineral" theories, and suggested that the relatively high potassium content of the antiscorbutic vegetables was only a coincidence.[69] (The review was unsigned, but Professor Parkes of the Army Medical School later acknowledged having written it.)[70] However, this was by no means the end of the potassium theory, and in 1862, Aldridge complained that he, rather than Garrod, should be receiving the credit for it.[71]

[66] Ibid., 143.    [67] Anderson (1847), 180–1.    [68] Garrod (1848), 458–62.    [69] Anonymous (1848), 467–8, 474.    [70] Parkes (1864), 445n.    [71] Aldridge (1862), 268.

In the summer of 1848, there was a normal potato harvest throughout northwestern Europe, prices of vegetables fell to their previous levels in Britain, and the scurvy epidemic was a thing of the past. The return of the potato was particularly fortunate because there was great public concern in Britain over the possibility that an epidemic of cholera would spread from the Continent; the recommendations for escaping the disease included the following: "Avoid the use of uncooked vegetables, unripe, sour or stone fruit . . . and acid drinks generally."[72] Presumably, these were considered dangerous because of their laxative properties. There was a serious and widespread epidemic of scurvy in Russia that winter, as in many years throughout the century;[73] in the next year, the disease was also to break out in epidemic proportions on the other side of the Earth.

## Scurvy in California, 1848–50

Early in 1848, gold had been found in a remote part of northern California where there were just a few pioneer settlers from other parts of the United States. The news caused great excitement in the main areas of population in the country, all in the East. In the next two years, some 100,000 set off to the gold fields, either by sea or overland, or by a combination of the two.[74] The last route involved a sea journey from an East Coast port to Panama, an overland journey of some 100 miles to the West Coast, and another voyage up the coast to San Francisco. (The Panama Canal was not, of course, to be constructed for another sixty years.) This was, in general, the quickest way to travel, with one party going from Boston to San Francisco in fifty days; it was also the route that was least associated with disease.[75]

The direct route by ship required the much longer journey around Cape Horn but it was taken by 16,000 passengers in 1849.[76] Ships seem commonly to have stopped at Rio de Janeiro and Valparaiso for refreshment, but even from the latter port it could still take several months to reach San Francisco. There are reports of scurvy developing among passengers on some ships during this time.[77] Also, it was noted that men leaving a ship in apparently good health would often develop the disease a few days later,[78] perhaps a result of the unaccustomed stress of manhandling their own baggage after a long period of inactivity on board.

By far the greatest privations were endured by those going overland. The distance to be covered from Ohio, for example, was some 2,500 miles. As far west as Kansas City, it was possible to make some use of trains and river steamers. But for the remaining 1,800 miles, the journey had to be made by mule carts or ox wagons, and involved crossing the Rocky Mountains in the

---

[72] Edinburgh Board of Health (1848), 485.      [73] Hirsch (1885), *II*, 521–6, 536; Mahé (1880), 60–4.      [74] Holliday (1981), 25–44.      [75] Lorenz (1957), 486.      [76] Ibid., 487.      [77] Ibid., 484.      [78] Praslow (1939), 45.

absence of any constructed roads. This part of the journey was expected to take six months. Despite its being so formidable, the records at Fort Laramie, Wyoming, an army post on the most popular northern route, indicate that nearly 45,000 people (of whom 40,000 were men) had passed there by August of 1850.[79]

Typical provisions loaded onto the wagons were similar to those taken for a long voyage at sea – flour and biscuits (crackers), sugar, and salt pork or beef.[80] In some places along the route, and at certain times of the year, there were berries to be picked,[81] but when the foothills of the Rockies were reached, vegetation became sparse.[80] Some travelers took pickles and vinegar with them as antiscorbutics.[80] A physician who published the diary of his trek recorded that one evening they picked some leafy plants that they called "lambquarters" and "ate these delightful greens with vinegar, a sure preventive of scurvy."[82] A physician member of another party encouraged his companions to eat wild onions for the same reason.[83]

Such precautions were probably exceptional. Other diarists saw pitiful scenes on the route: adults on crutches and children so crippled from scurvy that they could not move a limb;[81] and men, nearly dead with scurvy, abandoned in the snow at the roadside at the final stages over the mountains, with winter setting in.[84] Others who had reached California by sea recorded seeing overland groups arriving "with cases of scurvy in the most aggravated and shocking form."[81, 85] There is no record of how many died on the overland trek, many from dysentery and cholera. One diarist recorded seeing a grave marker: "Sacred to the memory of W. Brown – Died with Skervy Sep 19th, 1849, Aged 35 years"; and noted that with the first rain, this and all the markers written in pencil would be obliterated.[86]

Among those working in the gold fields, conditions were not necessarily better. One miner wrote:

I was again dreaming of fortune and success, when my hopes were blasted by an attack of a terrible scourge that wrought destruction through the northern mines during the winter of 1848/9 . . . land scurvy. The exposed and unaccustomed life of two-thirds of the miners, and their entire subsistence upon salt meat, without any mixure of vegetable matter, had produced this disease, which was experienced more or less by at least one-half of the miners within my knowledge. It was first noticed . . . about the middle of February, many persons were rendered unable to walk by swellings of the lower limbs, and severe pains in them. . . . Many, who could obtain no vegetables or vegetable acids, lingered out a miserable existence and died. . . . I noticed its first attack upon myself by swelling and bleeding of the gums, followed by a swelling of both legs below the knee; and I was laid up in my tent. . . . I believe I should have died, had not accident discovered a remedy. In the second week of my illness, one of our party found, strewn along a foot-track, a

[79] Lorenz (1957), 475.    [80] Ibid., 478.    [81] Ibid., 481.    [82] Geiger & Bryarly (1950), 91.
[83] Shaw (1896), 106.    [84] Bruff (1949), 241, 1010.    [85] Kelly (1852), 76; Comstock (1982), 218–23.    [86] Bruff (1949), 228.

quantity of beans which sprouted from the ground, and were in leaf. Some one had probably dopped them. He gathered a quantity and I had them boiled, and lived entirely on them for several days, at the same time using a decoction of the bark of the spruce tree. These seemed to operate magically, and in a week I found myself able to walk, and with two companions walked into Coloma, there living principally upon a vegetable diet, which I procured by paying three dollars per pound for potatoes; in a very short time I recovered.[87]

A second victim described a similar cure, with spruce boughs boiled to a strong tea and raw potatoes sliced in vinegar.[88] Another writer reported that the miners' diet at that period seemed to consist of "stewed beans and flapjack 21 times per week, though the latter was occasionally replaced by flour dumplings and molasses," and that those weakened by scurvy tried to obtain onions and vinegar but these were available only at very high prices.[89] Yet another diarist recorded that land scurvy was on the increase, "owing to the constant use of salt and greasy provisions without vegetables." He saw cases with deep purple limbs, contracted muscles, and gangrenous gums. Many quack doctors were selling patent medicines, but the only success he had seen was from an old mountaineer's recipe of giving up tea and coffee, and drinking only a decoction of sassafras and spruce leaves.[90] Some miners also resorted to the old treatment of burial up to the neck in earth; a whole camp would do it at once, "except a few who remained out to keep off grizzlies and coyotes."[91] It is understandable that sailors, who were impressed by their developing the disease at sea and recovering again so quickly when they reached land, would try to maximize the effect of *land* by immersing themselves in it, and there are many references to this method of treatment.[92] But it seems strange that miners who had *developed* the disease on land should have retained the idea.

A physician who spent some time in the area in 1850 also said that he had seen "terrible cases of scurvy" and attributed them to "the exclusive use of dried and salted meats . . . as vegetables and fresh meat were luxuries rarely obtained in the mining districts; it became necessary to guard against it by using stewed fruits, pickles, and acidulous drinks."[93] At the Sonora mining camp in November 1849, they established a hospital for the destitute sick, "of which there were large numbers, with land scurvy the most prominent disease – brought on by exposure and bad living but above all by the quantities of fat from salt pork eaten to make the bread taste better."[94]

The great demand for a more varied diet and the high prices being paid rapidly led to their increased supply. Oranges from Tahiti and limes from Acapulco were shipped in, and land owners in southern California were encouraged to begin the production of citrus fruit on a commercial scale.[95]

[87] Buffum (1850), 97–8.     [88] Ferguson (1948), 114.     [89] Shaw (1896), 189–90.     [90] Kelly (1852), 118–20.     [91] Sawtelle (1876), 5.     [92] Martin (1604), 199; Bennett (1832), 574; Coale (1842), 76; Knox (1914), 14; MacDonald (1927), 101–2.     [93] Tyson (1955), 3–4.     [94] Lorenz (1957), 490.     [95] Ibid., 473.

No more was heard of the epidemic after 1850. Anthony Lorenz, who had made an intensive study of the subject and read much unpublished material, estimated that at least 10,000 men died "of scurvy, or its sequelae, in the California Gold Rush. . . . Its victims outnumbered those of cholera." [96] Dr. Praslow, the German physician who was in the Sacramento area in the winter of 1849–50, testified to the weakening effect of the disease: "I frequently saw patients who had suffered from scurvy . . . die within a few days from an acute diarrhea." [97]

It is striking that only one article on this subject seems to have been published at the time in a professional medical journal. This took the form of a letter to the editor of a New Orleans journal from Dr. Thomas Logan, who had been practicing in that city before going around Cape Horn to seek his fortune in the gold fields.[98] He confirmed that scurvy had been "a source of widespread calamity amongst the overland immigrants and miners; these scenes sicken us with the extent of suffering." [99] His main conclusions were:

1. There was no difference between this land scurvy and the sea scurvy that he had seen in his earlier work.[100]
2. The disease had no essential connection with cold and moist conditions, as had often been suggested in the past, because it flourished in California when the environment was hot and dry.[101]
3. Scurvy was a disease of the blood caused by the deficiency of salts of potash and soda; however, giving potassium nitrate and sodium chloride was ineffective. The potash and soda had to be "in that state of chemico-organic combination in which they exist in milk and in fresh meat and vegetables." Where there was edema, potassium iodide had a useful exciting influence on the vital actions.[102]
4. Spoiled food could produce scurvy by being in a state of putrefaction. Such putrefaction could be brought about, for example, in sausages, by a yeast; this then resulted in a dissolution of blood and tissues similar to that in the food.[103]

The last point seems to contradict the previous explanation, but is interesting because it appears to be the first statement of a theory that was to gain a considerable credence by the end of the nineteenth century.

## The Crimean War, 1854–6

The next outbreak of scurvy on a large scale occurred as the result of warfare in southeastern Europe. In 1854, Britain and France allied themselves with Turkey and declared war on Russia, which was trying to increase its influence in the Balkans and Middle East. At the end of May, a joint expeditionary force landed on the Bulgarian coast of the Black Sea, and, during a summer spent in preparation, the armies became infected with cholera. At the beginning of September, some 30,000 from each country sailed and

[96] Ibid., 506.    [97] Praslow (1939), 47.    [98] Lorenz (1957), 498.    [99] Logan (1850), 468, 473.    [100] Ibid., 469–72.    [101] Ibid., 473.    [102] Ibid., 476.    [103] Ibid., 477.

landed on the Crimean Peninsula (on the north side of the Black Sea) with the intention of capturing the Russian naval base of Sebastopol. After two hard battles they began a formal siege of the base that was to last until September of the following year.[104]

The British Army had to get its supplies from Balaclava, a small port that was some eight miles away, but accessible only by an unmade road that turned into a deep quagmire with the winter rains, so that it was impassable by wheeled carts or wagons, and supplies had to be carried up by the men themselves. In November, a hurricane, in which twelve British supply ships were lost, compounded the hardships. Finally, soldiers were practically unable to obtain wood of any kind for for cooking, and cholera flared up again in the cold and wet.[105]

In the British Army, ominous signs had begun to appear as early as August. The chief surgeon of the First Division reported:

> Scurvy first began to show itself before embarkation for the Crimea, and soon after its arrival there spongy and bleeding gums were only too evident; spots appeared on different parts of the body which degenerated into troublesome sores, and were followed by the usual chain of symptoms, diarrhea and dysentery etc, which continued almost unchecked until good supplies of fresh meat, vegetables and lime juice were obtained.[106]

During the ensuing winter 1,600 were admitted to hospital with the disease. However, the official *Medical and Surgical History* of the war states that

> the returns convey but a very faint conception of the disastrous part which it acted among the troops; . . . in a vast proportion of cases, evident indications of it existed as a complication of other diseases – fever and infection of the bowels. Before the more specific signs appeared, the patient was apathetic, . . . and dull aching pains in the ankles and feet were complained of. . . . There was shortage of breath on slight exertion.[107]

The surgeons with the troops made urgent requests for supplies of vegetables and lemon juice.[108] One ship laden with vegetables reached Balaclava in November. According to the official *History,* they failed to reach the troops "because the transport had already broken down."[108] In another account, it was stated that they were finally thrown overboard because they were not consigned to anyone in particular.[109] Twenty thousand pounds of lemon juice arrived at the port in December, but did not reach the Army until February.[108,109] There is no explanation for the delay, but one can imagine that, each day, transporting the staples of meat and flour seemed to deserve priority. The chief reporter for the *London Times* wrote in his later reminiscences:

[104] Judd (1975), 33–91.    [105] Kinglake (1881), 125, 142, 145; Wood (1895), 174–9.    [106] Parliamentary Papers (1858), 171.    [107] Ibid., 172    [108] Ibid., 182.    [109] Wood (1895) 176–7.

A considerable number of men were sent down on the 10th [of February] from the camp to Balaclava. There were many bad cases of scurvy and scorbutic dysentery among the men: and yet vegetables of all sorts, and lemons and oranges, . . . could have been purchased in any quantities all along the shores of the Black Sea. . . . Balaclava contained ships which had been lying there for weeks . . . doing nothing.[110]

This was the first major war in which newspaper correspondents were able to send back uncensored accounts of conditions at the front by electric telegraph. Articles published in the *Times* produced such an outcry in Britain that the Prime Minister had to resign, and tremendous efforts were made to correct the deficiencies.[111] Best known is the work of Florence Nightingale in the main base hospital at Scutari, near Constantinople.[112] Once the supply situation improved, scurvy virtually disappeared from the British Army, with only a relatively small recurrence the following winter – 200 cases in hospital with 2 deaths, compared with 1,600 cases and 175 deaths the previous year.[106]

In great contrast to this account is the experience of the French Army. They began the war with much better supply and hospital organizations that had been developed during their recent campaign in Algeria.[113] However, their two-man bivouacs (pup tents) were inadequate for winter conditions so that many thousands were disabled by frostbite, and their rations seemed insufficient for the hard physical work required in both camps.[114] The rations included neither fresh vegetables nor citrus fruit in any form and, in the autumn of 1854, the French Commander in Chief issued an order that the men should pick dandelion plants, growing in abundance in the area, and use them for salads.[115] The official French Sanitary Commission thought that they made a pleasant salad, having a "salutary bitterness," and believed that they staved off scurvy for a while, until the plant disappeared with the onset of winter in November.[116]

The official French statistics of mortality and hospital admissions are incomplete for the first winter of the war. From November to March, the total recorded admissions into ambulances for all reasons were over 40,000. There had also been a very large inflow of reinforcements over this period so that there were still 95,000 men in the Army in March 1845.[117] In February, when more detailed statistics begin, there were 3,000 cases in the main field hospital classified as scurvy, and 1,800 more were received in the next two months.[118]

Thus far, the two allies had similar experiences, but they diverged in the next period. The epidemic of scurvy in the French Army continued and even worsened right through the summer of 1855 and into the following winter

---

[110] Russell (1858), 267.     [111] Baudens (1862), 20; Kinglake (1881), 302–3.     [112] Judd (1975), 124–33.     [113] Kinglake (1881), 130.     [114] Ibid., 131.     [115] Ibid., 134.     [116] Baudens (1862), 35; Maupin (1860), 205.     [117] Kinglake (1881), 136.     [118] Ibid., 138.

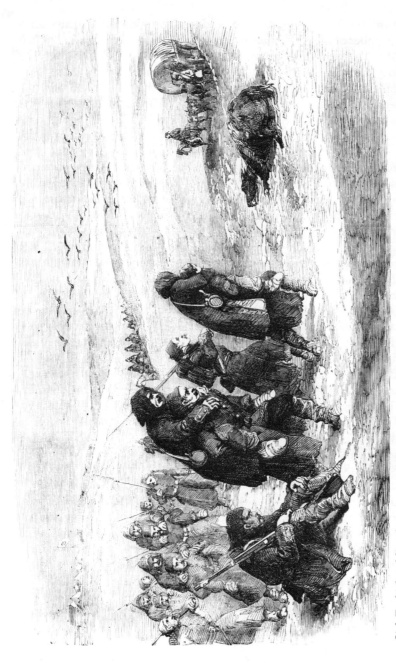

Sick Turkish soldiers being carried back to Balaclava by their comrades in the Crimean War. The many thousands of cases of scurvy were a major cause of the heavy losses in both the Turkish and French armies in this campaign. (From *Illustrated London News*, March 17, 1855.)

when hostilities were virtually at an end, so that even the statistics for a limited number of their hospitals recorded an extraordinary total of 23,000 cases. After the end of the fighting in March 1856, the Medical Inspector to the French Armies reported that they had 4,000 cases in hospital in Constantinople and 650 in field hospitals, and that "the disease still fills to a great degree our regimental infirmaries."[119] The Turkish Army, too, was very severely affected.[120] Another modern writer has quoted from a contemporary account that their hospitals were crowded to the point of suffocation, with scurvy accounting for five cases out of six.[121]

The British Fleet remained generally healthy, although there were nineteen cases of scurvy reported in May of 1854. In the same period there were twenty-five cases of night blindness. The surgeon reporting the occurrence considered the latter to be a premonitory sign of scurvy – appearing before the more palpable symptoms. All the signs – that is, both the night blindness and those of ordinary scurvy – cleared up when treatment with "lime juice, fresh vegetables etc" was instituted.[122] The French Fleet in the Black Sea suffered much more severely, as on many other occasions in the nineteenth century.[123] In November 1854, a fleet of six battleships, manned by some 4,000 men, had over 1,000 scorbutics, and some ships were said to be at the point of becoming unworkable because of the epidemic proportions of the disease.[124] The Chief Surgeon to the Fleet noted that the sailors in ships that returned to Turkish ports were given money to buy fresh vegetables and fruit, and that these had an almost instantaneous effect in eliminating the disease.[125] He then convinced his Admiral to continue the distribution of fresh vegetables and meat because these foods, "rich in digestible juices," were the only remedy and the best preservatives against the return of the disease."[126]

Medical opinion in the French Army did not hold the same view. In their analysis of earlier outbreaks of scurvy in barracks in France, they had implicated their bad situation in relation to neighboring marshland, and the inadequate ventilation.[52] A spokesman, writing after the war, said that a great number of wounded in the base hospital at Constantinople had arrived with no sign of scurvy but actually developed it there, even though they received a diet that was above criticism: It included vegetables, fresh bread, fresh meat, and wine, and on frequent occasions, even coffee or chocolate.[127] These were the foodstuffs considered antiscorbutic in Napoleon's armies.[128] A year later, scorbutics sent to the same hospital were still failing to show any improvement in a month, and only a change in locality could help them.[129]

---

[119] Baudens (1862), 189; Maupin (1860), 200.     [120] Buzzard (1866), 735.     [121] McCord (1971), 591.     [122] Rees, (1854), 234.     [123] Hirsch (1885), II, 533.     [124] Marroin (1861), 88–9, 93.     [125] Ibid., 95.     [126] Ibid., 127.     [127] Maupin (1860), 199.     [128] Larrey (1814), I, 16, 391.     [129] Ibid., 201–2; Perrin (1858), 146.

The same spokesman argued that one had to examine the totality of stresses laid on the French Army – their fatigue and lack of sleep, the unwholesomeness of confinement within one and the same place, the emotions inseparable from the knowledge that their lives were constantly at risk, and the influences of a capricious climate, as well as an inadequate, mediocre diet; all of these acting in combination weakened the nervous system and thinned the blood: It would be taking a very narrow view to attribute the severity and persistence of the epidemic to the lack of a few fresh vegetables, or, on the other hand, to think that a little cress or a few dandelions, an orange or a lemon could have made a substantial contribution toward mitigating its effects.[130] Something of this attitude may have survived right up to World War I, because there was quite a serious outbreak of scurvy in the French Army in June 1917, which was explained by a lack of fruit and fresh vegetables in the diet, whereas nothing comparable was reported for the British Army fighting in France.[131]

Baudens, the French Medical Inspector in the Crimea in 1855 made some interesting comments after the war:

The English physicians ascribe great anti-scorbutic virtues to the lemon juice, and say it is in a large degree owing to its use that their army was saved from the scurvy in the Winter of 1855/6. . . . The soldiers drew rations of lemon juice preserved in casks and they used it [three times per week] . . . with rum and sugar. Our field hospitals and regimental infirmaries were well provided with it towards the close of the campaign but our experience, although attended with good results, was not sufficiently tried to render it fully conclusive.[132]

Thus, in the French Army, they were making use of it as a cure, but still not as a preventive. It is not clear from Bauden's statement why the good results seen in the patients treated with lemon juice were not deemed conclusive: Perhaps it was because the patients were also receiving other antiscorbutic treatments at the same time. It was probably more difficult for the French doctors to accept the notion that a small quantity of lemon juice could have some special virtue because of their stronger background in contemporary French and German animal chemistry, and Liebig's conclusions that were drawn from it. Bauden himself indicates this. "The necessity of a varied nourishment has been established as a practical fact. The theoretical views by which it has been attempted to account for this necessity, do not seem to accord with the facts observed in late years . . . [and] ought to be abandoned."[133] The terms "lemon juice" and "lime juice" were used almost interchangeably at that time, as will be discussed later.

The official British report is almost as hesitant about the virtues of "lime juice," as they called their issue:

---

[130] Maupin (1860), 200, 203–4.    [131] Harvier (1917), 395, 398.    [132] Baudens (1862), 36, 39.    [133] Ibid., 34.

With regard to the value of lime-juice in the treatment of this affection [disease], as it occurred in the Crimea, some difference of opinion is expressed. . . . But when we recollect the decided influence which it undoubtedly possessed in rendering the food of the soldier . . . easily assimilated . . . and consider that the diet of the troops was defective in kind rather than quantity, we are obliged to claim for it greater consideration than it has received.[134]

The British surgeons also praised the value of preserved potatoes and mixed vegetables as antiscorbutic. Another Army surgeon made a similar evaluation at the same time on the basis of his experience in a troop ship sailing from Britain to India. Six cases of scurvy had developed, and in each case, the victims had failed to eat their ration of preserved potatoes. In other troop ships, there had been more cases despite the regular issue of lime juice, which he believed to be often adulterated and of dubious quality, so that potatoes were a more reliable supplement.[135]

The official British report also refers to the opinion of a Dr. Crawford that scurvy, as seen in the Crimea, often came from a deficiency of protein; and that this was confirmed by the failure of lime juice to alleviate symptoms in some cases which then responded to milk, eggs, and soups rich in gelatin.[136] This idea was revived eight years later by yet another surgeon who had seen scurvy develop in troop ships "despite the free use of lime-juice. . . . The salting of meat produces scurvy by removing all its protein materials into the brine which is discarded by men on board ship. . . . Preserved milk, meat and vegetables are inefficacious because their albuminous substances, by such means are rendered totally inert." [137]

## The American Civil War, 1861–5

The next outbreak of hostilities with its usual train of disease and suffering was in the United States. The U. S. Armed Forces had already had some experience of scurvy within the lifetime of the senior surgeons during the War, and we shall review that first.

In 1838, the U. S. Navy had sent a frigate on a cruise around the world with approximately 500 on board. The rations did not include lemon or lime juice, but were considered "ample and judicious" and included "500 cases of preserved beef and chickens, 600 gallons of preserved cranberries and 1,000 gallons of excellent pickles, which were deemed sufficient preservatives against any scorbutic affection." [138] They sailed in June, calling first at Rio de Janeiro, then at the Cape of Good Hope and Singapore. After fourteen months away from home, and while crossing the Pacific, "scurvy made its appearance and proved so disastrous." [139]

The sick list was over 120, and while at sea was only lessened by deaths, as none were cured. The deaths from scurvy alone, uncombined with any other disease were

---

[134] Parliamentary Papers (1858), 183.     [135] Morgan (1855), 587.     [136] Parliamentary Papers (1858), 180.     [137] Oliver (1863), 61.     [138] Coale (1842), 68.     [139] Ibid., 70.

23. . . . . It seized upon the old rather than the young. . . . . No post-mortems were made as it was deemed inexpedient to do anything that might increase the gloom amongst the crew. . . . . The effect of fresh diet after our return to port was remarkable. . . . . No ill consequences followed the uncontrolled indulgence in fresh diet . . . milk, eggs, chicken, bread and pumpkins and potatoes both sweet and Irish. . . . . After 3 weeks on the Sandwich Islands [Hawaii] the sick list was reduced to 62." [140]

The signs of the disease were characteristic of earlier descriptions except that some of the sick also showed nyctalopia (or night blindness), i.e., failure to see as well as normal subjects in dim light. Some men who had been regular grog-drinkers for years found it now produced immediate vomiting. "In all these cases the tongue was red but perfectly clean, and in one case it presented highly painful fissures of slight depth. . . . Longing after fresh food gave way to loathing of all food. . . . As the disease advanced the body became swollen, the face bloated." [141] This image recalls the descriptions of some very early voyages of crews victualed in the East Indies, as discussed in Chapter 1. The surgeon who described these events was modest in his conclusions:

I have not upheld any particular doctrine or another. . . . [Many factors] have been enumerated separately or in combination among the causes of scurvy. . . . each writer seems to be impressed with the effects of one single agent, and does not permit others to have due weight. . . . Lemon juice, pickles and citric acid, so long the sheet-anchor of naval surgeons, have all proved fallible.[142]

A second, serious outbreak occurred in 1846 in the squadron blockading the Mexican coast, "and for some months disabled several of the largest and most efficient ships. The Potomac with a complement of 500 . . . had 100 cases upon her sick report and with symptoms of the disease in most of the crew who still continued to perform their duty." The captain was forced to return to a home port for two months of refreshment.[143] Dr. Foltz, the surgeon who described the epidemic in this Fleet, was himself on the *Potomac's* sister ship, the *Raritan*, which fared even worse: "The Raritan, which has been so efficient for two years, with her powerful crew of young men, was now *hors de combat*. More than two hundred cases of scurvy were under treatment. . . . The more vigorous and active men's habits, in the same ratio were their liabilities to the attack, and the violence of the disease." [144]

Foltz felt that the symptoms, as they appeared on the *Raritan*, "varied materially from such as are laid down in the books. . . . Lassitude was not among the early symptoms; . . . frequently there was cheerfulness and good appetite for weeks after the teeth were loosened, . . . and the limbs discolored. . . . Where the disease was far advanced, the respiratory system was much involved." Nyctalopia was detected only in five cases.[145] He attributed the severity of the epidemic to (a) the imperfect ventilation of the

[140] Ibid., 74–6.     [141] Ibid., 72–3.     [142] Ibid., 76–7.     [143] Foltz (1848), 38.     [144] Ibid., 43–4.
[145] Ibid., 47–8.

berth deck in that class of ship, (b) the fact that the men received fresh meat and good vegetables only rarely, (c) the poor quality of the salt used, and (d) the despondency of the men when their period of service was extended.[146] The Navy suffered some further outbreaks,[147] and in one joint operation with British ships off the South American coast, they too had suffered from a combination of ordinary scurvy and night blindness.[148]

With regard to treatment, Foltz found raw potatoes to be "superior in all other remedies," but cooked potatoes did not show the same activity. He then attempted some surprising chemical explanations.

The basis of the potato is starch, and from the facility with which it is transferred into healthy nutritious matter, we may expect some of the same salutary effects from the use of starch itself, in the treatment of scurvy. . . . What years of experience have proved to be so serviceable, lemon juices and vegetables, analytical chemistry now . . . proves to contain just such elements as the body is deficient in. The discovery of protein in vegetables alone, and the part it performs in nutrition, only confirm . . . the simplicity and harmony of all the operations of nature. . . . The whole treatment of sea scurvy can be summed up in a few words. Supply the system freely with protein, by giving patients freely those vegetables in which it most abounds. . . . where the fruits and vegetables in recent state cannot be obtained, starch and lemon juice, both of which can be carried at sea in sufficient quantities, will give us all that is required, when combined with cleanliness, ventilation, abundance of water and cheerfulness.[149]

This seems complete nonsense, and one has to assume that Foltz's belief that protein was only to be found in vegetable foods came from a misunderstanding of Liebig's writings, where he argues that the sole and sufficient source of protein for the animal kingdom, considered as a whole, is the vegetable kingdom.

The U. S. Army also had suffered severe outbreaks of scurvy. In 1819, after the Louisiana Purchase, some 800 men were sent up the Missouri River to form a western outpost, Fort Atkinson (sixteen miles northwest of the present Omaha, Nebraska). By the end of January 1820, the rations were reduced to salted pork and beef (both evil-smelling), wheat flour, and corn meal. There was very little game as an extra source of fresh meat. Nearly 500 developed scurvy, and 160 died of it. None of the sick showed any improvement until the coming of spring, when a small wild onion was harvested.[150]

Dr. W. A. Hammond wrote that the disease was also "exceedingly prevalent" among troops stationed in New Mexico for eight months of the year. He described three individual cases that he had seen in 1850, showing ulcers and livid spots on the legs and swollen gums. The only treament that he ordered was five grains (0.32 gram) potassium carbonate four times a day for two of the cases, and potassium bitartrate four times a day for the third.

---

[146] Ibid., 52–3.    [147] Gihon (1871), 73–5.    [148] Bryson (1850), 436.    [149] Foltz (1848), 56–7.    [150] Forry (1842), 78–82; Reals (1949), 141–51; Levine (1955), 10, 13–4.

All three were discharged, completely cured in one to two weeks.[151] Hammond believed that his unit was less affected than were others in the territory because the stream from which they drew water was rich in potash, and he thus recommended that "a small portion of some salt of potash be issued to troops as a component part of their rations. . . . It would, I am confident, entirely prevent the occurrence of this affection among them."[151]

There was no other outbreak in peacetime at all comparable with that in Fort Atkinson in 1820.[152] However, the prevention of the "scorbutic taint" in isolated outposts during winter continued to be a worry for surgeons throughout the 1850s. There was still no regular issue of lemon juice. In 1858, at Fort Laramie, for example, there were no potatoes available either, and the surgeon prepared an extract of sliced cactus leaves which he administered with whiskey: "This affected a wholesome change in the whole system though not so rapid as that resulting from the use of potatoes."[153]

In 1858, Dr. Tripler, another Army surgeon, gave a general lecture on the cause and treatment of scurvy. He referred to the two outbreaks just discussed, and also to one in Florida and another at Fort Laramie.[154] The disease appeared after soldiers were exposed for some length of time to a comparatively low temperature. Qualitative deficiency of the diet was also an important stimulus. Salted meat was more difficult to assimilate than fresh, and the rest of a soldier's ration – beans, rice, and wheat flour – supplied an abundance of carbon and nitrogen but could not meet the requirements for potash and iron.[155] He acknowledged the priority of Garrod's recommendation of potash for the treatment of scurvy and expanded his arguments with further examples of rapid cures.[156] Lastly, he argued that nyctalopia was not in any way related to scurvy, though the two diseases were occasionally, by coincidence, seen in the same subject.[157]

The Civil War broke out early in 1861, though large-scale land operation began only in July. As one would expect, we have better records for the Union (or Federal, i.e., Northern) Armies, that won the war, than for the Confederate (Southern) Armies. In the first year, the largest forces were engaged in fighting south of Washington. The Union "Army of the Potomac," consisting of some 200,000 men, had Dr. Tripler as its Medical Director. The number seriously sick during the winter of 1861–2 was some 114,000, but scurvy was not reported.[158] However, it appeared in at least six regiments in that Army in June, 1862. The Surgeon of the Twenty-eighth Massachusetts Regiment, for example, reported "the usual marks of the disease – swollen and ulcerated gums, painful swelling of the muscles, languor, nostalgia, petechial eruptions. . . . Unless potatoes, onions and other vegetables are soon supplied in liberal quantities there is reason to apprehend its manifestation in more serious forms."[159] Tripler wrote imme-

---

[151] Hammond (1853), 103–4.    [152] Forry (1841), 321.    [153] *Med. Surg. His.* (1875–88), Pt. III, 683 n3.    [154] Tripler (1858), 133.    [155] Ibid., 137–8.    [156] Ibid., 143–7.    [157] Ibid., 147.    [158] Steiner (1968), 103–4.    [159] *Med. Surg. Hist.* (1875–88), Pt. III, 687.

diately to his superior, W. A. Hammond (now the Surgeon-General). He said that the men had been refusing to eat their "dessicated vegetables"; he had telegraphed immediately for a supply of lemons and was, in the meantime, issuing cream of tartar (potassium bitartrate) to affected units.[160] It is interesting that Tripler and Hammond were the two men who had written before the Civil War in support of the concept that scurvy was due to a potassium deficiency.

Tripler was relieved of his position a few days later and replaced by Dr. Letterman, who described, in a later report, what he had found:

> Scurvy had made its appearance. . . . it is not to be dreaded merely by the numbers it sends upon the reports of the sick. . . . The causes which give rise to it undermine the strength, depress the spirits, take away the energy, courage, and elasticity of those who do not report themselves sick, and who yet are not well. . . . Their energy, their powers of endurance, and their willingness to undergo hardship are in a great degree gone, and they know not why. In this way it had affected the fighting powers of the army.[161]

Later in July, 1,500 boxes of lemons were distributed to the hospitals and troops, as well as a variety of vegetables, and a month later the condition had disappeared.[162]

The official *Medical and Surgical History* of the Union Army quotes from over twenty surgeons' reports of the occurrence of scurvy in a number of other areas during the next four years.[163] Many of these came from the army in Tennessee, which, in 1863, had many cases of overt scurvy, and it was noted that even vaccination, in many men, produced ugly, slow-healing ulcers, thought to be due to their "scorbutic constitution." The voluntary Sanitary Commission organized the distribution of donated vegetables from farmers – 15,000 bushels in the first month – at a time when the official organization had been unable to obtain them, and the condition of the soldiers improved.[164] In the summer of 1864, the greatest problem occurred in the army operating against Atlanta, Georgia. The surgeon in charge of one division of 7,000 men believed that over 2,000 were suffering from "scorbutic affections."[163] Treatment, as already indicated, consisted usually of fresh vegetables and lemonade, but there are occasional references to the use of molasses, vinegar, and nitric or sulfuric acids.[165]

The statistics for the years 1864–6, when large numbers of black troops were in the field, indicate that these soldiers had an annual average of nearly 9% sick with scurvy – a rate six times the average for white troops over the entire period of the war. It has been hypothesized that the difference was partly due to the black recruits typically having had to subsist, for

[160] War of the Rebellion (1880–1902), *XI*, Pt. 1, 209–10.    [161] Ibid., 211.    [162] Ibid., 214.
[163] *Med. Surg. Hist.* (1875–88), Pt. III, 689–93.    [164] Rawson (1862), 42, 125; Stille (1866),
320–9.    [165] McBride (1863), 267–8; *Med. Surg. Hist.* (1875–88), Pt. III, 691, 696, 698–9;
Stinson (1966), 22.

some time prior to joining the army, on inadequate diets, as well as to their subsequent lack of vegetables.[166]

The total number of cases recorded as scurvy in the Union Armies was 47,000. Only 700 deaths were directly attributed to it, compared with a total of 200,000 deaths from diseases of all sorts.[166] This would make scurvy seem unimportant, except that so many surgeons felt that it contributed greatly to the 45,000 deaths from diarrheas and dysentery.[167]

The very worst conditions were to be found in the prisoner-of-war camps on either side.[168] There was particular indignation in the North at the conditions in which prisoners from the Union Army were kept at Andersonville, Georgia, and after the War, the camp commandant was tried for atrocities. The detailed reports make grim reading, but are available for those needing to know what can happen when 30,000 men are penned into an area allowing less than forty square feet per prisoner and are provided only with dirty water and a meager scorbutic diet.[169] Mortality rose to 9% *per month*, with 3,000 dying directly from scurvy. One charge of which the commandant was probably not guilty was that of deliberately having prisoners vaccinated with poisonous material; as we have seen, vaccination was followed by ulceration in scorbutic soldiers in the Union Army, even when it was performed by their own doctors.

It is difficult to conclude that all of this suffering resulted in any real advance in scientific understanding of the disease. We have no published analyses of blood or urine in scorbutics. After the War, Surgeon-General Hammond wrote that he no longer thought that scurvy was due to a deficiency of potassium; he still believed that potash was of great value in restoring scorbutic blood, but iron was equally valuable.[170]

## The Siege of Paris, 1870–1

The Franco-Prussian War was short, and casualties were few as compared with the two wars just considered. However, the scurvy that resulted deserves some attention because it involved civilians in one of the world's intellectual capitals and stimulated scientific discussion. The fighting began in early August 1870, and the Prussian Army advanced so rapidly that it began the investment of Paris by mid-September and then settled in for a long siege. At the end of January an armistice was effected, and the city received fresh provisions; peace terms were agreed by the end of February.[171] The actual siege had therefore lasted for 4½ months.

---

[166] *Med. Surg. Hist.* (1875–88), Pt. III, 684, 694–6.     [167] Steiner (1968), 8.     [168] War of the Rebellion (1880–1902), Ser. 2, *VI*, 473, 1039–41.     [169] *Trial of Henry Wirz* (1868); *Treatment of Prisoners of War* (1869); *Med. Surg. Hist.* (1875–88), Pt. III, 37–71; Breeden (1975), 178–98.
[170] Hammond (1865), 15, 26.     [171] Howard (1961), 120–44, 317–31.

Food quickly became scarce and very expensive: By the end of November, merchants were selling half-carrots, and potatoes had reached twenty-five times their normal price; later the severity of the winter weather made production of green vegetables within Paris impossible. Bread and meat were rationed, the latter being mostly horsemeat. Even the small rations could not always be obtained, and "from 3 in the morning, even in the coldest and wettest winter nights one would see lines of women, men and children queuing at the doors of the butchers and bakers who would open only at 7." Fuel was so scarce that the poor could cook only by burning their furniture.[172]

Two professors of clinical medicine wrote: "The investment of Paris and the state of want which resulted, provoked an explosion of scurvy and, at the same time, less well-defined states of debility that were even more serious."[173] They could not even estimate the number of scurvy cases in the general population, but they made particular studies of outbreaks in the Paris prisons and in a hospital where the rations and general conditions were well recorded. In the prisons the meat ration was eliminated at the end of October, and potatoes were replaced by a mixture of rice and beans. The ration of onions and fresh vegetables ceased at the same time. The work schemes, by which prisoners had been able to earn a little money to buy extra food items, were also stopped. Because the so-called "green vegetables" that the prisoners had received prior to the siege amounted to only 2½ ounces per head of onions, carrots, and cabbage, which disappeared in the preparation of soup, the writers felt that their omission could not explain the outbreak.[174]

They were impressed by the great differences in incidence of scurvy in the various prisons – from nil to nearly 90%. The most modern "model prison," with large airy cells and a benevolent director, had the highest incidence. With no heating during the winter, the cement had never dried out but remained dripping and glacial. On the other hand, even a pleasant bourgeois house converted to use as a "house of correction for young women" and run by nuns, was "gravely tainted by scurvy." Their final conclusion was that the incidence depended on the previous length of imprisonment; those who had been incarcerated for over six months were at high risk. This they attributed to the idleness imposed on the prisoners, which reduced both their physical condition and their morale. In addition, they considered that too much attention had been paid to the quality of the rations during the siege, and not enough to the reduction in their quantity.[175]

A naval surgeon attached to a group of 800 sailors manning one of the forts in the outer defenses of Paris took a rather different view. He attributed the appearance of scurvy in seventy of his men principally to their being *over*worked, short of sleep, and also to their having to live in cold, damp,

[172] Lasègue & Legroux (1871), 5–10.   [173] Ibid., 23.   [174] Ibid., 14–17.   [175] Ibid., 18–19, 700–1.

# A LIST

OF THE

# UNION SOLDIERS BURIED AT ANDERSONVILLE.

All Persons numbered below 12367, died in 1864; above that number, in 1865. All names with a *, denote Corporal; those with a †, Sergeant.

## ALABAMA.

7524, Barton, Wm, 1 cav, Co L, died Sept 1, scorbutus.
2111, Berry, J M, †, 1 cav, Co A, died May 17, diarrhea c.
4622, Belle, Robt, 1 cav, Co A, died Aug 8, dysentery.
5505, Boobur, Wm, 1 cav, Co E, died Aug 13, diarrhea.
8425, Brice, J C, 1 cav, Co L, died Sept 11, scorbutus.

8147, Guthrie, J, 1 cav, Co I, died Sept 8, scorbutus.

2514, Henry, P, 1 cav, Co F, died June 26, pneumonia.

996, Jones, Jno F, 1 cav, Co K, died Mar 15, anasarca.

4715, Mitchel, Jno D, 1, Co A, died Aug 4, scorbutus.

5077, Ponders, J, 1 cav, Co H, died Aug 8, diarrhea.
5763, Panter, R, 1, Co L, died Aug 15, diarrhea c.
6886, Patterson, W D, 1, Co A, died Aug 25, diarrhea a.
2504, Prett, J R, 1, Co F, died June 26, diarrhea a.

10900, Redman, W R, 1 cav, Co G, died Oct 14, scorbutus.

4731, Stubbs, W, 1, Co I, died Aug 4, bronchitis.

## CONNECTICUT.

2380, Anderson, A, 14, Co K, died June 23, diarrhea c.

3461, Batchelder, Benj, 16, Co C, died July 17, diarrhea a.
3464, Baty, John, 16, Co C, died July 19, diarrhea c.
7306, Brunkiaell, H, 14, Co D, died Aug 30, dysentery.
2833, Brennon, M, 14, Co B, died July 3, dysentery c.
3224, Burns, John, 7, Co I, died July 12, diarrhea.
10414, Blumly, E, 8, Co D, died Oct 6, scorbutus.
545, Bigelow, Wm, 7, Co B, died April 14, diarrhea.
11965, Ball, H A, 3, Co B, died Nov 11, scorbutus.
12082, Brookmeyer, T W, 8, Co H, died Nov 18, scorbutus.
12152, Burke H, 16, Co D, died Nov 24, scorbutus.
12209, Bone, A, 1, Co E, died Dec 1, scorbutus.
10682, Burnham F,* 14, Co I, died Oct 11, dysentery c.
10690, Barlow, O L, 16, Co E, died Oct 11, dysentery a.
10876, Bennett, N, 18, Co H, died Oct 13, scorbutus.
5806, Brown, C H, 1, Co H, died Aug 15, dysentery.
5919, Boyce, Wm, 7, Co B, died Aug 17, dysentery.
6083, Bishop, B H, 1 cav, Co I, died Aug 18, dysentery.
6184, Bushnell, Wm, 14, Co D, died Aug 19, cerebritis.
7763, Bailey, F, 16, Co E, died Sept 4, dysentery.
2054, Brewer, G E, 21, Co A, died June 16, diarrhea c.
5596, Burns, B, 6, Co G, died Aug 14, dysentery.
5632, Balcomb, 11, Co B, died Aug 14, diarrhea.
5754, Beers, James C, 16, Co A, died Aug 15, dysentery.
11658, Birdsell, D, 16, Co D, died Oct 23, scorbutus.
4296, Blakeslee, H, 1 cav, Co L, died July 30, anasarca.
3900, Bishop, A, 18, Co A, died Aug 24, dysentery.
1493, Besannon, Peter, 14, Co B, died June 2, diarrhea.
2720, Babcock, R, 30, Co A, died July 3, pneumonia.
2518, Baldwin, Thomas, 1 cav, Co L, died July 3, pneumonia.
2256, Bosworth, A M, 16, Co D, died June 21, diarrhea c.
5132, Bougin, John, 11, Co C, died Aug 8, dysentery.
5152, Brooks, Wm D,* 16, Co F, died Aug 9, dysentery.
5348, Bower, John, 16, Co E, died Aug 11, scorbutus.
5452, Bently, F, 6, Co H, died Aug 12, diarrhea.

5464, Bently, James, 1 cav, Co I, died Aug 12, scorbutus.
4830, Blackman, A,* 2 artil, Co C, died Aug 6, scorbutus.
7742, Banning, J. F, 16, Co E, died Sept 3, dysentery.
8018, Ballentine, Robert, 16, Co A, died Sept 6, dysentery.
12408, Bassett, J B, 11, Co B, died Jan. 6, '65, scorbutus.
12540, Bohine. C, 2, Co E, died Jan 27, '65, rheumatism.
12620, Bemis Charles, 7, Co K, died Feb 8, scorbutus.

3707, Chapin, J L, 16, Co A, died July 21, '64, fever intermittent.
3949, Cottrell, P, 7, Co D, died July 25, diarrhea c.
3941, Clarkson, —, 11, Co H, died, July 25, scorbutus.
4867, Culler, M, 7, Co E, died July 31, diarrhea.
4449, Connor, D, 18, Co F, died Aug 1, scorbutus.
4848, Carrier, D B, 16, Co D, died Aug 6, diarrhea.
6060, Cook, W H, 1 cav, Co G, died Aug 18, cerebritis.
6153, Clark, H H, 16, Co K, died Aug 19, cerebritis.
6846, Clark, W, 6, Co A, died Aug 25, diarrhea.
5799, Champlain, H, 10, Co F, died Aug. 15, dysentery.
336, Cane, John, 9, Co H, died April 2, diarrhea.
620, Christian, A M, 1, Co A, died April 19, dysentery.
775, Crawford, James, 14, Co A, died April 28, diarrhea c.
7316, Chapman, M, 16, Co E, died Aug 30, scorbutus.
7348, Cleary, P, 1 cav, Co B, died Aug 31, scorbutus.
7395, Campbell, Rob't, 7, Co E, died Aug 31, diarrhea.
7418, Culler, M, 16, Co K, died Aug 31, diarrhea a.
7685, Carver, John G, 16, Co B, died Sept 3, dysentery.
7780, Cain, Thomas, 14, Co G, died Sept 4, diarrhea.
9984, Crossley, B, 8, Co G, died Sept 29, scorbutus.
10272, Coltier, W, 16, Co D, died Oct 3, diarrhea.
11175, Callahan J, 11, Co I, died Oct 19, scorbutus.
11361, Candee, D. M, 2 artil, Co A, died Oct 23, scorbutus.

25, Dowd, F, 7, Co I, died March 8, pneumonia.
7325, Davis, W, 1 cav, Co L, died Aug 30, dysentery.
2813, Davis, W, 10, Co E, died Aug 3, anasarca.
3614, Damery, John, 6, Co A, died July 20, diarrhea.

The first page of a record of nearly 12,000 captured soldiers who died in Andersonville prison during the American Civil War. Approximately 3,000 (or 25%) are recorded as having died of scorbutus (scurvy). (Doe Library, University of California, Berkeley.)

and poorly ventilated quarters. "Their provisions were relatively good. . . . the bread was white, the meat though mainly horse was fresh, the wine ration was not reduced for a long time and was then supplemented with brandy; in a word there was no really appreciable privation." [176] This mirrors the view in the French Army during the Crimean War, that there could be nothing seriously wrong with a diet that included fresh bread, wine, and coffee, and which the men themselves were happy with.

[176] Grenet (1871), 279, 283–4.

A third writer, Professor Delpech, took still a different view. He had been called in to study the outbreaks of scurvy in the Paris prisons, but had seen the disease also in his private practice. He felt that it was of vital importance to disentangle all the various causes that had been advanced to explain such outbreaks and to determine which of them were always present, and which only occasionally accompanied them. Cold, humidity, depression, lack of fresh meat, and a reduction in the total quantity of food had all been possible factors in the institutions; however, he had seen private cases where none of these had operated.[177] For example, Madame M., a widow, was very well off, still quite young, and normally in good health. She did not have to endure fatigue or cold and she ate fresh meat regularly, but from the beginning of the siege, she had given up eating vegetables. Toward the end of January, she was developing all the signs of scurvy.[178] Another patient was a carter of age fifty-two, vigorous, with well-developed muscles. He had become too weak to work and showed all the signs of scurvy in his legs and gums. He had never gone hungry during the siege; in the first months he had eaten fresh horsemeat, bread, and dried beans, but no salted meat. Since January, he had subsisted on bread, soup, rice, and sometimes dried peas. From September on, he had dropped fresh vegetables completely from his diet.[179] The same change had been instituted in the rations in the Paris prisons; from the end of September, green vegetables and potatoes, and also meat, were entirely eliminated.[180] From his review of what had happened in Paris, and also from all the examples given by Lind and other writers on scurvy, he concluded that the only common factor was the exclusion of fresh vegetables from the diet, and that this must, therefore, by elimination, be considered the true cause of the disease.[181] This also fitted the circumstances of a serious outbreak in a French naval ship four years earlier.[182]

There is an interesting postscript to the events of the siege. Fourteen years later, another paper was published, pointing out that scurvy was still occasionally occurring in the prisons in the Paris area. The cases appeared in the summer months, from May to August, and coincided with the omission of potatoes from the diet, because of the gap between the end of the old crop and the appearance of the new crop.[183] The author's recommendation was that, in the absence of potatoes, other fresh vegetables should be given, and if this was impossible, then there should be a special distribution of meat, wine, or milk.[184] There is no mention of fruit or lemon juice as alternative supplements.

Obviously, there were still differences of opinion about the causes of scurvy after the Siege of Paris, and in 1874 there was a formal debate between two protagonists in the Academy of Medicine. It began with a

---

[177] Delpech (1871), 325.     [178] Ibid., 320.     [179] Ibid., 311.     [180] Ibid., 317–18.     [181] Ibid., 358–9.     [182] Léon (1868), 297.     [183] Lancereaux (1885), 300–1.     [184] Ibid., 303.

paper read by Dr. Jean-Antoine Villemin. He is remembered today for his demonstrations nearly a decade earlier that tuberculosis was an infectious disease which could be transmitted from humans to animals and then from one animal to another. At the time, it had been thought to arise spontane-ously as a consequence of the weakening effects of a poor environment, inadequate diet, and other debilitating conditions. For a long time, his work was either contested or ignored.[185] We can see the influence of his previous experience in his analysis of scurvy. He made extensive use of the published literature, and argued from it on the following lines (here condensed and paraphrased):

Scurvy is a contagious miasm, comparable to typhus, which occurs in epidemic form when people are closely congregated in large groups as in prisons, naval vessels and seiges. Admittedly, those in strongest condition are most resistant but it is ridiculous to suppose that a lack of fresh vegetables is the *cause* of the disease. It has been alleged that lack of potatoes was the cause of the outbreak in Western Europe in 1847; but some people must go without potatoes every year.[186] As Lind said, in refuting this kind of argument from Bachstrom, there are many parts such as the Highlands of Scotland where vegetables are unavailable for six months at a time. And how can one explain the health of people in Greenland where they do not grow vegetables at any time? I [Villemin] have also kept a variety of animals in good health without providing them with any of the types of food which are considered anti-scorbutic. The 1847 epidemic gradually spread eastwards, reaching Russia in 1848, killing 68,000 people in that year, and hanging on in small pockets after that.[187] Certainly, fresh vegetables and lemon juice have a certain curative value, but do we, just because quinine can cure malaria, conclude that the *cause* of malaria is a defi-ciency of quinine? We have many examples of well-fed sailors and soldiers going down with scurvy, while others less well fed to not.[188] Also, we have positive evidence of the spread of the disease by contagion – for example, the introduction of scurvy into French miliary hospitals by veterans returning from the Crimea, and the rapid spread of scurvy from one sailor to another in naval vessels.[189]

The respondent was Le Roy de Méricourt, a senior naval surgeon. He congratulated Villemin on being willing to make an independent and critical examination of an issue that seemed to have been settled. He pointed out that some of the evidence brought forward to suggest that servicemen contracted scurvy without any change in their rations was misleading be-cause at some periods they bought their own supplementary foods, and at other times they were unable to do so. It was unnecessary to hypothesize a "miasm" to explain why it was that large numbers in a group would all develop scurvy within a short time. Where they had all been exposed to the same diet for the same period of time, as in a voyage or a siege, it was only to be expected.[190] The practical danger in thinking of scurvy as a contagion was

---

[185] Dubos & Dubos (1952), 98–9;     [186] Villemin (1874), 710, 726.     [187] Ibid., 711, 731.
[188] Ibid., 729, 738, 768.     [189] Ibid., 773–90.     [190] Le Roy de Méricourt, (1874), 967.

that victims would have to be isolated and quarantined. Even the authorities whom Villemin had relied on for his evidence, had concluded that scurvy could not be a contagion.[191]

At the next session, Villemin said that he was not concerned with the *beliefs* of earlier observers but rather with their *observations*. There were many other diseases, generally accepted as infectious, which only rarely attacked medical officers in attendance on them, and this was another example of greater resistance because of better diet, hygiene, etc. He did not believe, therefore, that there was really much difference between himself and his opponent.[192] Le Roy de Méricourt was unwilling to compromise: All the evidence indicated that outbreaks could be attributed solely to faulty nutrition.[193]

Villemin was clearly one of a small minority. Hirsch, in his scholarly review, was outspoken: "The doctrine of the *contagious nature of scurvy* . . . lately revived by Villemin . . . is quite untenable . . . inasmuch as it goes against all clinical and historical experience."[194] Mahé, in his monograph and bibliography of the literature up to 1877, compiled for a French medical encyclopedia, found no good evidence that scurvy was contagious. However, he dissociated himself from the "monogenists," who considered lack of fresh vegetables the *only* causative factor. He was of the "polygenist" school, who believed that many factors, including environmental and psychological stress, combined to bring on the disease.[195] This was in agreement with a German monograph which stated that treatment of the disease could not be reduced to a single formula, and listed impartially all those that had been proposed, including mineral acids and creosote as well as potatoes.[196]

### The "diminished alkalinity" theory

In the 1860s and '70s, there was probably general acceptance in England of the statement in a newly published medical textbook:

Scurvy only occurs when fresh vegetable nutriment has been for some time partially or completely withheld. A variety of forms of impaired nutrition will follow the want of other descriptions of food, but this particular condition is only seen as a sequel of that special privation. . . . so abundant and conclusive are the proofs, that to assert less strongly would be to imply a doubt which cannot be allowed to exist.[197]

This was doing no more than to restate the position held seventy-five years earlier. And, there was the persistent problem, particularly in Britain, that fresh fruit and vegetables could not readily be supplied on long sea voyages or in remote parts of the British Empire, where army units were now perma-

---

[191] Ibid., 1036–7.    [192] Villemin (1875), 595, 636.    [193] Le Roy de Méricourt (1875), 703–4.
[194] Hirsch (1885), 560–1.    [195] Mahé (1880), 126–7.    [196] Krebel (1866), 201–6, 252–3.
[197] Buzzard (1866), 732.

nently stationed. Lemon juice (or lime juice) was the routine alternative issue, but there were continued complaints of its failure to prevent the development of scurvy at sea, particularly in troop ships[198] and, also on land, particularly in India, where this was generally attributed to adulteration by the merchant supplying it and possibly also to deterioration during storage at high temperatures.[199] There was, therefore, a strong incentive at the British Army Medical School to discover the antiscorbutic factor and to have it readily available for the men in their charge. It seemed that the spectacular advances in chemistry and physiology in the previous decades should be able to provide a solution to the problem.

Professor Parkes, the leader in this work, had already concluded that potassium was *not* the vital factor.[69, 70] Potassium nitrate, specifically, had been lauded in the 1790s, and was again favorably assessed by two surgeons in convict ships en route to Australia in the 1830s.[200] But when it was tested in some fairly well controlled experiments organized by the Admiralty, it had been found inactive and even injurious.[201] In 1863, the regular occurrence of scurvy among Canadian lumbermen had been associated with their eating large quantities of pork, heavily pickled with potassium nitrate; [202] this apparently ended the claims for its antiscorbutic value.

The other chemical compound for which claims had been made was citric acid,[203] but these had not been confirmed in the nineteenth century.[204] There had been an attempt to retest it, in comparison with lime juice, on convict ships. The surgeons could not distinguish between the effects of the two, but because the disease had developed while the men were already receiving lime juice, this did not really say much for either remedy.[205] The only firm conclusion drawn from the tests was that the quality of the lime juice needed to be improved. However, the idea that citric acid could be antiscorbutic had also been undermined on more theoretical grounds. Trotter, as we have seen, originally suggested that it as well as other vegetable acids (tartaric, malic, etc.) acted by *donating* oxygen to the tissues.[206] However, by the 1860s, it was accepted that when organic compounds (including the vegetable acids) that contained only the elements carbon, hydrogen, and oxygen were eaten, they were all largely combusted in the body to carbon dioxide and water. It now appeared, therefore, that, quite contrary to Trotter's suggestion, they *took up* oxygen rather than donating it, and that their only possible contribution was body heat.[207]

Given this concept, organic acids seemed incapable of making any specific contribution to health, but in 1864 Professor Parkes suggested one, reviving the seventeenth-century belief, discussed in Chapter 2, that scurvy

[198] Murray (1838–9), 367; Henderson (1839), 12–13; Burnett (1854), 635; Vaughan (1850), 269; Morgan (1855), 586; Wrench (1867), 317; Markham (1877), 7.    [199] De Lisle (1877), 302; Wright (1886), 142; Faulkner (1887), 198; Hickman (1888), 392.    [200] Cameron (1830), 752; Henderson (1839), 15.    [201] Bryson (1850), 213.    [202] Grant (1863), 213.    [203] Trotter (1804), 391–8.    [204] Budd (1842), 716.    [205] Bryson (1850), 213.    [206] Trotter (1792), 144–5. [207] Liebig (1842), 66–7; Wright (1904), 97.

could arise from an imbalance between acids and alkalies in the body.[208] He pointed out that neutral salts are formed from a base and an acid, but if the acid is organic and is oxidized in the body to carbon dioxide, it is lost, and what remains is only the base. Admittedly this could react with some carbon dioxide to form a carbonate. However, because carbonic acid (the gas in solution) is only weakly acidic, the carbonate salt is still basic rather than neutral. Thus a substance like lemon juice, although analysis shows it to be acid because it contains free citric acid as well as citrate salts, can really have an alkaline (basic) effect in the bloodstream with the rapid loss of the organic acid material.[209] Since some German experiments with animals had shown that acidification of their blood caused tissue damage and hemorrhages, he suggested that scurvy, too, was caused by "acidosis" (acidity of the blood) and that the true value of antiscorbutic foods lay in their "latent" alkalinity. From this it followed that they should be replaceable by salts of organic acids, such as potassium citrate. In 1869, a paper appeared, reporting the successful use of potassium binoxalate in treating scurvy at a military post in India.[210]

Parkes's idea was developed further by Dr. Ralfe in 1877. By then it was appreciated that the metabolism of foods also provided a source of acids. The sulfur and phosphorus present at low levels in proteins were converted (or released) to form sulfuric and phosphoric acids (so-called mineral acids). Also, the salts in meat, beans, and cereal grains were, to a large extent, phosphates, and were unchanged by metabolism.[211] Ralfe simulated the biological effect of oxidizing the organic matter in foods by heating them in a laboratory oven, so that the organic matter burned away, to leave just an ash, the mineral residue. As expected, the ashes of potatoes were more alkaline than those of meat or wheat flour. He also showed that the ash of the whole daily ration of the British soldier at the time was nearly twice as alkaline as that from the corresponding ration of a sailor, and it was judged that only the latter (if not supplemented with lime juice) was scorbutic.[212] He then related this to some indications that the blood of people with scurvy had "diminished alkalinity," i.e., it took more than the usual quantity of acid to make a sample sufficiently acid to turn blue litmus paper red.[213]

Ralfe's final discussion includes an important paragraph:

We will now proceed to the consideration whether the changes which occur in the blood and tissues in scurvy are due to the withdrawal of some special constituent required directly for their nutrition, or are brought about by some chemical alteration in the quality of the blood, which interferes with the processes of nutrition. . . . The chief argument which can be urged against the view that scurvy originates from [the first] cause , . . is that it is not a disease brought on by mere reduction in the amount of food. A starving man subsisting on roots and berries will

---

[208] Parkes (1864), 446.      [209] Leyden & Munk (1861), 238–9.      [210] Tayler & Tayler (1869), 778.      [211] Ralfe (1877), ii, 81.      [212] Ibid., ii, 82.      [213] Ibid., i, 869–70; ii, 83.

not have scurvy, whilst the most liberal allowance of meat will not prevent its occurrence if fresh vegetables are withheld; the amount, however, required of these is small, and out of all proportion to the immense protective influence they afford. [This] . . . supports the view that the disease is primarily brought about by some chemical alteration in the quality of the blood.[212]

This line of reasoning makes little sense to the modern reader, but it seems to have been accepted without question in the British Army Medical School, and Dr. Almroth Wright of their Faculty developed an ingenious micro-method for measuring the alkalinity of small samples of blood.[214] In May and June 1900, he found diminished alkalinity in the blood of a series of six soldiers who were brought home from South Africa after having been in the Siege of Ladysmith, which had ended by early March. The men had all suffered from dysentery, typhoid, or enteric fever, as well as having been classified as scorbutic, and were extremely ill; four of them died within a short period of the tests. It is difficult to believe that scurvy could still have been their primary problem after at least eight weeks of medical attention. Nevertheless, Wright's results convinced him of the correctness of the theory, and he concluded: "It [therefore] . . . seems probable that scurvy is a condition of acid intoxication. . . . the proper prophylaxis and treatment of the condition would consist in the administration of salts of easily oxidisable organic acids . . . to restore the normal alkalinity of the blood by the most direct means."[215]

The hypothesis was tested by a medical officer in India who measured the alkalinity of the blood in eleven cases of scurvy, and found that it did not differ from that of blood taken from healthy control subjects.[216] An outbreak of scurvy in South African native auxiliaries following the Boer War (1899–1902) provided another opportunity to test the hypothesis. Of twenty-two blood samples from scorbutics, only five showed diminished alkalinity as measured by Wright's test, and the army surgeon in charge reported that fresh meat juice seemed as valuable as fruit and vegetables in restoring the men to health.[217] But Wright became more dogmatic. In 1904, he stated

Nothing in pathology is to my mind more certainly established than that the essential essence of scurvy is to be found in a diminished alkalinity of the blood. . . . I have urged the substitution of the essential anti-scorbutic elements for the raw materials ordinarily administered. . . . I have employed, in particular, lactate of soda. . . . Lime juice ought to be eschewed [avoided] as containing citric acid.[218]

To quote MacRae, the surgeon who worked in South Africa: "The pendulum of scientific thought was thus suddenly swung to the other extreme – a not uncommon error in the history of human speculation; but it must be

[214] Wright (1897), 719–21.    [215] Wright (1900), 565.    [216] Lamb (1902), 11–14.    [217] MacRae (1908), 1839–40.    [218] Wright (1904), 95, 97.

admitted that the problem of the etiology of scurvy still remains unsolved." [217] In fact, the ideas about this disease were complicated even further in the early 1900s by quite different conclusions drawn from studies in two other areas, one of which was Arctic exploration, and the other a new infant disease seen by pediatricians. These will be the topics of the next two chapters.

# 6

## Problems in the Arctic and the ptomaine theory (1850–1915)

In the Victorian period in England, the exploration of unknown territory had a great fascination. The Arctic seemed to present a particularly challenging environment, which made unique demands on the human system. The whole subject was somewhat akin to space travel in the 1960s. Anyone joining an expedition to the Far North was a hero, and those returning alive were considered to have been lucky.

Nevertheless, by the second half of the nineteenth century, the British Navy was confident that with lime juice it had the answer to the particular problem of scurvy under any conditions for at least two years. It was therefore regarded as a serious scandal when a naval expedition returned in 1876 from only one year in the Artic, and it was learned that, out of 120 men, 60 had suffered from scurvy and 4 had died of it. The House of Commons called for a full-scale inquiry.[1] This, and subsequent experience in the Arctic, led to the development of a wholly new theory of the cause of scurvy, and one that was to become very influential by 1900.

We shall begin by summarizing some of the earlier, and apparently paradoxical, experiences of men who had wintered in the North. These were well known to the planners of the Victorian expeditions. The earliest voyages from Europe into the Arctic, for which there are records, were made at the end of the sixteenth century. Their purpose was to reach the riches of Asia by going north of either America or Russia. Because the seas were frozen for so much of the year, it was soon realized that ships would have to spend more than one summer season on the voyage, and to lie up in the ice for the intervening winter. Meanwhile, summer expeditions continued to fish and catch whales around Greenland, Spitsbergen, etc.

In 1633, the Greenland Society of Dutch merchants sent out a party of seven volunteers to overwinter in the north of Greenland as an experiment.

[1] Admiralty Committee on Scurvy (1877), xi.

They were provided with "all manner of necessaries, as meat, drink, physical preparations [medicines], herbs, etc." [2] The ships left them at the end of August. On October 10, the weather turned very cold; they stayed in by the fireside and noted a feeling of giddiness. They continued to go out on the better days and tried to shoot some of the bears that were in the vicinity. They finally shot two in early November and brought back the carcasses, and shot a third in December. Their next success came in early March, and their diary recorded: "We feasted upon part of the flesh, and sprinkled the rest with a little salt only, by reason we were exceedingly afflicted with the scurvy." [3] They continued to explore and look out from a nearby hill, but on March 22 they wrote: "For want of refreshments we begin to be very heartless [despondent], being afflicted with scurvy to that degree, that our legs are scarce able to bear us." [4] On April 16 there was the first death, and the remainder "grew worse and worse every day for, being scarce able in health to keep ourselves tolerably warm by exercise, we were but in little hope of doing it while we were sick," and all were dead by early May. When the relief ship reached their huts, it was to find the tragedy and the diary they had left. [5]

That same year, another seven volunteers were taken in a separate expedition to winter in Spitsbergen. They were left on September 11, and already by November 24, "the scurvy began to appear among them; they searched very earnestly after green herbs, bears and foxes, but could find none," [6] nor did they have any success later. Several of them took "potions against the scurvy," but three of them died in mid-January, and the rest were too weak even to try to hunt for fresh meat. All were dead by the end of February. [7] Lind suggested that the "potions" were strong laxatives, which would have "increased the malady and hastened their end." [8]

Another account from the same period stands out in contrast to those two tragedies, and was regarded at the time as an example of divine intervention. In May 1630, an English fleet left on its usual summer expedition for catching whales and seals off the east coast of Greenland. On August 8, at the end of their season, and nearly 78° N, they were preparing to return, and eight men with two dogs were sent ashore in a small boat to obtain fresh venison for the journey. They planned to row the four miles back to the ship next day. However, the wind changed, and pack ice drove down and carried the ship over the horizon. Then, following further mishaps that occurred while attempting another rendezvous, the men realized that they were stranded until the fleet could return the next summer.

Like men already metamorphosed into the ice of the country . . . , stood we with the eyes of pity beholding one another. . . . For we were not only unprovided both of clothes to keep us warm, and of food to prevent the wrath of cruel famine, but

---

[2] Churchill (1704), *II*, 414, 427.　　[3] Ibid., 417–18.　　[4] Ibid., 419–23.　　[5] Ibid., 424–6.
[6] Ibid., 427.　　[7] Ibid., 428.　　[8] Stewart & Guthrie (1953), 164.

utterly destitute also were we of a sufficient house wherein to shroud and shelter us from the chilling cold. . . . [But] it pleased God to give us hearts like men and to arm ourselves with a resolution to do our best. . . ." [9]

Rowing to another bay, they found a large wooden shed that had been set up by a Flemish company as a summer factory for extracting the oil from their catches and putting it into barrels. From this they made a smaller cabin, and used old casks and boards for a modest store of fuel. They killed some deer as well as bears and walruses with their lances and a harpoon, and used deerskins for bedding. From mid-October, they never saw the sun, and did not expect to obtain any more food until spring. They reckoned that they had enough meat for one meal, three days a week. On the other four days, they gnawed at the moldy whale "greaves" left behind around the shed; these were the residues remaining after extraction of oil from the whales' tissues. In the New Year, the cold intensified: "If we touched iron at any time it would stick to our fingers like bird lime." At the beginning of February, with their food almost finished, the sun returned, and they were able to kill a bear: "Upon this bear we fed some twenty days. . . . This only mischance we had with her, that upon eating her liver, our very skins peeled off: for my own part, I being sick before, though I lost my skin, yet recovered I my health upon it." Later they killed more bears and snared wild fowl. On May 25, the returning fleet found them, and "after fourteen days of refreshment, we grew perfectly well, all of us." [10]

We now know that a party of seventeen Dutch sailors, after eating bear's liver, had an experience similar to that of the English group. In the autumn of 1596, their ship was broken up in ice on the coast of Novaya Zemlya, lying north of Russia. On the following May 30, they were pleased to have shot a bear attacking their hut, but "the death cost them dear for . . . having dressed the liver and eaten it with pleasure they were all indisposed, three of them . . . thought they would die; nevertheless they recovered, having a new skin from the head to the foot.[11] They were weakened by scurvy, and two died, but the remainder got home eventually.[12]

Most extraordinary of all the survival stories is that of four Russian sailors stranded on the more remote eastern coast of Spitsbergen in 1743 for the next six years, with an abandoned hut but hardly anything else save an axe, a knife, a small kettle, and some tinder. Their treasured finds were a long iron nail and a board with a long hook in it.[13] They were able to kill reindeer, using contrived bows and arrows, but were unable to cook the meat. One of them had previously wintered in West Spitsbergen, and

he instructed them [for the prevention of scurvy] to eat raw and frozen meat cut into small pieces, and drink the warm blood of the reindeer, and lastly, to eat as much as possible *cochlearia* (scurvy grass), the only grass that grew on the island, and that

---

[9] Pellham (1744), 746–9.    [10] Ibid., 750–2.    [11] Pinkerton (1808), I, 111.    [12] Beke (1853), cii–ciii.    [13] Pinkerton (1808), I, 595.

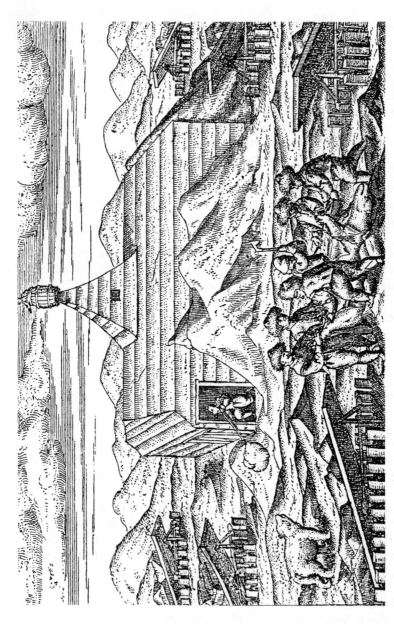

Woodcut of early Dutch explorers trapping and killing polar bears to obtain fresh meat and so ward off scurvy during a winter in the Arctic. (Doe Library, University of California.)

but sparingly. . . . Three of the sailors who made use of this regime kept entirely free of this complaint . . . [whereas] the fourth had an unconquerable aversion to the blood . . . and the malady made such progress that he was subject to cruel suffering . . . [eventually] without the power of moving his hand to his mouth.

He died, but the other three were eventually rescued.[14]

Arctic travelers usually refer to "latitude" as a measure of how far North they have been. This distance from the Equator to the North Pole is, of course, divided into ninety degrees, and one degree corresponds to sixty-nine miles (111 kilometers). Each degree is also divided into sixty minutes. The Arctic Circle, marking the area in which the sun does not rise above the horizon at midwinter, is at 66°17′ N and passes just north of Iceland. Spitsbergen lies between 76 and 81° N. Most of the sea north of 80° N is permanently frozen over with pack ice, and, to the north of Canada, navigation can be blocked by ice the whole year down to 70° N, and in winter much farther south. Latitude is not, of course, the only measure of the severity of winter weather. Thus, Cartier in his first winter in the ice and snow of Canada was actually some two degrees south of Paris! Even some of the trading posts on the Hudson's Bay are no further north than London at 51°30′. However, Canada does not have the moderating influence of the Gulf Stream. Also, to enter the Bay, ships had to go as far as 63° N through seas blocked by ice for much of the year.

Incidentally, the Hudson's Bay Company, although there were some cases of scurvy among their employees, never found it to be such a serious problem that it hampered their development.[15] From their beginning in the seventeenth century, they had shipped out small quantities of lime juice.[16] But even in the absence of fresh vegetables, they relied on their hunters' being able to catch fresh game throughout the year, and this would usually keep their men in good health. Thus, ". . . being informed that scurvy had made its appearance among the people [at Ungara], two active deer hunters were engaged to go thither this autumn." [17]

Coming back to nineteenth-century exploration, the British Government, in the era of peace following the Napoleonic wars, was urged to send official expeditions to explore the area of a "Northwest Passage," i.e., a possible sea route to the north of the America continent. It was argued that if they did not, the United States and Russia might claim the territories and outflank Canada; also that there were scientific discoveries to be made there, some possibly with commercial applications; and, lastly, that this was a way of testing naval equipment and supplies and of training officers and men in a rigorous school.[18]

The typical British experience in the subsequent voyages was that men could usually be expected in remain healthy for up to two years in the ice,

[14] Ibid., 601.     [15] Rich (1958), 109, 568–70; Smith (1919), 111–13.     [16] Rich (1946), 294, 309.     [17] Davis & Johnson (1963), 164–5, 176n, 304.     [18] Kirwan (1959), 77–9, 159.

but not much longer. For example, William Parry, the Commander of an expedition that had left in April 1821, wrote in his journal for July 1823:

. . . some slight, but unequivocal, symptoms of scurvy were this day reported to me by Mr. Edwards [the surgeon], to have appeared among four or five of the men, rendering it necessary, for the first time, to have recourse to anti-scorbutic treatment among the seamen or marines. . . . That a ship's company should begin to evince symptoms of scurvy after twenty-seven months' entire dependence upon the resources contained within their ship, (an experiment hitherto unknown, perhaps, in the annals of navigation . . .) could scarcely be a subject of wonder. From the health enjoyed by our people during two successive winters, unassisted as we had been by any supply of fresh anti-scorbutic plants or other vegetables, I had begun to hope that with a continued attention to their comforts, cleanliness, and exercise, the same degree of vigour might . . . [continue] at least as long as our present liberal resources should last. Present appearances however seemed to indicate differently.[19]

Parry was referring specifically to his "men." Contrary to the usual experience, he and some of his fellow officers had already been afflicted in the second winter and been treated with "a short course of additional lemon-juice necessary to restore them." [19] In September, a mate on one of his ships died, but Parry recorded that "it is proper for me, . . . in justice to the Medical Officers . . . , to state that he had taken so great a dislike to the various anti-scorbutics . . . , that he could seldom be induced to use any of them." [20] Because of the "impression of a strong predisposition to disease" as well as actual cases of scurvy, it was then decided to return rather than to stay in the Arctic for a third winter.[21]

The expedition that set out in 1836 was less successful. It sailed, with sixty men on board, on June 14, and by the end of December of that same year, scurvy had appeared: "Despite our efforts to keep the men active, they were seized with numbness and affection of the gums." By the end of April, three men had died, and the captain was perplexed because he had been issuing a variety of "anti-scorbutics" (cranberries, pickles, mustard, vinegar, spruce beer, and lime juice three times per week) and giving the men every day some amusement or exercise. He suspected that "a marine had brought the malady with him." [22] They were forced to return home that summer.

The provisioning of the ships in this period was similar to that in the eighteenth century except that it included "preserved" (i.e., canned) meat and vegetables.[23]

In 1845, another expedition led by Sir John Franklin set off to find the northwest passage from the Atlantic and were never seen again. Two years later, after nothing had been heard of them, and for the next five years, a whole series of rescue expeditions were set in train, many of them plagued by scurvy.[24] We shall follow the record of just one ship, the *Investigator*,

[19] Parry (1824), 462–3.     [20] Ibid., 479–80.     [21] Ibid., 472–3.     [22] Back (1838), 17, 172–3, 194–5, 208–9.     [23] Savours & Decan (1981), 131–41.     [24] Bellot (1855), 2, 259–65; Kane (1870), 484–6; Smith (1919), 191–203; Kirwan (1959), 161–74; Lloyd & Coulter (1963), *IV*, 110–13.

which took part in the second round of these expeditions. The surgeon of this ship, Alexander Armstrong, later wrote detailed accounts of the voyage and of their daily rations. He was issued two types of lemon juice and was asked to report on the quality of each. They were both prepared from fresh lemons processed at a dockyard in England; one batch had then been preserved with 10% brandy, and the other boiled and then bottled with a layer of oil to cover it.[25] The reason for the special concern was that one of the first relief expeditions, sent out in 1848, had returned the next year, following a severe outbreak of scurvy, and examination of their remaining stock of lemon juice revealed that it had only one-tenth of the expected acidity.[26]

In short, the *Investigator* sailed in January of 1850. They made their way around Cape Horn and, after a four-day stop at Honolulu to gather a relatively small amount of fresh food, went up the American coast, through the Bering Strait and along the north coast of Alaska, then forced a way east until, after three winters held in ice between 73° and 74° N, they were rescued by an expedition coming from the Atlantic.[27] In October 1851, when it became clear that they would be held in the ice for a second winter, "two-thirds rations" were introduced. By next spring, the men were looking haggard and complaining of weakness, but it was not until July 1852 that Armstrong could find evidence of the development of a general scorbutic taint.[28] Soon after this, two musk oxen were shot, yielding some fresh meat, and Armstrong found and organized the collection of sorrel and scurvy grass which seemed to improve the condition of the sick, but the Captain refused his request that rations be increased.[29] When it was realized that they would have to remain for a third winter, rations were further reduced, and there was real hunger. By April 1853, dysentery had further weakened those already scorbutic, and there were three deaths. Armstrong recorded that lime juice was then in such short supply that he could give it solely to allay urgent symptoms of the worst sufferers. He believed that they were saved only by the arrival of another rescue expedition.[30]

Despite all the problems of the last winter, Armstrong concluded that it was an excellent record for them to have kept in good health for the first two years, in which he was able to issue one ounce of lemon juice daily. He reported, therefore, that each batch was of excellent quality and added that his having an officer supervise its daily consumption, as a part of the experiment, also ensured that each man took his dose: In other expeditions some exchanging between sailors might have been responsible for scurvy cases developing earlier.[26,31]

For the next fifteen years, the British Admiralty was too concerned with other problems, including the Crimean War and the U. S. Civil War, to think of the Arctic. In the 1870s they were again urged, and they finally agreed, to

[25] Armstrong (1858), 17.   [26] Burnett (1855), 635–6; Smith (1919), 101.   [27] Neatby (1970), 159–94.   [28] Armstrong (1857), 524, 531.   [29] Ibid., 532, 538–40.   [30] Ibid., 554–6, 555–66.   [31] Armstrong (1858), 17–19.

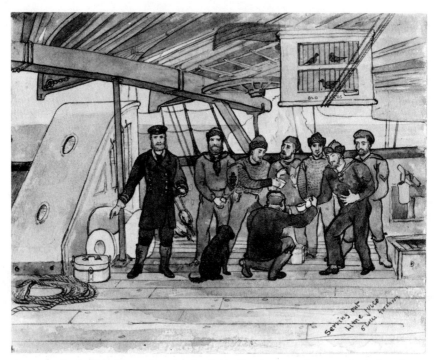

A watercolor by E. L. Moss showing the daily distribution of lime juice on the *Alert* in the 1875 expedition to the Arctic. Despite this distribution, scurvy forced their early return. (Scott Polar Institute, Cambridge.)

send an expedition to go even farther north and study conditions there. This was the expedition, led by Captain Nares, that was to be the subject of the parliamentary inquiry referred to at the beginning of this chapter. The two ships, *Alert* and *Discovery*, sailed at the end of May 1875 with altogether 122 people. The *Alert* had gone the farthest north up the west coast of Green-land, but finally, in early September, had to winter in the ice at 82° N. By then they had been able to kill some musk oxen on the neighboring coast. For six weeks they were able to carry out short sledging trips, laying food depots in preparation for the longer expeditions planned for the spring. Then the sun remained below the horizon from October 11 for the next twenty weeks.[32] Health remained good through the winter. Care was taken to ensure that the men got out onto the ice regularly and exercised, and there were weekly entertainments. The immediate problem seemed to be exces-sive condensation within the ship, leaving everything permanently damp.[33]

On April 3, 1876, Commander Albert Markham, the second in command of the *Alert*, began his sledging trip that was charged with getting as far as possible into the unknown area farther north. He had with him one other

[32] Markham (1880a), 9, 113, 122, 136–47.     [33] Ibid., 176, 182, 187.

officer (Lieutenant Parr) and fifteen men to drag their two sledges. They had planned on the basis that 210 pounds per head would be the maximum that they could drag over the very rough ice. As they set off, the temperature was −33° Fahrenheit, i.e., 65° below the freezing point of water. The dragging proved to be extremely tiring, and, as they progressed over the frozen sea, the ice grew rougher with occasional barriers over six feet high, through which they had to clear a path with pickaxes. On April 14, one of the men complained of pains in his ankles and knees. Three days later, a second man had the same complaint, and from then on, they had to be carried on the sledges. On April 19, still not much more than two weeks away from the ship, a third man could only stumble along.[34] After another two weeks of slow progress, and now with five men sick, Markham records:

Although we had been told that there was not the slightest chance of our being attacked with scurvy . . . the terrible idea forced itself on us that this fearful disease was slowly but surely laying its hands on us. . . . Parr and I spoke of this only when we were by ourselves . . . believing it of the utmost importance that the men should remain in ignorance as long as possible. . . . Our only hope was that the five men now afflicted might have been more prone to the disease than the remainder of our party.[35]

Although Markham realized the danger they were in, it seems not to have occurred to him to turn back.[36] It was only after another week, on May 10, and with only thirty days' provisions left to retrace a journey that had taken forty days, that he called a halt and made some magnetic observations and measured the depth of the sea beneath them. Then the ten of them who were still fairly fit walked on from the camp, carrying their flags, to ensure that they would be further north than had ever been reached by civilized man.

The walking was undoubtedly severe, at one moment struggling through deep snow-drifts, in which we floundered up to our waists, and at another tumbling about amongst the hummocks. . . . after more than two hours we had barely accomplished one mile! . . . Fortunatly the sun was favourable to us, and we were able to obtain a good altitude as it passed the meridian, although almost immediately afterwards snow began to fall, and the sun was lost in obscurity. We found the latitude to be 83° 20′ N., or three hundred and ninety-nine miles and a half [*sic*] from the North Pole.
The announcement of our position was received with three cheers, with one more for Captain Nares; then all sang the 'Union Jack of Old England,' . . . winding up, like loyal subjects, with 'God save the Queen.' . . . nought else but snow and ice could be seen in any direction. In spite, however, of these dreary surroundings,

---

[34] Ibid., 257, 275, 284, 286, 290.    [35] Ibid., 299–300.    [36] Markham was in the news in 1893, again for carrying out an order regardless of the consequence. When in command of a battleship in the Mediterranean, his admiral gave a clear but tragic order for Markham's ship to turn into what was obviously a collision course with the flagship. The flagship was rammed and sank with the loss of the admiral and 358 others.

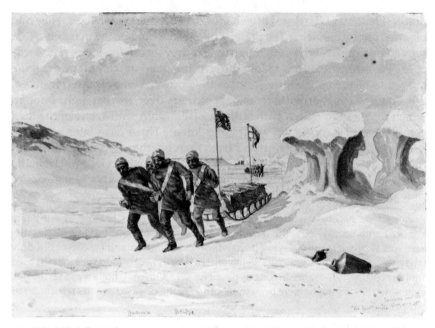

A watercolor by E. L. Moss, of the 1875 expedition, showing the return of the northern sledging party, which had suffered severely from scurvy. The artist shows in the foreground one of the ship's 60-pound containers of lime juice, which had been brought to them by the rescue party. (Scott Polar Institute, Cambridge.)

suggesting everything that was desolate and miserable, mirth, happiness, and joy seemed to reign paramount. . . . Even the sick, on our return to camp, prostrate and suffering as they were, participated in the general hilarity and rejoicing.[37]

What an extraordinary mixture of the truly heroic and the ludicrous; the kind of English occasion that Gilbert and Sullivan were beginning to parody in their operettas. "Trial by Jury" was first performed in 1875, and "H.M.S. *Pinafore*" in 1878. Yet we know that many pioneering achievements have had to depend on what seem like irrational obsessions to those who do not share such feelings.

As the party began to drag its way back, "the disease gradually gained mastery, so did the appetites decrease. . . . hunger was never felt but we all were assailed by an intolerable thirst. . . . The men begin to have an inkling of the nature of their disease. . . . having heard that tea leaves were a good vegetable, the contents of the tea kettle were eaten with avidity." By June 1, they were trudging through a sludge of melting snow, and only six were still able to help with the dragging. On June 7, with only four "effectives" left, Lieutenant Parr set off by himself to fetch help from the ship, and three days later, after one man had died, Captain Nares reached them with a relief party.[38]

[37] Markham (1880a), 307–11.     [38] Ibid., 314–16, 320–6.

Back on the *Alert*, Markham learned that the other sledge parties had also experienced scurvy, and that there had even been one definite case among those who remained on the ship. Later when they recontacted the *Discovery*, it was a similar story. Altogether there were sixty cases and four deaths. They had no alternative but to return home.[39] Markham ends by saying that, on their return, "the Lords of the Admiralty were pleased to express their satisfaction at the manner in which the expedition had been conducted by our leader."[40] This is rather a disturbing remark to find in a volume published three years after the report of an official inquiry that held Captain Nares to blame for the disease that cut the expedition short. As stated at the beginning of the chapter, the news that scurvy had broken out in the first year of an expedition by the Royal Navy was considered so serious that a full inquiry was called for by Parliament. The Committee consisted of three admirals and two senior surgeons. It issued its report in March 1877, together with the minutes of over 10,000 questions and answers from people called to given evidence.

One factor that they considered was that by wintering further north than any other ship, they had been longer in darkness. Witnesses agreed that this probably had a general debilitating effect, but they knew of no reason why it should have led to a "scorbutic tendency" in particular.[41] They also considered the possible effects of damp and "vitiated" air during the confinement of sailors to the lower decks through the winter. An analysis carried out in the *Alert* at the time showed a carbonic acid content of 0.33%, or five times the concentration in pure air outside, and this was considered to be confirmation of there having been inadequate ventilation and space per man. The extreme change in temperature (sometimes as much as 90°F) experienced by the men coming in and going out of the ship, acted as an additional stress. The very heavy physical labour of dragging sledges after a winter spent with much less physical activity was also judged to be an aggravating cause of the outbreak.[42]

Most time was spent considering the adequacy of the diet. There was general agreement that the men on board ship were very well fed through the winter, and that this was reflected by their gaining weight and remaining generally healthy.[43] The daily rations had included four ounces of preserved vegetables, one ounce of pickles, and one pound of meat. The meat ration was usually, on alternate days, "salted" or "preserved fresh meat" (i.e., canned), though on fourteen occasions during the winter, freshly killed meat was served.[44] Everyone also received one ounce of lime juice per day, and samples brought back were fully up to the chemical standards in use, i.e., for acidity and mineral content.[45] At this period, the terms "lemon juice" and "lime juice" were still being used almost interchangeably, as in

[39] Ibid., 321, 331–3, 337, 346.    [40] Ibid., 368.    [41] Admiralty Committee on Scurvy (1877), ii, ix.    [42] Ibid., iii, x.    [43] Ibid., xiv.    [44] Smith (1919), 110–11; Kendall (1955), 471. [45] Admiralty Committee on Scurvy (1877), 299.

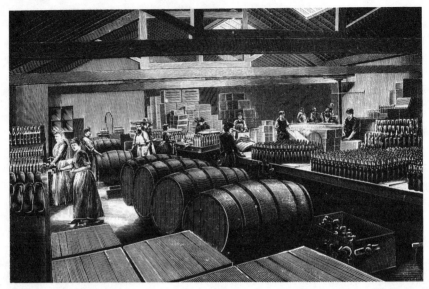

A Victorian print of the operation of an English factory bottling lime juice. There was a loss of faith in lime juice in naval circles after 1875. It is now thought that the vitamin C originally present was lost largely as a result of the long periods in settling tanks and pumping the juice through copper pipes. (Royal Album of Arts and Industries of Great Britain, 1887; Cambridge University Library.)

the reports of the analyst who headed his report "lemon juice," and then referred to the sample of "lime juice." However, another witness testified specifically that the Navy had been receiving its supplies from *limes* grown on the West Indian island of Montserrat, and two doctors gave it as their opinion that lime juice was probably the more antiscorbutic, though activity also varied with the ripeness of the fruit.[46]

The men who went on the sledging expeditions changed to a more concentrated diet based on pemmican. This was still judged to be adequate in quantity. However, its only "anti-scorbutic" was two ounces of preserved potatoes, and this was considered insufficient.[47] These were potatoes dried with heat, granulated and tinned; they were lightly boiled before being eaten.[48] The major point of controversy was that there had been no issue of lime juice for the sledging expeditions. The reason was that it would have been frozen solid on the sledges and could not have been thawed out on the overnight stops. Markham, giving evidence, described how he and Parr had, on their own initiative, each taken two beer bottles of lime juice with the thought of making refreshing drinks with it on the return journey when the thaw would have begun. When, in fact, scurvy did break out so unex-

[46] Ibid., 63, 201, 203.　　[47] Ibid., xix.　　[48] Ibid., 62.

pectedly on the outward journey, he tried to thaw out one bottle over their evening fire, and the glass broke. After that he tried to thaw his second bottle "in my sleeping bag by placing it between my legs. . . . I could only thaw in two or three hours a very small amount. . . . principally the spirit with which the juice was mixed. . . . Even this would have been impossible in the first three or four weeks. . . . the temperature inside my sleeping bag was one night below zero."[49]

The Army surgeons called to give evidence suggested that, for the future, lime juice should be evaporated to a solid and mixed with sugar to form lozenges that could be issued to sledgers.[50] Naval surgeons were skeptical of this, insisting that it would be unjustifiable to use an untried remedy, and that chemical analysis was an inadequate measure of antiscorbutic properties.[51]

The final conclusion of the Committee was that the outbreak of scurvy in the sledging expeditions was due to their not being provided with lime juice, and that Captain Nares was reponsible for this omisson.[52] There were immediate protests at the injustice of this decision. Two admirals with experience in the Arctic wrote to the *Times* that they had never supplied lime juice to their sledging expeditions.[53] The Secretary of the Royal Geographical Society published *A Refutation of the Report of the Scurvy Committee*, urging, on the one hand, that it had never been naval practice to try to use lime juice on Arctic sledging expeditions, and on the other, that there had been several recent instances of scurvy breaking out in naval ships in which lime juice was being taken.[54] Certainly it was clear that lime juice had failed to produce a rapid response in several cases on the Nares expedition.[55]

Another critic of the Admiralty Committee, a physician at one of the London teaching hospitals, pointed out that the Eskimos survived in Arctic latitudes "by an instinct which is successful; our imperfect knowledge leads us astray." He argued that the extreme cold required consumption of a particularly large quantity of "fuel" food whose combustion would maintain body temperature, and that the Eskimo obtained this by eating large quantities of fat as blubber.

A cup of lime juice will not satisfy this demand. . . . the doctrine of anti-scorbutics is untenable . . . the last remnant of an obsolete physiology. . . . All food is anti-scorbutic, though in most unequal degrees. Fat and oil stand at the head of the class. . . . Sugar has a high place in the scale. . . . Potato ranks high on account of its starchy elements. . . . Lime juice . . . stands very low indeed. . . . The chemistry of Liebig and of Liebig's time made physiology a new science. . . . it forged a weapon that gave the death blow to the doctrine of anti-scorbutics, just as the theory of Phlogiston fell before . . . the discoveries of Priestley.[56]

---

[49] Ibid., 27.   [50] Ibid., 170.   [51] Ibid., 246, 299.   [52] Ibid., *i*, 1137.   [53] Smith (1919), 108.   [54] Markham (1877), 6–7.   [55] Ibid., 330; Savours & Deacon (1981), 153.   [56] Black (1876), 13–16.

Indeed, right from the 1850s, there had been a succession of smaller, private expeditions that had tried to learn from the Eskimos and adopt their techniques of traveling light and living off the land. It had been observed earlier that Eskimos ate little or no vegetable food but remained, in general, free from scurvy. It seemed, therefore, that they were protected by eating large quantities of raw or very lightly cooked fish and meat.[57] *Meat* is, of course, very different from just *blubber*. Several explorers had already urged the antiscorbutic value of fresh game, and this had been generally accepted by witnesses at the 1877 inquiry.[58] However, Eskimos were not immune from the disease because they had been seen to suffer from it when living in the Danish settlements in Greenland.[59]

Some of the expeditions that attempted to live off the land ran into terrible trouble through scarcity of game, and suffered from a combination of scurvy and simple starvation.[60] However, in August 1881, one expedition of twenty-five men was shipwrecked and wintered successfully on Franz-Josef Land (81° N). They were unable to rescue any lime juice from the ship, but killed a great quantity of game. The surgeon recorded: "Whenever an animal was shot we collected as much blood as possible . . . : this became a solid mass in a few minutes. I tried to allow one pound of frozen blood in the soup every day."[61] For the first six months they had one to two ounces of vegetables per head per day and for the second six months none, yet all remained healthy and made an open boat journey before being rescued.[62]

This account was, of course, similar to some of the stories of early explorers, but, because the party included a physician whose report appeared in the contemporary medical literature, it made a greater impact. Another physician wrote from Argentina to point out that it was not just in cold climates that meat seemed to have antiscorbutic properties. He had practiced in a remote area where everyone lived almost exclusively on meat. A man would commonly eat four or five pounds at a meal. Fruit, vegetables, and even bread were all scarce and too expensive for the poorer classes. Yet, even though the meat was from animals killed only twice per week and not refrigerated, he had never encountered scurvy.[63] A surgeon, describing the diet eaten at the Hudson's Bay Company's posts, also affirmed that about eight pounds of meat per day was found to be protective.[64] A hypothesis that was tentatively proposed to explain the antiscorbutic property of fresh meat was that it contained a small but important quantity of lactic acid, which was comparable in activity to the citric, malic, and tartaric acids found in vegetables in natural combinations.[65] It was argued later that glycogen (the animal equivalent of starch) was the protective factor because both whale skin and raw seal's liver, the most potent of the animal antiscor-

---

[57] Kane (1870), 482–7, 554–7.     [58] Admiralty Committee on Scurvy (1877), 278–89, 478–80.     [59] Ibid., 71.     [60] Kane (1870), 512–17; Greely (1886), *II*, 221–4, 322–7.     [61] Neale (1883), *i*, 363–4; Neale (1896), 586.     [62] Ibid., 587; Smith (1883), 207.     [63] Greene (1883), 714.     [64] Rae (1883), 365.     [65] Colan (1883), 364.

butics, were richer in glycogen than ordinary muscle meat.[66] Another assertion was that salted meat was inferior to fresh meat in its protective value because the processing had leached out most of the phosphate,[67] or, according to others, that it had either removed the protein or made it indigestible, and so produced scurvy, which was due to protein deficiency.[68]

In 1893, a Norwegian expedition led by Fridtjof Nansen set out to test the theory that a ship caught in the pack ice north of Russia would move slowly westward and eventually come out into the Atlantic. The ship was provisioned for three years on the principle of avoiding any kind of deteriorated or infected food: ". . . such articles, even, as bread, dried vegetables etc., etc. were soldered down in tins as a protection against the damp." [69] Apparently they did not use lime juice, at any rate regularly, and, while on their ship, could not obtain much fresh meat. After nearly two years on board, Nansen and one colleague left the ship and sledged as far north as 86°13', then dragged their way back to spend the next winter in an improvised shelter on Franz-Josef Land, subsisting almost entirely on fresh meat. They were picked up in the spring by another party, and their ship also got safely home in 1896. None of them had experienced scurvy.[70]

Another expedition to Franz-Joseph Land provided an even more dramatic result. A small land party under Frederick Jackson, a British army officer and an experienced hunter and explorer, remained there in good health for three winters (1894–7). They lived largely on fresh bear's meat, together with only dessicated vegetables and very little lime juice (or none at all in the case of Jackson himself). In contrast, the crew of their transport ship, which was unexpectedly caught in the ice for the first winter, took their daily ounce of lime juice and lived largely on ship's stores that included tinned meat, but ate little or no fresh meat, and they did go down with scurvy.[71] Jackson compared this experience with what he had seen earlier amongst the Samoyod peoples of northeastern Russia. Those who wintered in the north ate fresh reindeer meat, but no vegetables, and remained healthy; those who went south ate cured fish that had developed a gamey, or "high" flavor, and many did have scurvy. He concluded: "the use of lime juice neither prevents nor cures scurvy. . . . [it] is a disease developed through eating tainted food . . . a slow poisoning. . . . as had already been suggested by Professor Torup in Christiana [Oslo].[72]

On his return home, he obtained the help of Vaughan Harley, Professor of Physiological Chemistry in London University, who agreed to help with an experiment to test the hypothesis, which he expressed in these terms:

If meat is not properly preserved, micro-organisms contaminate it, and as a consequence it goes *bad* – the bacteria chemically change the albumen, fat, carbohydrates in the meat, and the new chemical products formed (ptomaines) cause the change in

---

[66] Bertelsen (1911), 542–3.     [67] Morgan (1864), 349.     [68] Oliver (1863), 61; Tayler & Tayler (1869), 778.     [69] Nansen (1897), I, 73.     [70] Ibid., II, 403, 1023–4; Mirsky (1948), 202–12.     [71] Jackson (1899), II, 379–81, Koettlitz (1902), 343.     [72] Jackson (1899), II, 378–9.

colour, smell, etc. . . . . Before the meat has actually gone so bad as to be repugnant to the sense of smell and sight, bacteria may have done their work, and yielded their ptomaines. . . . It is such *tainted* meat, and not bad meat, that one must look to as the cause of scurvy. The greater prevalence of scurvy in the winter – which used to be argued in favour of the fresh vegetable theory of the disease – is in support of this theory; for in summer, if meat is kept, the bacteria would proliferate with such rapidity that the meat would soon smell bad and be rejected. In winter it would not taint so rapidly, and might be cooked and eaten without thought of danger. It must be remembered that, although cooking will destroy bacteria, the ordinary heat so used would have no action on their chemical products, or ptomaines. Again, if the meat were putrid, eating it would cause acute ptomaine-poisoning, with headache, violent diarrhoea, sickness, . . . if only slightly tainted meat were taken, the dose would cause no immediate symptoms, and the disease would gradually develop itself as we know scurvy does.[73]

They obtained a grant of research funds through Lord Lister, who was then President of the Royal Society. Lister had achieved fame, of course, for having greatly reduced the risks of surgery by using a germicidal, carbolic acid vapor spray, to minimize the infection of open tissues during the operation.[74] One can therefore understand the appeal for him of an inquiry based on an hypothesis related to bacterial contamination. To use Harley's own words: "No scientific investigation of the subject of scurvy has been prosecuted since the discoveries of Pasteur have shown us the havoc produced by bacteria as a cause of disease."[75]

Harley and Jackson did their experiment with monkeys, as the species closest to humans. As this was only the second controlled experiment, of which we have details, in the whole history of scurvy up to this time, it deserves some detailed attention. The monkeys used had to be newly imported ones that had not become acclimatized.[76] They were given a diet of soft, boiled rice and dry maize. Each day fifty grams (just under two ounces) of tinned meat was stirred into the individual portions of newly cooked rice, which were gently reheated, and finally the maize was added. The first group of animals received this diet made up with meat from a freshly opened tin; the second and third groups received their meat from tins of the same brand that "had been opened for a few days and had stood in the laboratory. . . . [It] was not what one would call bad but had a distinctly sour smell." The animals in the third group received each day, in addition, either an apple or a banana. They were all kept in individual cages.[77]

The results of the experiment are summarized from the author's charts in Table 6.1. Severe and fatal diarrhea developed in all the animals, save one in Group II, and all lost weight during the period of the trial. However, in Groups II and III the majority were reported to have shown blood and mucus in their feces, and half of them showed spongy gums; these signs

[73] Ibid., 382–5.    [74] Dolman (1973), 402–4.    [75] Jackson (1899), *II*, 387–8.    [76] Ibid., 386.    [77] Jackson & Harley (1900), 254.

Table 6.1. *Median results obtained with monkeys fed*
*on different diets in 1900*

| Diet variables | I. Freshly opened meat | II. Soured meat | III. Soured meat + fruit |
|---|---|---|---|
| Number of animals on each diet | 6 | 8 | 5 |
| Survival period on test diet, days | 57 | 54 | 31 |
| Weight at beginning of trial, kilograms | 2.23 | 1.80 | 2.00 |
| Weight loss on test diet, kilograms | 0.55 | 0.45 | 0.35 |
| Period on diet before diarrhea commenced, days | 10 | 6 | 16 |
| Period before blood seen in stools, days | (Not seen) | 27 | 18 |
| Proportion with spongy, bleeding gums | 0/6 | 5/8 | 2/5 |

were not seen in the animals in Group I.[78] Because space does not permit giving results for each animal, the table gives just the median weight and median observation period for each group. [The "median" is the midway value when the individual values are ranked from highest to lowest, and is preferable to an ordinary average (or "mean") where there are a few widely outlying values.] All the monkeys lost weight, and most developed severe diarrhea and died.

The authors reported that they saw no hemorrhages or evidence of pain and stiffness in the limbs. They concluded that the spongy gums were proof of the early specific signs of scurvy, even if blood in the feces was not characteristic of the human disease.[78] Monkeys are notoriously difficult animals to work with, and one can sympathize with the authors' problems in keeping the animals on any of their treatments in good health. However, the fact remains that they had no satisfactory "positive controls" on fresh meat. Also, the diagnosis of spongy gums was not something entirely "objective" (like body weight) and was made by investigators who knew which treatment each animal was receiving; thus, the evaluation was not done "blind." It is strange that the animals receiving tainted meat (Group II) lost rather less median weight than those receiving fresh meat. The fruits chosen, apples and bananas, were also not ones that were claimed by believers in the "fresh fruit and vegetables" theory to have strong antiscorbutic activity.

The paper containing these results was presented in 1900 in a way that would have lent it maximal prestige: It was communicated to the Royal Society by its President. I believe that this was the first communication on the subject of scurvy since Sir John Pringle's award of the Copley Medal to Cook. The results were regarded as supportive by those who already be-

[78] Ibid., 255–8.

lieved in the theory but were not sufficiently convincing to convert people with different opinions. The first published comment on the experiment, which came from a naval surgeon, drew attention to the fact that the tainted meat had only been "gently heated" before being given to the monkeys. Bacteria in the meat had not, therefore, been sterilized. The results, therefore, supported the writer's own theory which was that scurvy resulted from an infection of the mouth and gastrointestinal tract with organisms from decayed food. The likely action of lime juice was that it had an antiseptic action in the mouth from a combination of its acid and aromatic principles, and that fresh vegetables had similar but less concentrated activity.[79] Refreshingly, the author concluded his argument by drawing attention to one fact that he had not yet been able to explain: the antiscorbutic activity of both raw and cooked potatoes.

Another critic, later in the same year, made the point that "tainted meat" could not be the universal explanation for scurvy. In India it occurred among native soldiers who ate no meat and tried to save money by living on rations of flour, rice and dhal (cooked lentils and other dried legumes) and by not buying milk and fresh vegetables. When treated in hospital, "by the simple addition of fresh limes or potates to their original diet they will, in a fairly short time be quite fit for duty."[80] A physician writing from Rhodesia (Zimbabwe) said that scurvy was common there among the local population, but only at the end of a long, dry period when fresh vegetables (and milk and fresh meat, also) had been unobtainable. When animals had been killed for food, the locals would continue to eat the meat without apparent harm, even when tainted and, to a European palate, putrid.[81]

Two years later, the British Medical Association had a discussion on scurvy at its annual meeting. The opening paper was read by Inspector-General Turnbull, a retired naval surgeon. He said: "From extensive . . . researches in the literature . . . I am forced to the conclusion that . . . the presence of some toxic material in the food is the cause of scurvy . . . also that lemon or lime juice has been erroneously accepted as a certain preventative. . . . Fresh or pure provisions are the true antiscorbutic."[82] Other speakers disagreed, but the new line of thought clearly had influential support. It is not entirely surprising, therefore, that the next official British expedition, this time to the Antarctic, was provisioned in terms of the ptomaine theory. Reginald Koettlitz, the senior surgeon, had been with Jackson on Franz-Joseph Land. He wrote, as the expedition was about to sail:

The benefit of the so-called anti-scorbutic is a delusion. . . . That the cause of the outbreak of scurvy in so many polar expeditions has always been that something was radically wrong with the preserved meats, whether tinned or salted is practi-

---

[79] Home (1900), 321–2.     [80] Maitland (1900), 1164.     [81] Redpath (1901), 1444.     [82] Turnbull (1902), 1023.

cally certain. An animal food is scorbutic if bacteria have been able to produce ptomaines in it, . . . otherwise it is not.[83]

The expedition of altogether thirty-eight people, under Commander Robert Scott, sailed from New Zealand on the last leg of the outward voyage on December 21, 1901. This was, of course, mid-summer because of the reversal of seasons in the South. They brought their ship into McMurdo Sound (78° S) on the Antarctic land mass by February 8 and remained there for the winter.[84] They were able to practice sledging on short expeditions before the full darkness set in, and began longer trips with mainly man-hauled sledges in the spring. Their experience was then uncannily similar to that of the 1875 Nares expedition. After only a week out from the ship in September 1902, two men developed definite signs of scurvy; they took another week to return, and medical examination of the rest of the expedition then revealed widespread signs of the disease in an early stage.[85] Wilson, the junior surgeon, wrote in his unpublished diary: "We know what to expect from sledging work this summer – history is evidently going to repeat itself." [86]

During the winter they had all lived largely on tinned meat, inspected by Dr. Koettlitz on being opened, as "free from taint." Now, with Scott away sledging, his second in command ordered that seals, available in abundance in the area, should be killed and the fresh meat eaten in large quantities. Scott had previously forbidden killing on such a scale as being cruel.[87] Koettlitz also began to grow mustard and cress for the scorbutics, and lime juice was placed on the mess-tables at dinner.[88] Everyone appeared to regain his health.[85] Scott, writing after his return says: "We are still unconscious of any element in our surroundings which might have fostered the disease, or of the neglect of any precautions which modern medical science suggests for its prevention." [89]

After further short expeditions for the laying of food depots, Scott set off again with Shackleton and Wilson, on November 2, on the summer's main expedition to get as far south as possible. By December 24, Wilson saw that the gums of the other two were looking scorbutic. They finally turned back on December 31 at 82°17′ S and were then very short of food. By mid-January of 1903, all three were definitely scorbutic, and Shackleton, who had been the strongest and hardest working of them all, was breathless and coughing up blood. He still forced himself to struggle on, and they finally reached the ship on February 2.[88]

In his article for the *British Medical Journal*, written after their return home, Wilson attributed their subsequent recovery primarily to eating fresh seal meat "for breakfast as well as dinner six days in every week. . . . We at

[83] Koettlitz (1902), 343.    [84] Quartermain (1967), 77.    [85] Armitage (1905), 138–9; Wilson (1905), 77, 79.    [86] Wilson (1966) 192.    [87] Scott (1905) I, 544, 554; Huntford (1979), 165–6. [88] Scott (1905) II, 61, 101–3, 123; Fisher and Fisher (1957), 64–71.    [89] Scott (1905) I, 548.

no time forced lime juice, increasing instead the ration of jams and bottled fruits; but lime juice was freely taken by many of the men who liked it. In some cases, however, it appeared to disagree, and in my own case marked scurvy symptoms were dismissed and, the disease completely cured without recourse to lime juice."[90] Earlier in the same article, he had referred to "the free use of tinned foods having this result [i.e., scurvy]." It seems more likely, therefore, that he believed that they were the source of something toxic rather than that they lacked something present in the fresh meat. In any case, there was no more of the disease for their last fourteen months in the Arctic.[91]

In 1904, in London, there was another discussion on the etiology of scurvy. The main paper was read by Dr. Coplans on his experience as a medical officer attached to prisoner-of-war camps in South Africa. There was considerable scurvy in the native labor corps. He concluded that "scurvy is not due to the presence or absence of any particular kind of food, but rather to an infection for which food may act as a vehicle under conditions of dirty storage or preparation."[92] From the subsequent discussion it seemed that Coplans's arguments had not been convincing, but it was also clear that there was still no generally agreed alternative explanation for the disease. In 1907–9, Shackleton led another, even smaller expedition to the Antarctic; they reached 88°23' S, and there was no scurvy.[93] Shackleton had tried to improve the expedition's provisions by including large amounts of dried milk and bottled fruits.[94]

We now come to Scott's second and last expedition, which has become the most famous in British history, and has stimulated a number of most interesting character studies of Scott himself, his backers, and his colleagues.[95] This time a party of thirty-three sailed from New Zealand at the end of November of 1910, and again built a hut on the shore of McMurdo Sound. They hastened to lay depots farther south, using ponies and dogs, but lost many of their ponies in this work, before winter set in.[96] Calculations of their daily diet during the period in the hut have been made, using unpublished notes from the expedition's records.[97] The diet was more varied than in the first expedition but still had less milk powder and bottled fruit than were used by Shackleton's expedition; it is thought that they ate one to two pounds of fresh seal meat per day. Lime juice was available, but there was no insistence that it be taken regularly. It was thought important for maintaining health that everyone should try to take two hours of hard exercise each day.[98]

As part of the "entertainments" during the winter, there were regular debates and lectures. On August 18, Atkinson, one of the two naval sur-

---

[90] Wilson (1905), 77.    [91] Wilson (1966), 266, 278, 302.    [92] Coplans (1904), 91.    [93] Quartermain (1967), 136–88.    [94] Kendall (1955), 477–9.    [95] Huxley (1977); Thompson (1977); Huntford (1979).    [96] Huxley (1913) I, xix–xx; Quartermain (1967), 199, 206–10.    [97] Atkinson (1915), 12; Kendall (1955), 479–80.    [98] Atkinson (1915), 10.

geons in the party, lectured on "Scurvy," and Scott, now a captain, made the following notes in his diary:

. . . the disease is anything but precise. . . . Sir Almroth Wright has hit the truth, he thinks, in finding increased acidity of blood – acid intoxication – by methods only possible in recent years. . . . [This causes] the symptoms observed and infiltration of fat in organs, leading to feebleness of heart action. Lactate of sodium increases alkalinity of blood, but only within narrow limits. . . . So far for diagnosis, but . . . practically we are much as we were before. . . . [Atkinson] holds the first cause to be tainted food, but secondary or contributory causes may be even more potent in developing the disease. Damp, cold, over-exertion, bad air, bad light, in fact any condition exceptional to normal healthy existence. . . . Dietetically, fresh vegetables are the best curatives – the lecturer was doubtful of fresh meat, but admitted its possibility in Polar climate; lime juice only useful if regularly taken. He discussed lightly the relative values of vegetable stuff, doubtful of those containing abundance of phosphates such as lentils. He touched theory again in continuing [? attributing] the cause of acidity to bacterial action – and the possibility of infection in epidemic form. Wilson is evidently slow to accept the 'acid intoxication' theory. . . . He proved the value of fresh meat in Polar regions. . . . Scurvy seems very far away from us this time; yet after our *Discovery* experience, one feels that no trouble can be too great or no precaution too small to be adopted. . . . It is certain we shall not have the disease here, but one cannot foresee equally certain avoidance in the southern journey to come.[99]

Scott's notes are in general agreement with those made by another member of the party.[100] Atkinson later published results of his measurements of the alkalinity of the blood of everyone in the hut that winter; none was outside the normal range.[101]

Next spring, on November 2, the main party who were to make the attempt to reach the Pole left with their sledges. Their diet was the more or less traditional one based on biscuits and pemmican; no lime juice or fresh meat was carried.[102] Two motorized sledges that had been expected to help with more depot-laying broke down, but the party still had dogs and some ponies. The ponies were killed as they weakened and provided meat for the dogs. The weather was bad, with deep, wet snow and strong winds, and it needed heavy additional manhandling to help the dogs, but they finally got their sledges up on to the Beardmore Glacier (some 8,000 feet above sea level and 84° S) by December 10. The dog teams were then sent back. They were now a party of eight, and they reached 87°32' S on January 4, 1912. Here Scott sent three more men back. It had been planned that at this point four would go on and four would turn back, and there has been speculation as to Scott's reason for this last-minute change. Possibly he could not bear to deprive any of his last four companions of the honor of getting to the Pole, though he already knew from the logistics of dates, depots, and distances

[99] Huxley (1913) *I*, 264–5.     [100] Taylor (1916), 292–3.     [101] Atkinson (1915), 11.
[102] Rogers (1974), 576.

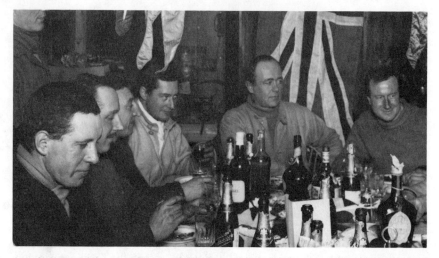

A midwinter celebration dinner at their base on Scott's last expedition. Oates, famed for crawling out to die in the snow so that his leg condition would not slow down the others' return from the Pole, is on the left. Scott and Wilson are at the right of the group. (Popperfoto.)

that they would need to have luck on their side if they were to complete the return journey.[103]

Of the three that returned, the leader was Lieutenant Edward Evans. They had a very difficult journey; there were blizzards, and, at one point, they were lost in a maze of crevasses on the edge of the Glacier. By the end of January, Evans had "a stiffness at the back of the legs behind the knees," then they turned "swollen, bruised and green"; soon he also had ulcerated gums and dysentery, and was passing blood. On February 13 he fainted, and the two sailors (Lashly and Crean) hauled him, tied to the sledge. Finally on February 16, they were thirty-five miles from the base hut but almost out of food. Crean walked on alone to try to reach the hut and fetch help, leaving Lashly to nurse Evans. He arrived there after 18 hours of trudging through deep snow, and a team brought back the two men.[104] Evans recovered, and proved to be one of the most successful destroyer captains in World War I; he was eventually to become Admiral Lord Mountevans in 1945.[105] It has been suggested that Evans's breakdown was due to his having been reluctant to eat seal meat when at the base hut during the preceding winter, but he had also been out for a longer period than the others on preliminary sledging journeys at the end of the winter, and he had had more days of tiring manhandling on the outward journey.[106]

---

[103] Quartermain (1967), 233–8; Huntford (1979), 472.     [104] Ibid., 261–5; Evans (1921), 223–6.     [105] Pound (1963), 155, 303.     [106] Quartermain (1967), 265; Huntford (1979), 472.

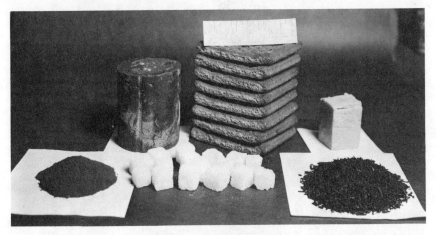

The daily ration for each man on Scott's polar party (pemmican, biscuits, butter, cocoa, sugar and tea). It was low in calories and lacked vitamin C. (Popperfoto.)

To go back to the party still heading south, they found the surface of ice crystals very difficult. They reached the Pole itself on January 16, only to find a Norwegian flag and a message from Amundsen who had arrived there three weeks earlier.[107] This was a very heavy psychological blow. By then, Petty Officer Edgar Evans had a nasty wound on his hand from a cut received some two weeks earlier, that was showing no sign of healing.[108] Evans continued to deteriorate and died on February 18 after two weeks of being "stupid and confused." It has been suggested that this stemmed from a fall not considered particularly serious at the time, but more liable to result in brain hemorrhage in someone in a state of incipient scurvy after many weeks on a scorbutic diet.[109] (Huxley's published version of Scott's diary had softened or removed some of his comments in this period.)

The remaining four continued to struggle back, on very short rations. On March 4, Oates, an army captain, admitted that one foot was giving intense pain and appeared gangrenous. This is known from Scott's diary. Wilson, Scott's old physician colleague, had given up writing his diary by this time. Oates continued to struggle on slowly, without pulling, but posed a serious problem for the others. On March 11, Scott records that he "practically ordered Wilson to hand over [from his medical supplies] the means of ending our troubles . . . 30 opium tabloids apiece."[110] Six or seven nights later (Scott had lost count of the exact date), when the others were in their sleeping bags, Oates deliberately walked out into a blizzard so that he would be frozen to death by morning. Scott noted that it was "the act of a

[107] Huxley (1913) *I*, 374–5; Huntford (1979), 516.    [108] Huxley (1913) *I*, 367; Wilson (1966), 230.    [109] Rogers (1974), 573–9.    [110] Huxley (1913) *I*, 406–7.

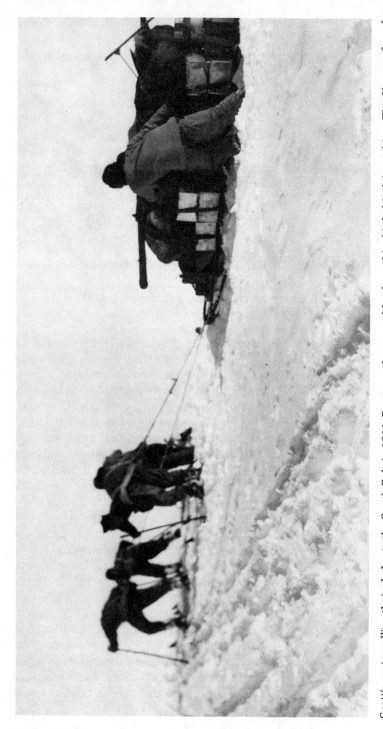

Scott's party pulling their sledge to the South Pole in 1911. Bowers, who was told to leave his skis behind, is pushing. The film was found with their frozen bodies. (Popperfoto.)

brave . . . gentlemen."[111] It has been suggested that he included Oates in the polar party at the last moment as a representative of the army.[112] Oates must have suffered a particular problem with his leg after such protracted dragging because the femur had been shattered in the Boer War, leaving it slightly shorter; in addition, the scar tissue of the old wounds may have been breaking up again after such a long period on a scorbutic diet.[113]

The three remaining men struggled on for three more days and then, after 4½ months out from base and nearly 1,800 miles of trudging, they were only eleven miles from the final depot, but another blizzard blew up and they were unable to leave their tent. There was no fuel left and very little food. Six and one-half months later, after the long Antarctic Winter, a search party led by Atkinson found the three frozen bodies in their snow-covered tent, with Scott's diary beside him.[114] One of the continuing points of discussion has been whether or not the disaster could be attributed to the scorbutic nature of the diet, although there is no mention in the diaries of any of the traditional signs of scurvy in the polar party.

The television series "The Last Place on Earth," shown in the United States, in 1985, was an impressive reconstruction of the Scott and Amundsen expeditions to the South Pole, based on Roland Huntford's book. Although great pains were taken to achieve authenticity, the conversations obviously had to be conjectured. When the bodies of Scott and his colleagues are discovered, a colleague says to Atkinson, the surgeon, "So this is scurvy." In his reports Atkinson made no mention of scurvy and referred only to hunger and frostbite. Huntford writes in his book: "There are stray hints that he [Atkinson] might have been concealing evidence of scurvy, which could not be revealed because it would have reflected on the whole conduct of the expedition." Certainly there had been no adequate precautions to protect against it. We will return to the question in the final chapter.

---

[111] Ibid., 408.     [112] Huxley (1977), 245.     [113] Rogers (1974), 578; Thompson (1977), 163.
[114] Huxley (1913), *II*, 237; Atkinson (1915), 12.

# 7

## Infantile scurvy: the new disease of affluence (1877 – 1917)

In the late 1870s, St. John's Wood, a newly developed suburb on the north side of London, was a fashionable neighborhood with the reputation of being a healthy area for bringing up children. One can imagine that a middle-class family living there would have read about the scandal over the outbreak of scurvy during the recent polar expedition, and possibly they would also have heard of its appearance in Paris during the privations of the siege, but they would surely never have dreamed that it would intrude into their own comfortable life. Yet for at least one such family it did.

In January 1877, Dr. Cheadle, a leading London pediatrician most famous for his studies of rickets, was brought out to St. John's Wood to see a firstborn child of sixteen months who had already been seriously ill for several weeks. He found the little boy so feeble that he could not even sit up. He obviously had rickets, with the long bones enlarged and the ribs beaded; in addition, he had extremely swollen gums, spongy and bleeding with an offensive smell; his legs were swollen and extremely tender to the touch. The child had no history of infection and was obviously well cared for. He was weaned when six months old, and for the next eight months was fed almost solely on oatmeal and rusks. The mother had tried giving him condensed milk but thought that it did not agree with him; from ten months on, he was given a little mutton broth.

The physician who had first seen the baby, at fourteen months, had prescribed potassium chlorate, iodide of iron, quinine bark, and, later, cod liver oil. He had also prescribed alum and "glycerine of tannin" for application to the gums, but the child's condition had worsened. Cheadle at once diagnosed "scurvy" in addition to rickets. He ordered fresh cow's milk, to replace the oatmeal and water, to be increased gradually to two pints a day as the child became accustomed to it; in addition he was to receive a table-spoonful of finely minced raw meat sweetened with a little sugar. By the

158

spring the child had greatly improved, and his parents received permission to take him away to the seaside to try the effects of saltwater bathing.[1]

Cheadle saw two more cases in the next three months. In each instance, the child, after weaning, had lived almost entirely on bread and butter with little or no milk. Neither had received potatoes or fruit and vegetables of any kind. Each responded rapidly to treatment, which consisted of fresh milk with potatoes mashed up into it together with a little raw meat and either orange or lemon juice. Cheadle commented that rickets was to be expected in children receiving such "farinaceous" (starchy) diets. However, to see scurvy in addition was most unusual.

Why did these particular rickety children out of all the number alone become scorbutic? I believe the explanation lies in the fact that, curiously enough, in each of these cases one factor usually present in the diet of children was omitted in addition to those ordinarily wanting in a simple rachitic diet – viz., *potatoes*. The common antiscorbutic element in the food of infants is milk; but after they are weaned, or if brought up by hand at an early age, the children of the poor get very little milk; it is too expensive. They soon begin to feed with their parents, and potatoes and gravy are almost invariably given them. This does not prevent them becoming rickety, but it seems to keep off scurvy.[2]

Four years later, Cheadle wrote again to the *Lancet*, reporting another case in some detail – a 10-month-old boy who had been fed for several months on nothing but a proprietary food, and who responded rapidly when fed on fresh milk and water thickened with fine potato gruel. He also argued that other cases being described as "periosteal cachexia," with swelling and hemorrhages at the ends of the long bones, were really scurvy and urged that they be treated with an antiscorbutic diet.[3]

## Early records of infantile scurvy

Was diagnosing scurvy in a young child something entirely new? No, for one thing, another London physician had published a note of a case in 1873. This paper referred to a 10-month-old child with legs very tender to the touch, spots on the legs, a sallow complexion, and spongy gums. The mother had been unable to suckle the child for more than three weeks, and had then given him nothing but condensed milk and water for five months, after which some wheat flour was added. She was told to give him plenty of fresh cow's milk and a little lemon juice, and in one week the signs had cleared up and the child was cheerful again. The physician commented that "a peculiar feature of the case was the early age in which the disease appeared," but he had consulted a standard dictionary of medicine and had read that "scurvy may occur at any age from childhood upwards."[4]

[1] Cheadle (1878), 685–6.     [2] Ibid., 686–7.     [3] Cheadle (1882), 48–9.     [4] Jalland (1873), 248.

However, to find earlier specific references to infantile scurvy, one has to go back 200–300 years. In 1596, William Clowes, while describing the scurvy that he had seen in sailors, mentioned in passing that earlier in his career, he had seen the same condition in twenty to thirty children in the London hospital where he had worked.[5] From the same period, there is a letter written to the German physician Fabricius Hildanus, requesting advice about the treatment of the fourteen-month-old child of a nobleman, with the signs of scurvy.[6] Between 1590 and 1640, frequent episodes of scurvy were recorded in a French charitable institution for abandoned children. In 1640, the directors of the charity called in an eminent physician for advice. He gave his opinion in writing and began by saying that he had seen a similar condition, with inflammation and ulceration of the gums and feebleness of the legs, in sailors in the navy. He recommended a whole series of treatments, which included gentle purging and a decoction made with lemon juice, which would help the gums and the general corruption of the tissues.[7] These children were probably not truly "infants" (i.e., of age when they could have been suckling); and the same would be true of scorbutic children in a Russian foundling home in the next century.[8]

As pointed out by Hess, Francis Glisson, the Cambridge Professor whose classic book on infantile rickets was published in 1650, also said: "The scurvy is sometimes conjoyned with the affect [i.e., rickets]," and added that it can be "produced from the indiscreet and erroneous Regiment [diet] of the infant," though he also included heredity, infection, and a bad climate as other causes. He referred specifically to "tumors" appearing on the gums, "pains running through their joynts" on any kind of movement, and sometimes "palpitations of the heart . . . soon mitigated by laying them down to rest."[9] Rickets itself was characterized by soft, distorted bones with swollen ends.

Dr. Shipley, who reviewed the subject in the 1920s, wrote:

The wonder that the occurrence of scurvy among children should have remained unnoticed and undescribed, save by Glisson, for so long a period of time . . . is susceptible to easy explanation. . . . the physicians of the sixteenth and seventeenth centuries did not feel the necessity of describing separately the occurrence in children of a malady that also affected adults. . . . Scurvy in a child was to them only scurvy; it was not Barlow's disease. Another and more tragic explanation is found in the enormous infant mortality during the period. It may almost be stated as an aphorism that . . . hand-fed children did not live to develop scurvy.[10]

The "Barlow" referred to in the quotation was another physician at the London's Hospital for Sick Children: Thomas Barlow. He followed Cheadle in writing about infantile scurvy in 1884, and, in addition to confirming Cheadle's clinical observations, was able to describe the findings from three

[5] Starnes & Leake (1945), 42–3.    [6] Shipley (1929), 6–7.    [7] Colly (1956), 36–7.
[8] De Mertans (1778), 669–76.    [9] Hess (1920), 10–11.    [10] Shipley (1929), 6.

postmortem examinations. The most characteristic finding was subperiosteal hemorrhage, i.e., effusion of blood, into the space between the epiphyses (ends) of the long leg bones and the cartilage layers coating the bones. The femur was usually the most affected. There was also effusion of blood into the deep muscles.[11] This was quite different from anything seen in ordinary rickets, but exactly what had been described by Lind in his postmortems, a hundred years earlier, of scorbutic sailors.[12] He also found the separation of rib bones from their connecting cartilage, which had been described even earlier still by Poupart.[13] Finally, within the bones there were characteristic changes, with the bony tissues in some cases being reabsorbed, or eroded, to "a mere shell," which explained the fractures that had been seen; separations were found between the ends of the long bones and the shaft, with the normal cartilaginous connecting zone being absent.[14] This contrasted with rachitic changes, in which cartilaginous tissue proliferated and the bones softened from inadequate mineralization. The bulging of the eyes that was seen in scorbutic children was again explained by effusions of blood between the bone and cartilage inside the eye socket. Changes in the gums were not the most consistent sign because they were usually found only when teeth had already erupted. Barlow argued that although most of these children also showed signs of rickets, the special changes he described in the bones were not "rickets in more severe form," nor congenital syphilis, but an entirely different condition, that is, scurvy.[15]

German medical scientists, who were, at that time, foremost in relating clinical disease to pathology, were impressed by Barlow's study and agreed that the fairly common condition that they had been diagnosing as "acute rickets" was, in fact, something outside their previous experience and, therefore, they called it "Barlow's disease." In other words, they, along with Scandinavian pediatricians, accepted the description of the disease without acknowledging Barlow's own argument as to its cause.[16] We shall return to this point shortly.

## American experience

In the meantime, from the early 1890s, physicians in the United States were beginning to realize that they, too, had been seeing infants with this condition. Professor Northrup, of New York, recalled that in 1889 he had failed to diagnose scurvy in an infant who later died, and that it was "only post-mortem findings that revealed the true nature of the disease." It was, he believed, "the first case of undoubted scorbutus [scurvy] in an infant recorded in the medical literature of the United States."[17] He then tried to search out

---

[11] Barlow (1883), 179–85; 196–7.     [12] Lind (1772), 496–8.     [13] Poupart (1708), 223–32.     [14] Barlow (1883), 185–7.     [15] Ibid., 198–9.     [16] Hirschsprung (1896), 1–3, 42–3.
[17] Northrup & Crandall (1894), 641.

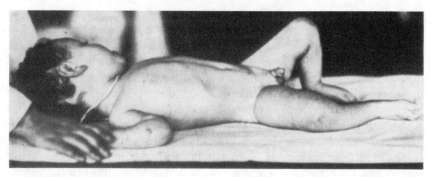

A child with scurvy, lying in the so-called frog position to minimize pressure on a swollen painful leg. (Cambridge University Press.)

other similar cases. The Surgeon-General's records revealed only one possible case; however, by 1891, eleven had been found, and, at a meeting of the Academy of Medicine in 1894, he could report 116 cases. At the same meeting two doctors from other cities also contributed 23 case histories.[17]

From a table giving 36 cases in more detail, it appeared that boys and girls were equally affected. Pain was the commonest symptom of the disease, and some children appeared to be paralyzed, simply because of their extreme reluctance to move their limbs. They typically had their legs bent and separated in what has been described as the "frog position." It was concluded that the disease was probably increasing, but that it was not a new one, having previously been misdiagnosed, most often as acute rheumatism, infantile paralysis, or some form of rickets.[18] Rapid recovery occurred when antiscorbutics were given. In nearly all cases, the children had been living exclusively on proprietary foods and/or evaporated or condensed milk.[19] "Condensed" milk had been evaporated to about one-quarter of its original weight and heavily fortified with sugar before being canned. The extra sugar made it less subject to spoilage when the can was left open.[20] Whether or not particular brands of processed, sterilized milks were associated with scurvy seemed to depend on exactly how they had been processed. Milk was "sterilized" by being heated and held near its boiling point in a sealed container, until it was judged to contain no live bacteria.

One story with a happy ending was reported by a New York pediatrician in 1894.

A little girl, eleven and a half months of age, was brought to me last August from a southern city for treatment. The baby had been ill about four months with a disorder so peculiar that it had been variously taken for Pott's disease of the spine, disease of the hip-joint, and rheumatism, by some of the physicians who had seen her, while others confessed that they were unable to make a diagnosis. The child had grown steadily worse in spite of careful treatment, and . . . her condition had become critical. The child evidently suffered . . . acute pain if she was touched or moved.

[18] Ibid., 644–6.     [19] Ibid., 642–4.     [20] Hunziker (1946), 133–5.

In crying, she exposed a set of purplish swollen gums, ulcerating around the bases of the teeth, . . . giving an offensive discharge. . . . the lower limbs were never moved, even in the frantic efforts of the child to resist examination; . . .

The child had always been nourished on a particular brand of condensed milk, diluted according to the printed directions, which appeared to agree with her, as she had been free from stomach and bowel trouble. As I was desirous of noting the effect of a simple change of diet, without medication, the baby was, the next day, put on pasteurized milk, 4 oz. with 2 oz. water, every three hours, and no drugs were exhibited [prescribed]. I ordered, however, the juice of one orange, daily, given in small amounts at a time, and also a teaspoonful, twice a day, of raw beef juice. I know of no better word than "magical" to describe the effect of these simple measures. . . . [After 3 days] she had ceased to cry and fret, and lay quietly on her cot, apparently free from suffering; the gums were half their former size, and had lost their congested look. . . . [After 9 days] it was noticed that she moved both legs quite freely. . . . She went home fully restored in all respects, in less than four weeks from the time of the first examination.[21]

We have no way of knowing how many other children may have suffered in this way without having the condition diagnosed. One physician referred to artificial methods of feeding having largely superseded natural breast suckling. He agreed with earlier writers that "the disease prevails chiefly among the children of well-to-do people who have the means to purchase the various commercial artificial foods. The poorer classes . . . , too frequently allowing their offspring to have the run of the table, as it is called, seldom offer us cases of the disease."[22] It seems strange that he should have said "too frequently" of the practice which he admitted was the cause of the children keeping healthy.

In 1897, the *Index Catalogue to the Library of the Surgeon-General's Office* listed over fifty papers under the heading of "Barlow's disease," with the greatest number coming from the United States.[23] By the following year, the American Pediatric Society had completed a collective investigation of the problem. Inquiries led to the collection of 379 cases recognized as infantile scurvy. All but 5 of these children were white, with almost exactly equal numbers of each sex, and the great majority were between seven and fourteen months old. It was confirmed that most were from families with better than average incomes and hygienic conditions, and typically the children themselves previously had had a good health record. In over half the cases, rickets was specifically stated to be absent, which differed from the typical case description from Europe.[24]

## Was "cooked" milk responsible?

With regard to the children's diet, there were records for 356 cases: 154 had been receiving mainly sterilized or condensed milk, 110 had been receiving

---

[21] Fruitnight (1894), 493–6.  [22] Ibid., 487.  [23] U. S. Surgeon-General (1897), 2, 105–6.
[24] Griffith, Jennings, & Morse (1898), 482–4, 492.

various proprietary foods (i.e., powders to be suspended or dissolved in water), and 36 had been eating mixed foods (oatmeal, gruels, etc.). Of the remainder, 12 were listed as having received breast milk, 5 raw milk, 20 pasteurized milk, and the remainder "cow's milk" with nothing said as to whether it was raw or processed. Twenty of the children died, and the other 336 were cured. The usual treatment was to transfer the child to raw cow's milk and to give orange juice in addition, and, in many cases, raw beef juice as well. Fifty-eight children also recovered on being switched to raw milk without any fruit juice.[25]

The conclusions drawn in the report, signed by three members of the original committee, were extremely tentative. They were that (a) the disease resulted from an unsuitable diet continued over a prolonged period, (b) certain forms of diet were particularly likely to lead to scurvy, particularly the various proprietary foods, and (c) apparently "the farther a food is removed in character from the natural food of a child the more likely its use is to be followed by the development of scurvy."[26] Even this was not acceptable to the fourth member of the committee who annexed a minority report in which he said that he believed scurvy to be "a chronic ptomaine poisoning due to the absorption of toxins," and that abnormal intestinal fermentation was a predisposing factor. "Sterilizing, pasteurizing or cooking of milk food was not *per se* responsible."[27]

The report was presented to a meeting of the Society for approval of its publication, and a summary of the ensuing debate was printed. One view was that the report, which was to be published on behalf of the Society as a whole, should contain no conclusions because not every member would agree with them: "It looks like establishing scientific truth by legislation."[27] One of the committee members replied that he had already received letters from doctors wanting to know what the conclusions were. "We were not summarising the opinions of individual physicans but the actual records of cases. . . . We do not say diet is the cause, but we say from the reports of these physicians diet *seemed* to be the cause."[27] A third member said that "if the evidence is accepted, there is only one conclusion that can possibly be drawn and that is, the sterilization of milk has something to do with the production of scurvy."[28]

Clearly, this presented a very difficult dilemma for the Society, which was not going to be resolved on that occasion. The very next speaker in the debate set out the problem:

The sterilization of milk is one of the greatest advances that has been made in infant feeding. . . . The most important diseases which we have to deal with among infants are the digestive disorders in summer time. The sterilization of the milk offers more advantages in checking or preventing those diseases than any other method which as yet been offered. . . . It is possible that sterilization of milk may

[25] Ibid., 485–6, 495–8.    [26] Ibid., 498.    [27] Ibid., 500.    [28] Ibid., 502–3.

injure its nutritive properties to a slight extent. . . . But the injury done by this is far outweighed by the greater advantage offered in preventing disease.[28]

Another paper being considered by the Society on the same day was entitled "Should all milk used for infant feeding be heated for the purpose of killing germs?" The author said: "It does not seem fair to put into an infant's stomach a food containing thousands of bacteria in each drop, these bacteria being of unknown quality and very possibly dangerous and pathogenic nature." [29]

The infant mortality in New York especially was a serious cause of concern. In the districts crowded with poor immigrants struggling to adapt to conditions that were strange to them, some 20% of the babies died before they were a year old. Mortality was particularly high when they could not be breast-fed, and the death rate increased 50% in the summer months; in some years, during July and August the death rate rose to two or three times the winter rate. There were about 15,000 deaths of babies each year in New York alone, and about half of these were attributed to either wasting or diarrheal diseases.[30] If the infant mortality rate could be reduced by even one quarter, this would mean that nearly 4,000 lives were saved per year in just one city. Because reducing the bacterial content of milk by sterilization gave promise of such a decline in mortality, it was natural that pediatricians would be very reluctant to weaken their support of sterilization unless, or until, the necessity to do so was demonstrated beyond any doubt.

One characteristic of the American papers was that they included no reference to, or acknowledgment of, earlier work done in other countries. A very similar debate over the sterilization of milk had already occurred at the British Medical Association's meeting in 1896. The opening speaker had referred to the great infant mortality in England, and its association with the feeding of unsterilized cow's milk. He acknowledged that there was some evidence to support "the belief that rickets, and specially scurvy rickets, may be induced by the use of sterilized milk." However, he believed that the changes brought about by the heat of sterilization were that the casein (the principal protein) was made less digestible and that the calcium salts precipitated. The delayed digestion of the casein coagulum in the stomach, in most cases, rendered it necessary for the intervals between meals to be longer. This, he believed was the cause of the association of sterilized milk with scurvy rickets; thus the condition was due to ". . . insufficient food . . . rather than . . . a subtle change in the milk as a result of sterilization." He pointed out that the milder "pasteurization" of milk, i.e., holding it at 155°F for fifteen minutes, was sufficient to kill all the pathogenic bacteria including the tubercle bacillus, and had little effect on the digestibility or flavor.[31] The discussion again referred to the danger that tuberculosis could be spread by raw milk, and it was agreed that there was no serious

[29] Freeman (1898), 513.     [30] Van Ingen & Taylor (1912), 20–3.     [31] Campbell (1896), 625.

risk of scurvy from feeding boiled milk.[32] Writers in England continued to warn against the danger of raw milk, "drawn through unwashed hands into a pail placed under the dung-spattered udder and belly of a cow."[33]

One argument put forward in 1902 to explain the scorbutic effect of commercial sterilized milk was that it might well already have accumulated bacterial toxins before the milk was processed, and also that if it were kept for a long period afterward, a few surviving pathogenic bacteria might again multiply, which would not be detected because the normal "souring" bacteria would not be present to provide the usual indicator of heavy bacterial growth. This paper cited the recent writing of Jackson and Harley, which had argued for the ptomaine theory of scurvy.[34] With regard to the best method of processing, there seemed to be a growing consensus that simple scalding at home gave adequate protection against infection and was unlikely to result in scurvy.[35]

## Parallel debates in France and Germany

In France also, the cause of Barlow's disease was debated by the Paris Pediatric Society in 1902. There was no disagreement that it was being encountered. Dr. Netter reviewed a series of French papers as far back as 1894, as well as Swiss, Dutch, Scandinavian, and German papers, and argued that the disease represented the infantile form of scurvy and arose directly from the use of sterilized milk.[36] Raw milk was known to be antiscorbutic, but this quality was lost during sterilization.[37] He accepted the recently published hypothesis that the sterilization process resulted in the precipitation of calcium citrate from the milk, and that the antiscorbutic value of uncooked milk and of other foods came from their content of the alkaline salts of citric acid, and probably of some other organic acids.[38] The disease had nothing to do with rickets.[39]

Dr. Ausset disagreed, believing that Barlow's disease was a hemorrhagic complication of rickets, but of the same character; this signified for him that it represented a pasteurellosis (toxic infection) of the gastrointestinal tract.[40] The disease could *not* be said to be "*due* to sterilized milk," because in at least one-quarter of the cases sterilized milk had not been given to the child. The important feature was that it was always preceded by gastrointestinal disturbances, which were often caused by overfeeding. It was true, however, that the ailing child had often been receiving sterilized milk, but the reason for this association was that it was no longer a living food. The destruction of

---

[32] Ibid., 626.   [33] Ransom (1902), 440.   [34] Ibid., 442.   [35] Ibid., 441; Barton (1897), 14.
[36] Netter (1902), 300–5.   [37] Ibid., 306–7.   [38] Corlette (1900), 573–4.   [39] Netter (1902), 315.   [40] Ausset (1902), 330.

its ferments (enzymes) meant that the casein remained a long time in the digestive tract and gave rise to breakdown products which caused the gastroenteritis. The chemical environment in the gut was then so changed that pathogenic organisms could multiply and invade the bloodstream.[41]

Ausset then argued that the role of the alkaline calcium citrate in raw milk had been misunderstood. Its only function was the physical one of assisting in keeping the calcium phoshate salts in solution. Citric acid certainly had a role to play in the treatment of Barlow's disease, but it was purely as an intestinal antiseptic, acting against the organisms responsible for the gastroenteritis. This was the mechanism of action of lemon juice, which he had given with good effect in his own cases. With regard to prevention of the disease among infants who could not be breast-fed, the best solution was to use pasteurized milk. This should have been heated to 75°C, but no higher (or the "ferments" would be inactivated), and then rapidly rechilled to reduce growth of any surviving bacteria. Although, in his opinion, adult scurvy was not to be equated with Barlow's disease, it was interesting that a professor in St. Petersburg (now Leningrad), in an unpublished work, had shortly before reported the isolation of bacteria from the liver and spleen of adults who had died with scurvy, and found that they were of the *Pasteurella* type.[42]

In Germany, as mentioned already, the term "Barlow's disease" was in common use in the 1890s, though writers agreed that it was the same condition that had first been described in 1859 by Professor Möller of the University of Königsberg (then in East Prussia, but now in the Soviet Union and renamed Kaliningrad), who characterized it as "acute rickets." [43] (During World War I, German physicians revived the designation "Möller's disease" or "Möller–Barlow disease," perhaps because it seemed more patriotic.) A representative paper from Berlin in 1896 expressed concern at the increasing incidence of the disease, and surprise that it seemed to occur only in well-situated families and typically in children five to seven months old. The physician did not allude to any relationship between that disease and scurvy, stating only that its cause was unknown. However, he warned his colleagues against recommending the use of a well-known brand of modified cow's milk that was on the market, because he found it to have been given to many of the children who had developed the disease.[44]

A speaker in the subsequent discussion argued that this was an unwarranted criticism. As early as 1892, one clinician had been able to assemble eighty case records of the disease and that was *before* this particular type of processed milk had been on the market. Between 400 and 500 children must have been fed on the product condemned by the first speaker, and only a very few could have developed the disease. The way to proceed was to

[41] Ibid., 331–2.     [42] Ibid., 332–5.     [43] Meyer (1896), 23.     [44] Ibid., 24.

initiate discussions with the manufacturers. In his opinion, if the milk was
being overheated, this could have resulted in a precipitation of alkaline
calcium salts. Adding calcium salts back to the final product would prevent
its having this scurvylike effect.[44]

At another meeting of the Berlin Medical Society in 1903, Dr. Heubner
said that he had certainly seen an increasing number of cases of Barlow's
disease: no more than three or four per year up to 1900, fifteen in 1901,
thirty-two in 1902, and already a whole series in the first two months of
1903. As others had said previously, it occurred typically in well-to-do
families, and never in children being breast-fed. He had seen cases where
the milk had received only a short cooking. He was of the opinion that there
were important differences between the disease seen in infants and classical
scurvy, but from the point of view of treatment, the same antiscorbutic diet
cured both.[45] In the discussion, Dr. Jacusiel strongly disagreed. There only
*appeared* to have been an increase in the incidence of scurvy because diagnosis had improved. The most important point was that total infant mortality in Berlin had greatly *decreased*. Most infant deaths were due to diseases
of the digestive tract, and the use of pasteurized or sterilized milk had led to
a great reduction in these. He agreed that overheating could have a deleterious effect on milk, but that great progress had been made by the dairy industry in the quality of their products.[46] We see, therefore, that the medical
communities were in the same dilemma in both the Old and New Worlds.

In this period, the most sophisticated analysis of the cause of the disease
in Germany was made by Dr. Neumann of Berlin. He considered it to have
been proven that the disease occurred only among children who had been
receiving sterilized or doubly pasteurized milk products; a simple boiling of
the milk at home before use did not seem to be harmful.[47] He then went on
to speculate as to the nature of the injurious changes in the milk. It could not
be a loss of enzyme activity because that occurred also with simple boiling,
as did the denaturation of "the specific serum bodies whose role as carriers
of immunity we are beginning to understand." He measured the freezing
point of different milks, because it seemed well established that the depression of this measurement below the freezing point of pure water was proportional to the number of independent molecules in a given volume of an
aqueous solution. He found that milk, when cooked for sixty-five minutes in
a Soxhlet apparatus, gave approximately 20% greater depression than the
corresponding raw milk, whereas milder treatments caused no significant
change. He also measured the electrical conductivity of different samples, in
order to obtain a measure of the relative quantities of dissociated salts that
they contained, because it was these ions that were the means whereby
electricity was conducted through an aqueous solution. In short, milk
heated for sixty-five minutes in the Soxhlet cooker had no greater conduc-

[45] Heubner (1903), 109–10.     [46] Jacusiel (1903), 117.     [47] Neumann (1902), 628–9.

tivity than raw milk. He therefore concluded that the additional molecules present in the severely cooked milk, as indicated by the greater depression of freezing point, could *not* be dissociated salts, but rather organic compounds of some kind.[48] (The Soxhlet cooker was arranged so that a number of small bottles of milk could conveniently be immersed in boiling water, typically for a forty-minute period.)[49]

Neumann then considered the significance of another worker's finding of the presence, in heated milk only, of a phosphorus compound that appeared to have broken off from a larger organic molecule. However, he concluded that the harmful effects of such milk could not be explained by the possible degradation of large, phosphorus-containing compounds because he had known cases in which Barlow's disease had developed despite the infant's having received regular quantities of egg yolk, which was a rich source of such compounds. The second possibility was that heating resulted in a change in the form of the iron present in the milk, so that it was no longer so usable by children. He did not believe that this could be the cause of the disease because inorganic iron preparations failed to cure the condition, and he had also seen it develop in an infant who had been receiving an organic iron preparation, "haematogen." In addition, he had observed that there was no relation between the severity of a particular case and the degree of anemia, the latter being the specific effect of a deficiency of iron.[50]

His argument, slightly paraphrased, continued as follows: One might think that if we could definitely categorize Barlow's disease as infantile scurvy this would settle the question as to whether or not it was brought about by intoxication. However, that would be a mistake, for the same question is similarly undecided for scurvy itself. With regard to the rational treatment of the disease it would, of course, be of the greatest importance to establish whether or not it was the result of chronic toxicity. If it were, then the first action would be to cut out the source of the trouble. On the other hand, if one believed that, as a result of heating, the milk had only lost some specific positive quality, we could continue to give it and only supplement it with recognized antiscorbutic materials. In the latter case, one would then have to discover what it was that the milk had lost through heating.[50]

From his own experience, once more, he could say that he had known at least four children with Barlow's disease, who continued to receive the processed milk on which the condition developed but, in addition, were given asparagus, spinach, and various other vegetables or apple puree, and none of them had improved. To restore the children to good health, it had always proved necessary to change them to a better milk. Of the other items mentioned in the literature as suitable supplementary foods, such as eggs, meat broth, and starchy materials, it was certain that they were quite worthless. The undoubted value of vegetables was apparent only in the very

[48] Ibid., 629–30.    [49] Judson & Gittings (1902), 224.    [50] Ibid., 630, 647.

earliest stage of the disease, before the state of chronic intoxication had developed.[51]

He then explained how *his* "intoxication" theory of poisonous substances that were formed in the heated milks differed from those previously advanced:

The authors of the American enquiry accepted, according to von Starck, that it was a chronic auto-intoxication of the intestines resulting from the continued use of unsuitable food and that sterilization, pasteurization and cooking were not responsible. On the other hand, Johannessen believes that Barlow's disease is caused by poisoning from bacterial toxins which had arisen through the growth in the milk of bacteria which survived a short period of heating. I refer to these theories only to argue against them for I have seen children get ill while receiving the best Berlin milk, which had received the most thorough heating.[51]

In his final summing up, he suggested that the toxic substance formed during heating most probably was produced from chemical reactions involving the protein fraction of the milk, and that the frequency of the disease in Berlin could be attributed to the use of a mass-produced milk that had received extensive heating in a Soxhlet apparatus. He again affirmed the necessity of changing to raw or very carefully pasteurized milk, and that the purpose of giving vegetables in addition was "to correct the disorder in the blood more quickly." [52]

Neumann's study, with its use of physicochemical methods of analysis to measure very small changes in cooked milk, must have seemed very advanced and modern at the time. However, while going into the details, he had overlooked one obvious fact, which was that the very great majority of the infants in Berlin who were receiving processed milk must, as Dr. Jacusiel had said, have remained free from Barlow's disease. Yet, Neumann had explained why *everyone* receiving such milk should be poisoned by it. In this respect, his analysis of the problem was inferior to that put forth twenty-five years earlier by Cheadle who asked very early on: "Why have these particular children developed the disease when so many others are free from it?" Cheadle had speculated that the others had remained healthy because they had been given potatoes as well; he had then put his hypothesis to the test.[2] Neumann made no attempt to discover what the healthy babies drinking processed milk in Berlin were receiving in addition.

From all accounts, the incidence of the disease continued to grow. In a retrospective analysis of cases seen at the Children's Hospital of Philadelphia, sixty-five had been diagnosed as having Barlow's disease in the period 1911–15, compared with twenty-one in the period 1901–5, and thirty-three in the period 1906–10.[53] Similar findings were reported from Boston over the same period, and a correlation with the increased use of pasteurized milk was suggested.[54] The 1920 edition of the *Index Catalogue to the*

[51] Ibid., 648.    [52] Ibid., 649.    [53] Gittings (1923), 510.    [54] Morse (1918), 161.

*Library of the Surgeon-General's Office* cited over 300 papers on Barlow's disease; these reports came from twenty-two countries as far apart as Japan, Australia, Norway, and Brazil.[55] Strangely, although Russia was a center of endemic adult scurvy,[56] Barlow's disease did not seem to occur there, and this may have been one of the factors that made less plausible any arguments in favor of a relationship between the two diseases. It was explained by the universality of breast feeding, and other evidence was collected indicating that breast-fed children escaped illness when a community was suffering from adult scurvy.[57]

One factor that may have had a deleterious effect in the United States was a report issued by the New York Milk Commission in 1912. It was the stated aim of the Commission to provide national standards of milk quality. They had collected a group of twenty selected experts in different fields, principally bacteriology, chemistry, and dairying.[58] Their unanimous conclusion was that all milk not coming from specially inspected and certified farms should be pasteurized, and the majority felt that all milk, regardless of its source, should be pasteurized. They also stated that pasteurization led to no destruction of chemical constituents of the milk.[59] One cannot find fault with the recommendations for pasteurization, but it seems to have been taking a narrow view not to have included even one pediatrician on the Commission. He or she would have been able to represent the client most at risk and, at the very least, to have ensured that a warning be included in the report regarding the evidence as to the need of infants for supplementary antiscorbutic foods when given processed cow's milk with only starchy supplements.

In the winter of 1913–14, the Jewish Orphanage in New York stopped giving orange juice to their infants. The doctors felt that they should thrive without it because the pasteurized milk now being supplied had been heated only to 145 °F, "which is claimed by many (including the Commission on Milk Standards) not to destroy its chemical constituents."[60] Numerous cases of scurvy developed, though the signs were quite variable in their order of appearance. Almost any region could be involved in hemorrhage, and it was suggested that the femur was commonly predominant only because it was so frequently handled in the changing of diapers.[61] Hess and Fish, in their report, also confirmed that freshly cooked potato was an excellent antiscorbutic and recommended it to be added, instead of barley-water, to the pasteurized milk. However, commercially prepared potato flour did not show the same activity. Cod liver oil was also inactive, and malt soup seemed, if anything, to be positively harmful.[62] "Malt soup" was apparently in common use for infant feeding at that time, and was made

[55] U. S. Surgeon-General (1920), 351–5.     [56] Berthenson (1892), 128–9; Comrie (1920), 209–11.     [57] Hess (1920), 37–8.     [58] Commission on Milk Standards (1912), 673.     [59] Ibid., 676.     [60] Hess & Fish (1914), 386–7.     [61] Ibid., 397.     [62] Ibid., 400–1.

from fresh or pasteurized milk with added wheat flour and a rediluted commercial malt extract; the mixture was brought to the boiling point for six to ten minutes.[63] Presumably this would have been prepared in batches that would then take more than one day to be consumed, especially in a single family. Hess and Fish also suggested that it was not only the severity of heat treatment that led to loss of antiscorbutic activity in milk, but also the period of subsequent storage before it was consumed, and, in a paper published in 1917, Hess gave further evidence for this. A second heating of pasteurized milk was particularly deleterious.[64]

By this time it had become clearer that Barlow's disease and adult scurvy were essentially the same affliction. This came about in part from more detailed work in Germany on the pathology of the adult disease in Russian prisoners of war.[65] Scurvy was prevalent in the Russian Army during World War I,[66] as it had also been in the Russian Army during its war with Japan ten years earlier.[67] Postmortem examinations of bones showed that there were not only subperiosteal hemorrhages but also spontaneous fractures at the epiphyseal line. With regard to the condition of the gums, it was concluded that the characteristic changes in adults were really due to irritation around the base of teeth as a result of eating hard food or the presence of bacterial decay on the teeth, sufficient to initiate ulceration in the scorbutic gum tissue. These changes were not normally found in toothless infants eating soft food, nor in men who had lost all their teeth. There was thus no real difference between infantile and adult scurvy.[68]

The year 1917 by no means saw the end of infantile scurvy, but from this time on, the advances in treatment and understanding of the condition increasingly depended upon the results of animal experiments which must be dealt with in a separate chapter. As a postscript to the present discussion, in 1933 the International Paediatric Congress was held in London. At that time, a senior pediatrician, say, fifty years old, might first have learned about Barlow's disease in 1904, which was already twenty years after the appearance of Barlow's famous paper on the subject. Judge the amazement of the pediatricians, therefore, at seeing Sir Thomas Barlow himself at the Congress as one of the British delegation! He was then eighty-eight years old, still full of interests, and was to live on until nearly the end of World War II.[69]

---

[63] Judson & Gittings (1902), 112–13.      [64] Hess & Fish (1914), 400; Hess (1917), 340–2.
[65] Aschoff & Koch (1919).      [66] Hoerschelman (1917), 1617–19.      [67] Sato & Nambu (1908), 151.      [68] Hart (1912), 394.      [69] Barlow & Barlow (1965), 1.

# 8

## Guinea pigs and the discovery of vitamin C (1905 – 1935)

From 1875 to 1905, there was, as we have been seeing, growing confusion over the cause of scurvy. At first, it had seemed straightforward – the true cause of the disease was the suppression of fresh vegetables from the diet. Yet by the end of the period, the most prestigious medical textbook ended its discussion of the etiology of the disease with the following:

Summing up all the evidence, it seems probable that whilst a deficiency of fresh vegetables, i.e., of organic salts of potash, plays a part in the production of the disease by reducing the alkalinity of the blood, yet this does not afford a complete explanation of the occurrence of all the symptoms, and it is not unlikely that upon the soil so prepared there is grafted some specific infection which finds access to the body by the mouth. Insanitary surroundings, overwork, mental depression, and exposure to cold and damp, facilitate the development of the disease by lowering the resistance of the patient.[1]

And as we have seen, there were others, in responsible positions, who attributed it to ptomaine poisoning from bad meat, or, in the case of infantile scurvy, to poisoning from products formed during the sterilization of milk. But now, in a very short time, all these views were to be swept away.

The year 1907 saw the publication of what I judge to have been the most important single paper in the whole history of this subject.[2] Its importance came not from its having any immediate practical result, but because it provided an animal model for systematic study of the preventive value of different substances, so that the identification of the antiscorbutic factor would now become almost inevitable. The authors were two Norwegians working at the University of Christiana (Oslo). The first author, Axel Holst, was forty-seven years old and Professor of Hygiene and Bacteriology; he had studied in various European laboratories including the Pasteur Institute

---

[1] Hutchinson (1907), 893.    [2] Holst & Frölich (1907).

173

in Paris and was with Koch in Berlin when the latter was working on tuberculin. A few years earlier, he had visited Eijkman's laboratory in the Dutch East Indies to learn more of the pioneering use of chickens as animal models to study the dietary deficiency responsible for the disease beriberi.[3]

For the previous ten years or so, there had been concern in Norway at the increase in incidence among the crews of their sailing ships, of a disease described as "ship beriberi." The increase seemed to date from Govern- ment-imposed changes in the rations issued to sailors, which were having an effect opposite to that intended. In particular, the ship owners had been ordered to supply "soft" bread, baked from white wheaten flour in place of the traditional, hard rye bread.[4] In practice this "soft" bread was made with baking powder rather than yeast. The meat ration was also reduced, and salted meat and peas were largely replaced by canned meat and fish.[5]

Holst began his work with pigeons, because they were more convenient than chickens, and responded to a beriberi diet with essentially the same condition of polyneuritis that Eijkman had demonstrated. However, he felt that the condition was very different from the disease of sailors and that he might find something closer to it if he used a mammalian species.[6] For us, eighty years later, if an investigator had no a priori reason to prefer one species to another for a nutritional experiment, the rat would usually be the first animal chosen, because it breeds rapidly and is therefore cheap to produce.[7] But at that time, rats were regarded as biting, infection-carrying pests, and McCollum, a few years later, had to fight prejudice at the Wisconsin Agricultural Experiment Station in order to establish the first colony for use in nutritional experiments.[8] In contrast, the guinea pig had been accepted as a children's pet in Victorian Europe and was at least more economical, as regards space and food requirements, than dogs, which had been used in most French and German feeding trials up to that time. It was, therefore, not really surprising that Holst chose the guinea pig as his first mammalian model for producing ship beriberi. For those interested in scurvy, it was a fortunate choice. He enlisted the help of Theodor Frölich, a pediatrician with a special interest in infantile scurvy, when his animals began to show something that resembled that disease.[9]

## Guinea pig scurvy

So much for the background to the experiments; what did they acually show? In the first series of tests, sixty-five animals were fed just a single grain, either whole, or milled to remove the outer layers, and baked into bread. All the animals died on these diets, on average after thirty days and

[3] Johnson (1954), 3–4.    [4] Holst (1911), 76.    [5] Ibid., 77.    [6] Holst (1907), 633.    [7] Carpenter (1984).    [8] McCollum (1964), 118–21.    [9] Johnson (1954), 8.

weighing 40% less than at the beginning. When the carcasses were opened the majority showed

*pronounced hemorrhages,* most frequently in the muscles of the hind-limbs . . . some haemorrhages in the ribs . . . and in tissues inside the lower jaw. . . . We further found a pronounced fragility of the bones . . . due to a fracture of the shafts just below the intermediate cartilages. . . . There was always looseness of the molar teeth, usually most were affected. . . . They were also somewhat greenish-gray instead of the normal pearly white.[10]

Microscopic examination of the tissues failed to show the kind of damage found in pigeons fed on the same diets, and comparable to the polyneuritis of beriberi. Several, but not all, of the guinea pigs showed a fatty degeneration of the heart muscle. The authors paid greatest attention to the "osseous system" (bones and cartilages) because these had shown quite specific changes in infantile scurvy, as discussed in the previous chapter. In short, they found the same characteristic changes in the animals.[11] Another pathologist described these in something approaching layman's language:

Roughly what happens is that the preparatory changes in the cartilage, before it is turned into bone, do not come off, or occur in some irregular way which . . . prevents it performing its ordinary function. The result is, that at the growing ends of bones – and it is particularly well seen at the junction of the bony to the cartilaginous parts of the ribs – instead of there being an orderly conversion of cartilage into bone, there is disorder. The end of the medullary cavity, instead of being active tissue, forming periosteal bone and being filled with bone-marrow, is filled up with a lot of connective tissue. . . . That wad of connective tissue is what gives the gross appearance [in x-ray photographs] . . . that at the ends of these bones there is a clear area.[12]

One obvious question was whether such changes could result from inadequate food intake (i.e., semistarvation), which occurred perhaps because the simplified diet became unpalatable. The authors, to test this hypothesis, gave three animals a ration of a good diet, but in much reduced amounts. They died after ten to twelve days, and their bone marrows showed changes of the type seen in humans who had died of wasting diseases, but quite different from those seen previously in the guinea pigs.[13]

In the next series of trials, various grains were fed with supplements of foods regarded as antiscorbutic – fresh cabbage, lemon juice, or apples. These supplements did not prolong the animals' life, but on postmorten examination the guinea pigs showed little or none of the signs characteristic of scurvy. The most common abnormality was edema, which was more characteristic of beriberi.[14] Next, they investigated the possibility that the condition arose because the grains were deficient in calcium salts and/or

[10] Holst & Frölich (1907), 635–9.    [11] Ibid., 647–50.    [12] Boycott (1917), 179.    [13] Holst & Frölich (1907), 654–5.    [14] Ibid., 659–61.

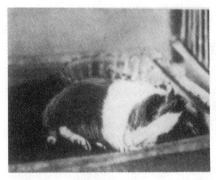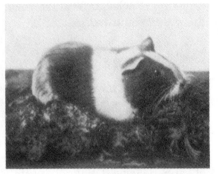

Typical postures of *(left)* a scorbutic guinea pig, lying so as to take the weight off a hind limb, and *(right)* a healthy guinea pig in the normal sitting position. (Cambridge University Press.)

had an ash that was too acid (i.e., the line of thought propounded by Almroth Wright). However, guinea pigs receiving grains liberally supplemented with calcium carbonate showed no protection from the scorbutic symptoms.[15] In view of the similarities between human scurvy, particularly as seen in infants, and the disease in guinea pigs, and of the similarities of dietary components that did or did not protect against the disease in each case, their final opinion was that the disease in guinea pigs was identical with human scurvy.[16] Also, as pointed out by L. G. Wilson, "They had shown that scurvy could be produced by diet and . . . cured by diet. Of the three theories of scurvy then existing, infection, toxication, and faulty diet, only the last was supported by their findings."[17]

A report making such bold and important claims is bound to be scrutinized on two counts: Is it correct, and if so, is it really original? We shall take the second point first. Ironically, Holst and Frölich were certainly not the first to produce guinea pig scurvy. In the early 1890s, a group in the U. S. Department of Agriculture's Bureau of Animal Industry had been using guinea pigs as model animals to study the nature of bacterial diseases in swine. In their annual report for 1895–6, they reported the death of an animal that had been inoculated and then added, in terms of an apology:

To explain the death of this guinea pig [No. 254] it will be necessary to record some facts which have been observed for some years in this laboratory. When guinea pigs are fed with cereals (bran and oats mixed), without any grass, clover, or succulent vegetables, such as cabbage, a peculiar disease, chiefly recognizable by subcutaneous extravasation of blood, carries them off in from four to eight weeks. The death of 254 was undoubtedly due to the absence of such food, as the attendant had neglected to provide it after the disappearance of grass in the fall of the year. Furthermore, No. 255 was weakened by the restricted diet and succumbed to an inoculation which otherwise might have had no visible effect.[18]

[15] Ibid., 663.    [16] Ibid., 669.    [17] Wilson (1975), 50–1.    [18] Smith (1895–6), 356.

One cannot help but feel that if this paragraph had been seen by any of the group of people engaged in the controversies in England at that time over the cause of scurvy, it would have aroused their interest in experimenting further with this species. But there was no systematic abstracting of scientific papers at that period, and even now it is uncertain that the contents of an annual report would be regarded as original material, especially whether such a peripheral issue unrelated to the title of the title of the report would be even mentioned in an abstract.

In 1902–3, another paper appeared in Germany, reporting the successful use of guinea pigs as models for Barlow's disease, which the author considered to result from the toxic effect of consuming strongly heat-sterilized cow's milk. He reported that animals receiving unheated cow's milk remained healthy for a full three months, whereas those receiving milks heated for ten minutes or more were dead within two weeks.[19] No details were given as to how the experiment was conducted, but another German scientist, who attempted to repeat the work, cited a letter from the first author that provided more information.[20] Even following these instructions, the second worker found that all his animals died. The survival time was twenty-nine days on average, and showed no relation with whether or not the milk supplied to them had been heat treated.[21] He also gave more detailed accounts of the changes in the bones of the dead animals. Holst and Frölich were doubtful as to whether these changes really corresponded to those seen in scurvy; when they themselves fed similar milks as the sole food of guinea pigs, they too found alterations in bone that differed from those seen in the animals receiving cereals.[22]

In a sense, therefore, Holst and Frölich's work was not entirely novel. However, they were not copying the German workers because they had not set out to produce scurvy, and began with quite different diets. Second, and most important, they were the first to relate the condition of guinea pigs to scurvy in general, as opposed to the supposed toxicity of cow's milk (of certain kinds) to infants. They were still perplexed by the relationship between the beriberi, as seen in Norwegian ships, and classical scurvy. In 1912, they considered that cabbage, which prevented both experimental neuritis in pigeons and experimental scurvy in guinea pigs, might be active in this way because it contained two different compounds, one preventing each disease.[23]

Between 1907 and 1912, they continued to be very active. I refer to just some aspects of their results. They studied the stability of the antiscorbutic factor in cabbage and cow's milks, and tried to develop methods of processing those foods so that they would retain their activity. They found that the presence of even small amounts of residual moisture in dried cabbage led to

---

[19] Bolle (1902–3), 356.    [20] Bartenstein (1905), 10.    [21] Ibid., 12.    [22] Ibid., 13–16; Holst & Frölich (1907), 653–4.    [23] Holst (1911), 80.

an increased loss of activity during storage.[24] They also found that milk heated at or above 100°C lost most of its antiscorbutic activity.[25] Finally, another member of Holst's group reported that fresh yeast and malt extracts were both inactive, but that germination of grains or peas resulted in their developing considerable activity.[26] These papers are in German, but in a later review, Holst also summarized most of the findings in English.[27]

After 1913, this group did no more experimental work. Holst says in his last review, in terms of an apology for not having applied a particular test, ". . . we have had nobody to assist us."[27] Frölich, in a memorial address after Holst's death in 1931, is reported to have said: "It engendered much bitterness in Holst's mind that the wretched economic conditions under which Norwegian science had to work in pre-war years, made it impossible to carry on a continuous programme within this most significant field of study."[28] Professor Torup, also of the University of Christiana and still attached to his ptomaine theory, was apparently hostile to Holst's ideas, and this may have hindered his receiving support. In any case, both Holst and Frölich went on to do important work as teachers, administrators, and clinicians, and they had already done enough to show clearly how the problems of preserving and identifying the antiscorbutic factor could be tackled, at last, in a systematic way.

In retrospect, it seems surprising that no other group was to follow up the Norwegian work for nearly a decade. There was, however, a whole group of other studies which, in combination with the work of Holst and Frölich, was beginning to form a definite pattern. In 1912, Gowland Hopkins, working in the University of Cambridge (and later to become its first Professor of Biochemistry), reported that rats stopped growing when fed a diet containing only purified protein, fat, carbohydrate, and minerals, but responded rapidly when given quite small amounts of cow's milk.[29] This was by no means the first time that such purified diets had failed, but this was the first appearance of such a result in a major, widely read scientific periodical, and the first to be accompanied with a discussion of the evidence of the need for small quantities of specific, though still unknown, compounds in a complete diet.[30] Ironically, later workers were unable to repeat Hopkins's specific experiment, but that did not affect its impact at the time. In the same year, Casimir Funk, a young Polish chemist working at the Lister Institute in London, made the startling proposal that four diseases – scurvy, pellagra, rickets, and beriberi – were due to a dietary deficiency of different factors, each of which was a nitrogen compound with an "amine" (basic) nature, so that the four could collectively be called "vitamines," as an abbreviation of

[24] Holst & Frölich (1912) 79–91; Holst & Frölich (1913), 338–41.     [25] Frölich (1912), 172–80.     [26] Fürst (1912), 129, 151–4.     [27] Holst & Frölich (1920), 261–3.     [28] Johnson (1954), 12.     [29] Hopkins (1912).     [30] McCollum (1957), 204–5, 211; Guggenheim (1981), 156–60.

"vital amines." [31] This again was not to stand up to later criticism, but the name "vitamine," (later changed to "vitamin") focused attention on the issue. Belief that there were indeed such compounds was strengthened by findings published in the United States in the following year. Both McCollum and Davis, in Wisconsin, and Osborne and Mendel, at Yale University, reported that *some* fats, but *not* others, contained a factor necessary for the growth of rats. [32]

Then, finally, in 1916 and 1917, there were reports from two groups, again in the United States, of experiments with guinea pigs, but each of them disagreed rather fundamentally with the conclusions of Holst and Frölich. First, a group in Chicago, Jackson and Moore, published two papers. (The "Jackson" here was *not* the coauthor of the earlier British experiment with monkeys.) They produced the disease in animals by feeding both raw *and* heated cow's milk, though not raw goat's milk. The lesions seen on post-mortem examination of the animals were virtually identical with those described by Holst and Frölich. However, these investigators were also able to colonize bacteria from minced tissues of their joints or muscles. These varied in their properties but were of the *Streptococcus* type. When cultures were grown and then inoculated into healthy guinea pigs, the animals lost weight and developed some lesions resembling mild scurvy. [33] However, they could not find bacteria in blood taken from live guinea pigs that were seriously affected by scurvy; nor was it possible to transfer the disease by passage of blood from one animal to another. [34] Later workers in the field did not consider their data to be really persuasive that guinea pig scurvy was caused by a bacterial infection, and no further evidence was to appear in support of the idea. Apparently some Russian physicians still regarded adult human scurvy as an infectious disease; [35] there was also one suggestion in this period that the disease was spread by lice. [36]

## The autointoxication theory

The next paper on the subject appeared in 1917, from McCollum's laboratory in Wisconsin, and it was a surpise indeed. McCollum had, of course, been a pioneer in developing the experimental evidence that unidentified trace factors were required for diets to be complete, and had characterized what he called "fat-soluble factor A" and "water-soluble factor B" as the outcome of his experiments with rats. [37] However, the conclusion drawn from his experiments with guinea pigs was that the scorbutic animals were suffering from *constipation* rather than from lack of an unidentified factor in

[31] Funk (1912).    [32] McCollum & Davis (1913) 174–5; Osborne & Mendel (1913).    [33] Jackson & Moore (1916), 480–6, 493–4.    [34] Jackson & Moody (1916), 512–14.    [35] Hess (1920), 30.    [36] Much & Baumbach (1917), 854.    [37] McCollum & Kennedy (1916), 497.

the diet: "The significance of this interpretation is far reaching. It removes from the list one of the syndromes [scurvy] which has long been generally accepted as due to dietary deficiency."[38]

Such a conclusion from a nutritionist as eminent as McCollum obviously requires detailed examination. In their introduction, the authors reasoned that, since rats did not show signs of scurvy on what for humans and guinea pigs would be a "scorbutic diet," one was faced with two alternatives: *either* guinea pigs and humans required something in their diet that rats did not *or* scurvy was not really a deficiency disease in the ordinary sense.[39] They obviously preferred the second: "As a working basis the assumption seemed warranted that all animals as highly developed as mammalia should require the same chemical complexes in the diet if growth and well-being are to be maintained."[40]

On a diet of rolled oats and fresh whole milk ad libitum (unrestricted), two of their guinea pigs lived and gained weight for three months whereas two others died with signs of scurvy after four and seven weeks respectively. For the authors, the survival of the first two was evidence that "nothing can possibly be lacking in the mixture of milk and oats," and it must therefore have been something else about the diet which made it difficult for the two others to tolerate it. On postmortem examination, very little food was found in their stomachs and small intestine, reflecting, as one would expect, the fact that an animal would eat very little in its last few hours of life. On the other hand, "the cecum was greatly distended with putrefying feces." This, it was suggested "resulted from the diet leading to pasty feces which the animal is unable to remove from its delicate cecum." This, in turn, could lead to "the absorption of toxic products of bacteriological origin which possess the peculiar pharmacological property of destroying the walls of the capillaries in those regions where hemorrhage is observed in scurvy."[41] The idea that intestinal autointoxication could result from constipation was commonly held at the time.[42]

In further experiments, McCollum and Pitz gave various supplements to the basic "oats and milk diet." Of the seven animals given the laxative, phenolphthalein, three survived. The remaining four, which developed scurvy, were younger and smaller. In another trial, six guinea pigs were fed on "oats and milk" for thirty-one days. The three survivors were then given liquid petroleum as a laxative, and two of these three then gained weight and survived for a long period.[43] Autoclaved carrots had much less protective activity than raw carrots. McCollum and Pitz attributed this to the change in physical properties with cooking, such that the fibers no longer had the laxative properties that they had in the raw state.[44] In experiments with supplements of orange juice, a higher proportion of the animals re-

[38] McCollum & Pitz (1917), 238–9.    [39] Ibid., 231.    [40] Ibid., 230.    [41] Ibid., 232–3.
[42] Alvarez (1924), 352–4; Whorton (1982), 216–23.    [43] McCollum & Pitz (1917), 248–9.
[44] Ibid., 237–8, 253.

ceiving raw juice remained free of scurvy as compared with those receiving autoclaved juice or a mix of citric acid, salts, and sugar made up to imitate the flavor of orange juice. These differences were not regarded as significant: "There is such great variation in the vitality of guinea pigs . . . to experimental diets that uniform and consistent results cannot be expected."[45] In another paper, describing work done in the following year, when McCollum had left Wisconsin, Pitz reported that adding lactose to "grain + milk" diets also prevented the development of guinea pig scurvy, and he attributed this to a modification in the intestinal flora to a more acidic, and therefore less "putrefactive," one.[46] He also mentioned that some animals recovered from scurvy without a change in their treatment.

We know that McCollum had not altered his opinions in the year following their joint paper, because he re-presented its argument at a symposium organized by the American Medical Association, and added that, along with "stagnation of the contents of the colon, the absorption of abnormal decomposition products of proteins may be responsible for the change observed."[47] Hess, the New York pediatrician, was converted to this view, and in the conclusions to his next paper wrote: "Infantile scurvy is not, however, a simple dietary disease. . . . [It] is an intestinal intoxication or an autointoxication . . . , the product of an unbalanced flora which is no longer controlled by a proper dietary."[48] However, he dropped this idea in the following year, after failing to find any characteristic changes in the flora of either guinea pigs or infants with scurvy.[49]

In the meantime, the group at the Lister Institute in London had begun to publish their extensive studies. This large group, led by Dr. Harriette Chick, consisted almost exclusively of women because nearly all their male colleagues had gone overseas to staff army medical laboratories dealing with problems arising in different combat areas during World War I (1914–18). Their priority was to provide practical advice for ensuring that soldiers on army field rations would not develop a deficiency disease.[50] They found that the response of guinea pigs to a "grain + raw milk" diet depended entirely on how much milk an individual animal drank.[51] Their assessment was that raw milk was only feebly antiscorbutic and that a consumption of more than 50 ml per day was needed to keep an animal free from scurvy. If milk went at all sour while in the cage, the animal would no longer touch it. In their opinion, it was essential that the daily consumption by each individual should be measured, for a proper interpretation of the findings. The variability in response of the Wisconsin animals could well be explained by their variable milk consumption, but this had not been measured.[52] When Chick and her colleagues gave their animals a diet of "oats, bran and autoclaved milk," there was a more uniform production of scurvy, and the addition of

[45] Ibid., 236–7, 250–2.    [46] Pitz (1918), 475.    [47] McCollum (1918), 939.    [48] Hess (1917), 353.    [49] Torrey & Hess (1917–18), 78.    [50] Chick, Hume, & MacFarlane (1971), 143–60. [51] Chick & Hume (1917), 159.    [52] Chick, Hume, & Skelton (1918), 146.

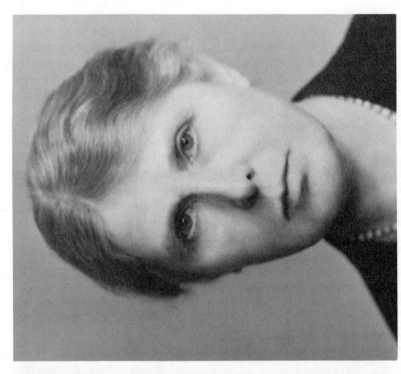

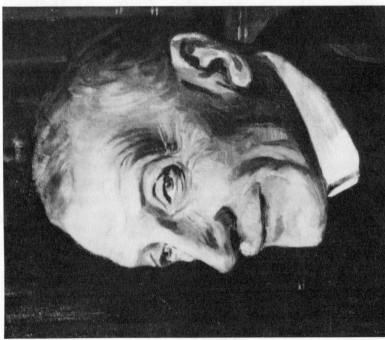

Portraits of Axel Holst (1860–1931), who first recognized that scurvy could be induced in guinea pigs by manipulation of their diet (Dr. Richard Forbes, University of Illinois); Harriette Chick (1875–1977), who made use of guinea pigs to assay the relative potencies of different "antiscorbutics" (Dr. Neige Todhunter, Vanderbilt University).

laxatives failed to prevent it.[53] Another study from the Yale Nutrition Laboratory also led to the conclusion that the "constipation theory" was totally mistaken: ". . . the cecum being full or partly full of semifluid feces is the natural condition for the guinea pig"; it was true that milk had a constipating effect on the guinea pig, yet it was the animals that drank the *most* raw milk that kept themselves free from the disease.[54] Hess and Unger, working in New York, came to the same conclusions, and both groups also directed their attention toward improving the basal assay diet so that the antiscorbutic factor would be its only deficiency.[55]

McCollum, in his scholarly *History of Nutrition*, published some forty years after these events, made no mention of his own incursion into the field. He merely said that "Holst and Frölich's description in 1907 of the experimental production of scurvy in guinea pigs fed dry or cooked diets, and its cure by feeding fresh vegetables or fruits, was a highly important contribution. It not only confirmed the vitamin hypothesis, but made available experimentally-induced scurvy in animals for study of the nature of the anti-scorbutic vitamin."[56] Why, then, did he seem, at the time, so determined to find alternatives to the hypothesis that scurvy (and also pellagra) was a vitamin deficiency? I suggest that it stemmed from the implicit assumption, in all his work up to that time, that the rat could be used as a model for mammals in general. If this were not the case, then the broader significance of his "fat-soluble A" and "water-soluble B" factors for rats would be cast into doubt. Yet he was confronted by his own observations that rats failed to develop characteristic deficiencies when given diets associated with either pellagra or scurvy. We know now, of course, that the sharp differences among single-stomached species in regard to whether or not they require a particular vitamin are confined solely to the antiscorbutic factor, and that the difference between rats and humans with respect to their requirement for pellagra-preventive factor(s) is a matter of degree only.[57] Therefore, the rat has, in fact, retained its general usefulness as a model in the study of human dietary deficiency, despite these two differences, but it cannot have seemed so at the time. McCollum's paper may therefore be considered now as an example of a scientist trying unconsciously to interpret new data in a way that would not disrupt the thread (or paradigm) that formed the basis of his previous work and perhaps, in turn, of his scientifc reputation.

## The biological assay of foods

Over the period 1912–19, there had been several demonstrations that the monkey was another species susceptible to scurvy if kept on an unsuitable

[53] Ibid., 147–8.      [54] Cohen & Mendel (1918), 427, 441.      [55] Hess & Unger (1918), 485.
[56] McCollum (1957), 217.      [57] Carpenter (1981), 240–3.

diet and was responsive to the usual antiscorbutics.[58] It was also confirmed at the Lister Institute that dried milk showed the same loss of antiscorbutic activity for monkeys as it had for guinea pigs.[59] Obviously, it was not practical to use these expensive animals for routine assays, but the fact that similar results could be obtained with a species so much closer to humans gave more confidence in the significance that could be attached to results obtained with guinea pigs.

With this new tool a whole series of different questions could be answered. One of the first to be addressed was how to minimize the loss of antiscorbutic activity in the cooking and preservation of vegetables. The experiments all showed how easily activity could be lost, and that, in general, a brief treatment at a high temperature was preferable to a slow process at a lower temperature.[60] Home canning of vegetables gave products of quite disappointing nutritional value.[61] On the positive side, it was discovered that juices expressed from vegetables, and particularly from swedes (turnips), could be quite potent.[62] This finding was soon to be made use of in Central Europe during the blockade that followed World War I, when many children were scorbutic and had to be given improvised, substitute diets.[63] The nutritional value of germinated pulses (peas and beans) prepared in different ways and assayed in the laboratory was also confirmed in 1918 among Serbian troops who had a scurvy problem.[64] They were also used successfully by a British Occupation Force in North Russia in 1919.[65]

The results from a series of assays with different types of citrus juice were particularly interesting in a historical context, and also extremely surprising. With freshly squeezed lemon juice a daily dose of 0.5 ml (milliliters) gave a small but definite degree of protection, 1.5 ml gave almost complete protection, and 2.5 ml gave full protection from scurvy in the four animals used for each assay. In contrast, the same three ascending grades of protection were given by 2.5, 5, and 10 ml, respectively, of fresh lime juice. The authors concluded that lime, when fresh, had something like one-quarter the activity of lemon juice. Samples of lime juice that had been "preserved" with 14% rum before they were issued to the Army and Navy, were also assayed, and with these neither 5 nor 10 ml was found to give protection to the guinea pigs. Of six commercial samples of lime juice, without added rum, only two gave any protection at a dose of 5 ml per day. One could only conclude that the lime juice available at that time had, in general, less than 10% of the activity of fresh lemon juice.[66] Part of this difference could be explained by losses that occurred during processing and storage, but a large part was also apparently due to a great, and previously unrecognized, dif-

[58] Hart (1912), 387; Harden & Zilva (1919), 246–51.     [59] Barnes & Hume (1919), 321.
[60] Delf & Skelton (1918), 462.     [61] Campbell & Chick (1919), 321.     [62] Chick & Rhodes
(1918), 775.     [63] Chick & Dalyell (1920), 268–9.     [64] Wiltshire (1918), 811–12; Chick &
Delf (1919), 213–17.     [65] Comre (1920), 209.     [66] Chick, Hume, Skelton, & Smith (1918),
735–6.

| Antiscorbutic material. | Dose c.cm. daily. | Age of juice (months). | Preservative. | Result. | Degree of protection against scurvy. |
|---|---|---|---|---|---|
| **LIME JUICE.** | | | | | |
| *Preserved.* | | | | | |
| 1. Army sample, Nov., 1916. | 5 | Uk. | Rum, 14% | Animals died of scurvy. | 0 |
| 2. Navy sample, March, 1917. | 5 | ,, | Rum, 14% | ,, | 0 |
| 2A. Navy sample, March, 1917.* | 10 | ,, | 0 | ,, | 0 |
| 3. Bombay samples (Willcox brand), Oct., 1917. | 5 | 2 to 4 | Alcohol and sal. acid. | ,, | 0 |
| *Crude.* | | | | | |
| 1. From Lewis and Peat, Feb., 1917. | 5 | Uk. | None. | Animals died of scurvy. | 0 |
| 2. From A. Riddle and Sons, April, 1917. | 5 | About 14 | ,, | ,, | 0 |
| 3. From L. Rose and Co., May, 1917. | 5 | 6 to 7 | ,, | Some protection in 2 cases out of 4. | + |
| 4. From L. Rose and Co., Sept., 1917. | 5 | 3 to 6 | ,, | Scurvy, but considerable degree of protection. | ++ |
| 5. Bombay crude juice, Oct., 1917. | 5 | 2 to 4 | ,, | Animals died of scurvy. | 0 |
| 5A. Bombay crude juice, Oct., 1917. | 10 | 4 to 5 | ,, | ,, | 0 |
| *Fresh juice.*† | 2·5 | 0 to 2 | ,, | Scurvy in all cases, but some protection. | + |
|  | 5 | 0 to 2 | ,, | Scurvy in 4 cases out of 6. | ++ |
|  | 10 | 0 to 2 | ,, | No scurvy. | +++ |
| **LEMON JUICE.** *Fresh juice.* | 0·5 | 0 to 2 | None. | Scurvy in all cases, but definite protection. | + |
|  | 1·5 | 0 to 2 | ,, | Protection almost complete in 2 cases out of 4. | ++ |
|  | 2·5 | 0 to 3 | ,, | No scurvy. | +++ |
| **FRESH RAW CABBAGE LEAVES.** | Grm. 0·5 | Fresh | — | Scurvy symptoms, but definite protection. | + |
|  | 1·5 | ,, | — | Protection. | +++ |
|  | 2·5 | ,, | — | ,, | +++ |

\* Without addition of rum.
† Limes imported monthly from Dominica, squeezed in laboratory, and preserved in refrigerator.
Uk., Unknown. Sal. acid., Salicylic acid.
+++ = Complete. ++ = Definite. + = Slight. 0 = No protection.

The responses of guinea pigs on a scorbutic diet to different supplements, showing the extremely low value of preserved lime juice. (From Harriette Chick's paper sent to the *Lancet* in 1918.)

ference between the activity of lemons and limes. Because of the importance of this last point, the comparison was repeated, this time with fourteen monkeys as subjects. Again the lime juice showed about one-quarter the activity of the lemon.[67] As the authors pointed out, these results threw a new light on the scandal of the outbreak of scurvy on the 1875 Arctic expedition. As we saw in Chapter 6, the trouble had followed the changeover from lemon to lime juice by the Navy.[68] We shall return to this matter in the final chapter.

The work at the Lister Institute on citrus juices also had an immediate, wartime application. The most serious dietary deficiency conditions had appeared in the British Army fighting in Mesopotamia (Iraq). The long supply lines and poor communications made it difficult to bring fresh fruit and vegetables up to the fighting lines. The British soldiers were beginning to show beriberi, whereas the Indian soldiers in the Army, who had different rations were free from beriberi but were seriously affected by scurvy – in 1916 alone there were over 11,000 cases among them.[69] The lime juice issued to the Army proved useless in practice, and the chief medical officer arranged a fresh supply from fruit grown locally that was more effective. By the following year, a better supply of vegetables had been organized.[70] Surprisingly, a partial failure of the potato crop also led to a small epidemic of adult scurvy in 1917 in Britain itself, mostly among men living in lodging houses.[71]

Experiments were also carried out with guinea pigs to test Almroth Wright's "acidosis" theory. None of a number of tests with sodium citrate, or with other salts yielding an alkaline ash, produced any improvement;[72] however, it was not until 1934, when an experiment was run on his own terms, that Wright finally conceded that he had been in error.[73]

The last application of the guinea pig assay in this research, and the one to have given the most important results in the long run, concerned the isolation of the antiscorbutic factor from active materials as a preliminary step toward its chemical identification. The quarry now needed a name. Because McCollum had already called the factors needed for growth in his rats "A" and "B," it seemed natural to call the antiscorbutic factor "accessory food factor C."[74] However, this was a clumsy phrase, and people had already become used to the term "vitamines." The chemists did not like the term because there was no reason to believe that these factors really were "amines." The suggestion was finally made that the "e" be dropped to leave "vitamins," which retained the idea that these factors were "vital," without implying a particular chemical structure.[75] There now began a series of

---

[67] Ibid., 736–7.    [68] Ibid., 737–8.    [69] Willcox (1920), 73, 75.    [70] Ibid., 74–5.    [71] Harlan (1917), 46.    [72] Holst (1908), 725; Lewis & Karr (1916–17), 21–22; Faber (1920), 140–1; Lepper & Zilva (1925), 588.    [73] Holt (1972), 48.    [74] Drummond (1919), 80.    [75] Drummond (1920), 660.

races – one for each of the vitamins – to be the first to isolate the pure chemical.

## The isolation of the vitamin

As early as 1675, Andreas Moellenbrock, a pharmacist in Leipzig, had attempted to isolate the antiscorbutic principle from the leaves of scurvy grass. He obtained crystals from the pressed juice, but was unable to prove their activity.[76] But now there was an animal model, and the first step in the attempt to concentrate vitamin C was made by Funk in 1913.[77] From 1918 on, the challenge was taken up in a systematic way by Zilva and a series of colleagues, working in the Biochemistry Department of the Lister Institute. Their first finding was that when the citric acid in lemon juice was precipitated with calcium carbonate and alcohol, the activity still remained in solution.[78] This was confirmed in infants.[79] The problem was that when the solution was evaporated to dryness, the activity was easily lost. Various techniques were tried, but the work proceeded slowly because a new, sixty-day feeding trial was required after every step.

In fact, the isolation was first achieved by a Hungarian scientist, Albert Szent-Györgyi, who was working for a short period in Hopkins's laboratory at Cambridge on a problem with quite a different objective.[80] He was interested in the individual biochemical reactions that allowed the oxidation of nutrients in both plant and animal tissues and their release of energy. This requires some amplification: The final products of oxidation of foods are carbon dioxide ($CO_2$) and water ($H_2O$). A sugar such as glucose ($C_6H_{12}O_6$) is gradually oxidized in a long series of steps. Some of these consist, not in the addition of oxygen, but rather the removal of hydrogen, which, in another series of steps, finally reacts with oxygen to yield water. Oxidation can therefore take the immediate form of dehydrogenation. Putting this in diagrammatic form, we might have:

(a) $$AH_2 + B \rightarrow A + BH_2$$

(b) $$2\,BH_2 + O_2 \rightarrow 2\,B + 2\,H_2O$$

In this series of reactions, when one compound is "dehydrogenated" (or oxidized), another is "hydrogenated" (or "reduced"). In the first reaction, B is "reduced" to $BH_2$; in the second, oxygen is "reduced" to water. In the 1920s, there was an obvious interest in discovering what compounds, like B in our scheme, could act in living tissues as both donors and acceptors of hydrogen. Szent-Györgyi had observed that there was a particularly high concentration of a powerful "reducing" (i.e., hydrogen-donating) chemical

[76] Lorenz (1953), 322–3.  [77] Funk (1913), 81–2.  [78] Harden & Zilva (1918), 259–62, 267–8.  [79] Harden, Zilva, & Still (1919), 17–18.  [80] Szent-Györgyi (1928), 1387–94.

in the adrenal cortex.[81] This is the core (or cortex) of the small gland that lies just above the kidneys in most animals. For this reason it is also known as the "suprarenal" (above the kidney) gland. He measured the amount of "reducing factor" in samples by their power to decolorize iodine. A well-known property of reducing agents was that they converted the bright yellow iodine to a colorless iodide:

$$A \cdot H_2 + \quad I_2 \quad \rightarrow A + \quad 2\,HI$$
$$\text{(iodine)} \qquad \text{(hydrogen iodide)}$$

He could therefore follow the factor through different procedures by a reaction that required only a few minutes rather than the months needed for Zilva's guinea pig assays.

After a study of the properties of the "reducing factor" (r.f.), its final isolation from all the other chemicals present in living material was achieved by the following steps:[82]

1. It was extracted from chilled and minced adrenal cortex by shaking with methyl alcohol, and bubbling through with carbon dioxide to prevent its having contact with oyxgen.
2. The filtered extract was then mixed with a solution of lead acetate, which precipitated r.f.
3. The precipitate, separated by further filtration, was suspended in water, and sulfuric acid was added. The r.f. dissolved, and lead sulfate was precipitated.
4. The filtrate was evaporated to dryness in a vacuum.
5. The solids were reextracted with methanol, and steps 2, 3, and 4 were repeated.
6. The solids were dissolved in acetone, and when an excess of light petroleum was added, crystals of r.f. gradually precipitated.

The yield was 300 milligrams (mg) per kilogram of starting material, with a total reducing activity about one-half of that originally present. He also obtained the same product from orange juice and from extracts of cabbage.[83]

Szent-Györgyi then studied the chemical nature of his crystals. First he determined their equivalent weight, that is, the weight combining either with one gram (g) of hydrogen *or* with the weight of another compound that, in turn, will combine with 1 g of hydrogen. The equivalent weight of iodine is 126.9 g. In his test, to 4.99 mg of the crystals dissolved in water, an iodine solution was added until no more iodine was taken up. At this point, 7.18 mg iodine had been added.[84] By proportion, therefore, 126.9 g iodine would react with 88.2 g r.f. This would be the relative weight of the molecule compared to that of hydrogen *if* the molcule donated only one hydrogen atom. If it donated two or three atoms, the molecular weight would be approximately 176 or 265, respectively, and so on.

To discover the correct multiple, Szent-Györgyi used Barger"'s micromethod for determining molecular weights. This method took advantage of

[81] Ibid., 1393.    [82] Ibid., 1394–6.    [83] Ibid., 1399–1401.    [84] Ibid., 1397.

a phenomenon found to be generally true – that the vapor pressure of water (or any other solvent) above a solution is reduced by having another compound dissolved in it, but that the exent of this decrease depends on the *number* of molecules dissolved, and *not* on their character. Also, if two solutions are separate but have a common enclosed space above them, vapor gradually distills from the solution with a lower concentration of molecules to the one with a higher concentration.[85] He therefore dissolved 9.0 mg r.f. in 0.5 ml water and distributed this into four very fine glass tubes; he arranged that above an air gap, a further length of a "comparison" solution was added, and that the ends were sealed. The four comparison solutions contained, respectively, 1.5, 3.0, 6.0, and 12.0 mg urea per 0.5 ml water. With solution 1, the r.f. solution gained volume, whereas with solutions 3 and 4, the urea gained volume; with solution 2, no movement was detected. Therefore, it was concluded that 9 mg r.f. had approximately the same number of molecules as 3 mg urea. But the molecular weight of urea was known to be 60, thus, by proportion, that of r.f. was close to 180. From the previous information, we can see that this corresponded most closely to twice the equivalent weight of 88.2, that is, to 176.

Other analyses had detected only the elements carbon, hydrogen, and oxygen in the crystals. The actual quantities of carbon and hydrogen were measured by burning 4.6 mg of the crystals in a stream of dry air and trapping the water vapor and carbon dioxide that evolved with separate absorbents and measuring their increases in weight. The values obtained were 40.7% for carbon and 4.7% for hydrogen; and by difference, this left 54.6% for oxygen. Carbon and oxygen atoms were known to have, respectively, twelve and sixteen times the weight of a hydrogen atom. Therefore, on the assumption that the molecular weight was 176 times that of hydrogen, he could calculate that each molecule had the following number of atoms:

$$\text{Hydrogen:} \quad \frac{176 \times 4.7}{100} = 8.3$$

$$\text{Oxygen:} \quad \frac{176 \times 54.6}{16 \times 100} = 6.0$$

$$\text{Carbon:} \quad \frac{176 \times 40.7}{12 \times 100} = 6.0$$

Within the expected limits of experimental error, especially when such small amounts had to be used, and knowing that even a trace of residual moisture in the crystals would raise their apparent hydrogen content, these results indicated a molecule containing six atoms of carbon (C), eight of

[85] Reilly & Rae (1939), 630–2.

hydrogen (H), and six of oxygen (O).[84] In the usual chemical terminology, this was written $C_6H_8O_6$.

Several very common sugars, including glucose and fructose, had the molecular composition $C_6H_{12}O_6$ and were classified as "hexoses," the "hex" referring to the *six* carbons, and the "ose" to their being sugars. Because he did not know the actual structure of his molecule, Szent-Györgyi wanted to call it "ignose" or even "godnose," but the editor of the *Biochemical Journal* objected, and he had to give it the alternative name of "hexuronic acid."[86]

The paper contained no claim that hexuronic acid might, in fact, *be* vitamin C but, as one would expect for someone working in Hopkins's laboratory, the question had arisen. In his discussion, Szent-Györgyi said: "The reducing substances of lemon juice have been made the object of a thorough study by Zilva, who established relations between vitamin C and the reducing properties of the plant juice."[87] Hopkins is reported to have said, around 1930: "We sent a sample to Dr. Zilva in London and were told that it had been proved not to be vitamin C. He never told us what specific tests he made but his report was accepted as reliable since he had been very active in vitamin C research for several years."[88] Certainly, Zilva repeatedly said in his papers that the reducing factor could not be the actual vitamin, though it seemed to act as a protective factor for it. The reasoning behind this was that when his concentrates, prepared from lemon juice, were oxidized under most conditions, they lost their reducing activity and, when tested with guinea pigs, also their antiscorbutic activity. However, under some conditions of mild oxidation within a plant juice, the reducing activity would disappear rapidly, whereas the antiscorbutic activity would remain for a short time thereafter.[89]

For Zilva it would, of course, be a terrible blow if hexuronic acid were to prove to be the compound he had worked for fifteen years to isolate. Here was someone else, who in one year, and without a single animal experiment, had isolated and characterized a compound, whereas he, Zilva, had proceeded systematically step by step for fifteen years, and had continually emphasized in his papers the difficulties of obtaining such an unstable material. After the work on hexuronic acid had been published, Zilva again argued that it could not be vitamin C, partly because he had made extracts that were still impure but that were at least as antiscorbutic as hexuronic acid could be – when one calculated how much could be present in the original juice on the basis of its reducing power.[90] Also, there was a feeling from the work in progress at that time on other vitamins that they would all be found to be present in foods in even smaller concentrations than that of hexuronic acid in orange juice (i.e., 100 mg recovered from 1 liter). There had already been examples of investigators who claimed to have a pure vitamin, the

[86] Szent-Györgyi (1963), 7–8.     [87] Szent-Györgyi (1928), 1401.     [88] King (1979), 2681.
[89] Connell & Zilva (1924), 638.     [90] Zilva (1932), 690.

activity of which was later traced to a small contaminant of the main product.[91]

In the next period, from 1928 to 1932, Szent-Györgyi spent a year in the United States at the Mayo Clinic where he prepared a larger quantity (25 g, still less than 1 oz) of his crystals from the adrenal glands supplied to him by large slaughterhouses. On returning to Cambridge, he sent one-half of his stock to Professor Haworth of the Department of Chemistry at the University of Birmingham in England, who had a special interest in the conformation of the atoms within molecules of carbohydrate (i.e., compounds of C, H, and O, only). Szent-Györgyi used the remainder to study its role in both plant and animal tissues. In 1932, he returned to Hungary to take up a professorship, and, just when his store was nearly exhausted, he found another rich source of the compound in paprika (Hungarian red pepper) and was able to prepare over one kilogram, and distribute supplies to other laboratories.[92]

In the same period, Dr. Glen King, at the University of Pittsburgh, had also been wrestling with the problem of the isolation of vitamin C from lemon juice.[93] After five preliminary papers reporting advances in its concentration and characterization, King and Waugh published a note entitled "The Chemical Nature of Vitamin C" in an issue of Science dated April 1, 1932, reporting that they had obtained crystals from lemon juice which showed all the characteristics of Szent-Györgyi's hexuronic acid, and that feeding 0.5 mg per day to guinea pigs protected them from scurvy.[94] Then, two weeks later, a note appeared in Nature entitled "Hexuronic Acid as the Antiscorbutic Factor," authored by Svirbely and Szent-Györgyi, that gave almost the same information resulting from a fifty-six-day assay with guinea pigs.[95] Svirbely had moved some months earlier from King's laboratory to Hungary.

At the time there was quite a flurry as to who and which country should be given the credit for "discovering vitamin C." Fifty years later, this seems unimportant. In his recollections published in the Annual Review of Biochemistry in 1963, Szent-Györgyi made this comment:

One day a nice young American-born Hungarian, J. Svirbely, came to Szeged to work with me. When I asked him what he knew he said he could find out whether a substance contained Vitamin C. I still had a gram or so of my hexuronic acid. I gave it to him to test for vitaminic activity. I told him that I expected he would find it identical with Vitamin C. I always had a strong hunch that this was so but never had tested it. I was not acquainted with animal tests in this field and the whole problem was, for me too glamourous, and vitamins were, to my mind, theortically uninteresing. "Vitamin" means that one has to eat it. What one has to eat is the first concern of the chef, not the scientist.[92]

[91] Harris (1933), 264-5.    [92] Szent-Györgyi (1963), 8.    [93] King (1953), 220-2.    [94] King & Waugh (1932), 357-8.    [95] Svirbely & Szent-Györgyi (1932), 576.

This is a very strange final statement. In any case, he received the Nobel Prize for Physiology and Medicine in 1937, "in recognition of his discoveries concerning the biological oxidation processes with special reference to vitamin C and to the fumaric acid catalyst." [96]

## The synthesis of ascorbic acid

The next problem was to determine the actual arrangement of the atoms in hexuronic acid – now renamed ascorbic acid. This would , in turn, provide a guide to the synthesis of the compound. As far back as the 1860s, it had been appreciated that chemical compounds seemed to obey prescribed rules,[97] one of which was that each element behaved as if it had a certain number of "hands" ("valency bonds"), each of which had to be joined to a "hand" of another atom in a compound formula: hydrogen had one, oxygen had two, and carbon had four. Thus we have the simple compounds:

$$H-O-H \qquad O=C=O$$

$$\begin{array}{ccc} H & H & H \\ | & | & | \\ H-C-C-C-H \\ | & | & | \\ H & H & H \end{array}$$

　　(Water)　　　(Carbon dioxide)　　　(Propane, gas)

It was gradually worked out that certain groupings conferred characteristic properties on compounds.[98] Thus, an "—O—H" grouping, added to a hydrocarbon (C and H only) to form an alcohol, reduced its boiling point and made it more soluble in water. Thus:

$$\begin{array}{ccc} H & H & H \\ | & | & | \\ H-C-C-C-O-H \\ | & | & | \\ H & H & H \end{array}$$    (Propyl alcohol or 1-propanol, liquid)

Also, logically, there should be two propyl alcohols and, in fact, there was a second one with slightly different properties:

$$\begin{array}{ccc} H & H & H \\ | & | & | \\ H-C-C-C-H \\ | & | & | \\ H & O & H \\ & | & \\ & H & \end{array}$$    (Isopropyl alcohol or 2-propanol)

However, there were no other possible models because other versions that appeared to be different could be superimposed on each other by turning the model left to right or by inverting it, for example:

[96] Hammarsten (1938), 45.　　[97] Leicester (1956), 181–8; Ihde (1964), 304–9.　　[98] Ihde (1964), 324–8, 1270–5.

$$
\begin{array}{ccc}
 & \mathrm{H} & \mathrm{H} & \mathrm{H} \\
 & | & | & | \\
\mathrm{HO} - & \mathrm{C} - & \mathrm{C} - & \mathrm{C} - \mathrm{H} \\
 & | & | & | \\
 & \mathrm{H} & \mathrm{H} & \mathrm{H}
\end{array}
\quad \text{or} \quad
\begin{array}{ccc}
 & \mathrm{H} & \mathrm{O} & \mathrm{H} \\
 & | & | & | \\
\mathrm{H} - & \mathrm{C} - & \mathrm{C} - & \mathrm{C} - \mathrm{H} \\
 & | & | & | \\
 & \mathrm{H} & \mathrm{H} & \mathrm{H}
\end{array}
$$

(with an additional H above the O in the right-hand structure)

And, in fact, no more than two alcohols having three carbon atoms could be found. The only other compound with the formula $C_3H_8O$ had quite different properties, and these were consistent with the formula:

$$
\begin{array}{cccc}
 \mathrm{H} & \mathrm{H} & & \mathrm{H} \\
 | & | & & | \\
\mathrm{H} - \mathrm{C} - & \mathrm{C} - & \mathrm{O} - & \mathrm{C} - \mathrm{H} \\
 | & | & & | \\
 \mathrm{H} & \mathrm{H} & & \mathrm{H}
\end{array}
$$

(Methyl ethyl ether)

There are also many examples which fitted a model in which atoms were joined by *two* valency links (or a double bond):

Propylene          Acetone

It had also been a common observation that where a model required a double bond between two carbon atoms, the compound was very reactive and would readily add on two other atoms. It was therefore described as an "unsaturated" bond. A $C=O$ bond did not seem to show this property, but the explanation, in terms of electrical charges, would take us too far from the point at issue. "Acetone" is an example of a traditional (nonsystematic) name, given to a substance before its structure was known. The systematic name is 2-propanone, because the $C=O$ group is a ke*tone*, which in this molecule is found on the second carbon, numbering the carbons from either end of the chain. To go one step further in this series of examples, three-carbon compounds containing more than one oxygen atom were known. One compound, glycerol, had all the properties of an alcohol, whereas the other, propionic acid, was an acid:

Glycerol          Propionic acid

One argument for the idea that both oxygens were attached to the same carbon in the model for propionic acid was that even formic acid ($CH_2O_2$), with only one carbon, showed the same acidic properties, and the only possible model for it was:

$$H-C\begin{array}{c} \diagup\!\!O \\ \diagdown O \\ \phantom{xx}\diagdown H \end{array}$$

The "—COOH" group is called a "carboxylic" group. The —OH group here is acidic, meaning that a positive hydrogen ion (proton) can dissociate or break off because the negative charge left on the oxygen can be "shared" (to put it crudely) with the second oxygen attached to the carbon.

Another complication was that two-dimensional representations (i.e., flat pictures) were not fully realistic. Evidence accumulated that the carbon valency "arms" were better represented as pointing out symmetrically in space as though three of them formed the legs of a tripod and the fourth pointed vertically upward (i.e., a tetrahedron). Even for oxygen, there were reasons to believe that models would be more realistic if the arms were not pictured as being opposite (i.e., at 180°) to each other, but rather much closer, that is, at an angle of approximately 105°. These two changes accorded with the evidence that organic compounds frequently formed rings.

One of the great achievements of organic chemists over the period 1875 – 1930, was to work out the structures of sugars from studying what reactions they underwent, and successively fitting different possible models.[99] For example, the structure of the sugar fructose ($C_6H_{12}O_6$) was worked out as:

The convention in drawing such structures was that the ring was to be viewed slightly from above, as a flat table, with the thicker bonds representing the near side of the table. Where there is no doubt of their position, the connections of the hydrogen atoms are not shown. Rings with one oxygen and either four or five carbon atoms were common and seemed to be stable;

[99] Ibid., 344–57; Haworth (1938), 1–9.

It is interesting that such rings also did not unduly strain the valency angle in three-dimensional models.

It was with this sort of knowledge that chemists began to study ascorbic acid. Like fructose, and also glucose, it had six carbons and six oxygen atoms, but had only eight hydrogens. It was, therefore, more oxidized (or dehydrogenated) than common sugars; yet paradoxically, it was still a reducing agent, i.e., readily giving up two more hydrogens. For a short time, it was thought that the structure might be:[100]

However, it was found that the mild oxidation of ascorbic acid (so that it lost two H atoms) also resulted in its losing its acidity. Yet the whole structure remained intact because the two hydrogen atoms could be added back to re-form the ascorbic acid. In the model above, the carboxylic acid group would still be present in the oxidized form. Therefore, in 1933 the Birmingham group, on the basis of many additional pieces of evidence, proposed the following structure:[101]

The acidity comes from the —OH group that is indicated with an arrow.[102] The structure at this point is similar to that of the acidic —OH group in phenol (carbolic acid), though at that time, there was no known example of a compound that had such a grouping which gave an acid with the strength of ascorbic acid.[103] After very mild oxidation (loss of 2H) to give dehydroascorbic acid, the potential acid group on this model disappeared:

[100] Micheel & Kraft (1933), 274.    [101] Herbert et al. (1933), 1270–5.    [102] Tolbert et al. (1975), 55.    [103] Hirst (1953), 416.

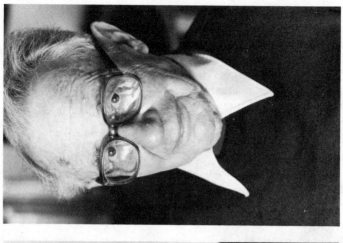

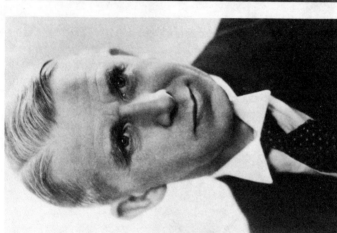

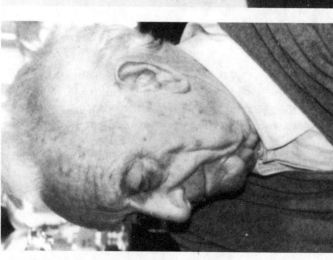

Three scientists associated with the isolation of vitamin C and its synthesis. *Left to right*: Albert Szent-Györgyi (1893 –   ), who first isolated the pure compound (National Foundation for Cancer Research); Sir Norman Haworth (1883 – 1950), who led the team that discovered its chemical structure (University of Birmingham); Tadeus Reichstein (1897 –   ), who first developed a method of synthesizing the vitamin on a commercial scale (*Roche Magazine*, Basel, Switzerland). Szent-Györgyi and Reichstein were each quite young when they did the work referred to, and their photographs were taken at least 50 years later.

It was this latter compound that had misled Zilva because it no longer had reducing activity, but guinea pigs were able to convert it back to the vitamin form. Under stronger conditons of oxidation and even in the presence of dissolved oxygen, if there were copper salts present to act as a catalyst, the change went further and was irreversible.

Because no one could actually *see* a molecule, the designing of models may have seemed like a game with no relation to reality, but not for long. Still in the year 1933, and using the model as their guide, both the Birmingham group and a Swiss group reported that they had achieved the synthesis of ascorbic acid,[104] and, furthermore, that the synthetic products were as active for guinea pigs as the natural vitamin.[105] This result can be stated so briefly that one can miss both its practical importance and the magnitude of the scientific achievement. It exemplifies the extraordinary advances made in twenty-five years, as compared with the previous two centuries. A writer in the 1950s went so far as to suggest that "the development of organic chemistry in the last 100 years may represent the most remarkable use of logical reasoning of a non-quantitative type that has ever taken place."[106] The speed with which this was done may also give a misleading impression. Haworth and Hirst, in their short communication, acknowledged the contributions of nine other chemists at different stages of the synthesis.[107] Also, of course, they still had intact the team that had gained so much experience from working out the structures of the sugars.

In 1937, Haworth was awarded a Nobel Prize in Chemistry for his work on both carbohydrates and vitamin C.[108] This was the same year in which Szent-Györgyi was similarly honored. Reichstein, the leader of the Swiss group, took out a series of patents with the pharmaceutical company Hoffman–La Roche for the commerical production of the vitamin, which yielded a considerable financial reward.[109] Holst, who made it all possible, died in 1931 without any special honors and is not even listed in the *Dictionary of Scientific Biography*.[110]

---

[104] Haworth & Hirst (1933), 645; Reichstein, Grussner & Oppenheimer (1933), 1019. [105] Haworth, Hirst, & Zilva (1934), 1155–6. [106] Leicester (1956), 187–8. [107] Haworth & Hirst (1933), 646. [108] Haworth (1938), 1. [109] Reichstein (1984), 14–15. [110] Johnson (1954), 15.

# 9

## Needs and uses for vitamin C (1935–1985)

One obvious change in scientific activity in the past fifty years, as compared with earlier times, is the extraordinary growth in the rate of publication of scientific papers. Even in 1934, L. J. Harris, in his review of one year's work on vitamins, apologized for being able to refer to only one-quarter of all the papers published, though he still had seventy-seven references relating to vitamin C.[1] *Chemical Abstracts*, in its collected index of papers for the five years ending 1981, had some 5,000 entries under the heading of "ascorbic acid." If this chapter is to retain the interest of the nonspecialist reader, it will have to be highly selective. There are, in any case, several excellent and easily available volumes that review recent advances in knowledge of the biochemistry of ascorbic acid.[2]

At the beginning of the period, many of the studies were making use of the newly developed method of chemical analysis for vitamin C. This was done, at first, by very simple measurement of the reducing power of solutions. In general, such values still seem to be close to the truth in most cases. However, various refinements were developed for particular types of foods.[3] One class of chemicals that reacted like true vitamin C in the original procedure were the "reductones," which are formed when carbohydrates are strongly heated, as in the frying of potatoes. The true loss of the vitamin that occurs with this sort of cooking was not, at first, appreciated.[4] Chemical analysis was quick and easy, but there was always the danger of error, so that guinea pig assays remained a "court of appeal."

Most of the analyses have been applied to foods, and to determining the possible effects of different kinds of food production and processing on

---

[1] Harris (1934), 247, 289–91.     [2] King & Burns (1975); Counsell & Hornig (1981); Hughes (1981a); Basu & Schorah (1982); Seib & Tolbert (1982).     [3] Olliver (1954), 253–6.     [4] Steele, Jadhav, & Hadziyev (1976), 240–1.

the vitamin. For example: Is the vitamin C content of tomatoes lower when the yield is increased with high levels of artificial fertilizers? It seems from the literature that it can be.[5] Does a rapid pasteurization process for cow's milk at a relatively high temperature cause less damage to the vitamin than a longer procedure at a lower temperature? In general, the answer has been that it does.[6] An unexpected finding was that the vitamin in milk could be destroyed quite rapidly with exposure to light.[7] Many studies also showed the great destructive effect on the vitamin of foods coming into contact with even very small amounts of copper or copper salts.[6] This last point may have been of significance in the controversies over the value of heated milks for infants, if some of the equipment used included copper parts. It must also have lowered the antiscorbutic value of lemon or lime juice that had been pumped through copper pipes.

Chemical analysis was also used to study why it was that most animal species did not need the vitamin. Every land animal tested was found to have ascorbic acid in its tissues. The animals that did not "need" it – that is, did not need to have it in their diet – were found to have a mechanism for making it for themselves. The exact mechanism for vitamin C production was traced in rats by feeding glucose and other compounds that had been "labeled" by replacement of some of their ordinary carbon atoms with radioactive carbon (which has a molecular weight of 14 rather than 12). Then ascorbic acid was later extracted from the tissues, isolated by modern methods, and tested for radioactivity. With feeding of labeled glucose, there was considerable conversion to ascorbic acid; with glucuronic acid, there was even more.[8] These and many other observations led to the conclusion that in rats (later, the same observations were made for other species as well) the sequence of reactions involved in the biosynthesis of the vitamin was:

Gulonolactone    Ascorbic Acid

Those species that cannot make ascorbic acid can make gulonolactone; however, they lack just one final enzyme, L-gulonolactone oxidase, which is

[5] Erdman & Klein (1982), 505.    [6] King & Waugh (1934); Hartman & Dryden (1965), 68–9. [7] Kon & Watson (1936), 2275–8; Hartman & Dryden (1965), 66–8.    [8] Gupta, Chaudhuri & Chatterjee (1972), 890; Chatterjee, Majumder, Nandi, & Subramanian (1975), 24–6.

required to remove two hydrogen atoms and so form the vitamin.[9] It has been suggested that the common ancestors of humans and primates on the evolutionary tree lost this enzyme some 25 million years ago. Fruit-eating bats and many birds have also been found to require the vitamin in their diet, and so have the fish and insects studied so far. Therefore, these species have all relied, as we humans have, on the synthetic powers of the plant world in order to obtain it. Among those species that have the enzyme, it is strange that in the more primitive ones it is found in the kidneys, whereas in the more advanced species it is found in the liver.[10] There has been speculation as to why and how this change could have occurred on at least two occasions in the course of evolution. At any rate, these findings do support the idea that ascorbic acid is of uniform importance in animal tissues.

The compound may, of course, prove to have many additional functions, but the best defined at present is its role in the final stages of the production of collagen, the principal protein in connective tissue. The protein is first synthesized with the usual range of amino acids. Then some of the proline and lysine units in the peptide chains are oxidized so as to contain a hydroxyl group. This is then of service for the final cross-linking between individual molecules to provide a strong, elastic sheet. The enzyme proline hydroxylase has been extracted and isolated from animal tissues, and has been found to require both ferrous ions ($Fe^{2+}$) and ascorbic acid in order to act on the proline units.[11] Such a function for ascorbic acid, is, of course, consistent with the observed abnormality of connective tissue in cases of scurvy. Other workers have drawn attention to the increased level of histamine in the blood of both humans and guinea pigs deficient in ascorbic acid. Because stress can also cause such an increase, it has been suggested that the increased histamine level could explain the historical association between scurvy and stress, and also some of the hemorrhagic effects of scurvy.[12]

### Experimental scurvy

Another question of obvious interest was to what extent could human scurvy, as seen clinically, be explained purely by a deficiency of ascorbic acid? It was surmised that, in practice, if a diet were poor enough to result in overt scurvy, it was likely to be deficient in other nutrients also. Fortunately, there have been volunteers willing to eat a deliberately unbalanced diet to the point of inducing disease.

The forerunner of this kind of experimentation was an eccentric young English physician, William Stark. He had studied in Glasgow and Edinburgh, and presumably attended William Cullen's lectures on the application of chemistry to medicine. He came to London in 1765 in search of a hospital appointment, but was not successful in this. He became acquainted

[9] Sato & Udenfriend (1978), 34–5.    [10] Ibid., 36–8.    [11] Tuderman, Myllylä, & Kivirikko (1977), 345.    [12] Clemetson (1980), 665–7.

with Benjamin Franklin, who was there as Agent for the Pennsylvania Assembly and already well known for his scientific work. Franklin may have impressed Stark with his arguments for a simplified diet. At any rate, in June 1769, and at age twenty-nine, Stark began a series of experiments on himself to test the effects of simplified diets on health. For the first twelve weeks he lived on bread and water with a little sugar. By then he was "dull and listless," and his gums were swollen and bled easily. For the next three weeks he took a more varied diet and "quite recovered." Then he returned to bread or flour with various supplements in turn – olive oil, butter, suet, a little cooked lean meat, and then honey. By the end of December, his gums were again purple and swollen. Apparently he consulted Sir John Pringle about his condition and was advised to reduce his salt intake. On February 23, he died, presumably of scurvy.[13]

The twentieth-century volunteers were more fortunate. In October 1939, John Crandon, a resident surgeon attached to Harvard Medical School placed himself on a diet of bread, crackers, cheese, eggs, beer, pure chocolate, and sugar with supplements of yeast and all the known vitamins other than vitamin C. For the first two months only, he also ate seven ounces of well-cooked meat per day and a little cream. At the beginning of the trial, chemical analysis of his blood plasma for ascorbic acid gave a value of 1.0 mg/100 ml. After three weeks, the value had fallen to 0.1 mg, and from six weeks on, none could be detected. The "white cell + platelet" fraction of his centrifuged blood gave a value of 28 mg/100 g when first measured, eight days into the experiment, and fell to a nondetectable value only after eight weeks without vitamin C.[14]

Crandon had continued his surgical work all this time. After twelve weeks, he began to develop a feeling of fatigue, but no physical signs developed until the nineteenth week. Then his skin became dry and rough and hair follicles on the buttocks and the back of the calves began to show little hard lumps or "plugs" at the base. This "hyperkeratosis" had previously been thought of as a sign of vitamin A deficiency, but other tests showed a normal level of vitamin A in the blood and no night blindness (loss of visual adaptation to low illumination) – the first sign of mild deficiency of this vitamin. After twenty-three weeks on the diet, and seventeen weeks with no detectable vitamin C in his plasma, Crandon first began to show small hemorrhages on his lower legs. However, there was still no obvious change in his mouth and gums; nor did he have even mild anemia or edema, or show heightened susceptibility to infection.[15]

The subject also had two wounds deliberately inflicted in his back. The first, made after thirteen weeks on the diet, showed normal healing ten days later, but the second, made after twenty-six weeks, showed no healing after

[13] Drummond & Wilbraham (1935), 459–62.     [14] Crandon, Lund, & Dill (1940), 353–4.
[15] Ibid., 355–8.

ten days. At this point Crandon was given a fatigue test, and he found that he could run at seven miles per hour for only sixteen seconds, and showed rapid exhaustion in other tests. He was then given 1,000 mg of ascorbic acid by intravenous injection each day for a week. A subjective improvement was noticed in the first twenty-four hours, and the second wound healed rapidly in the following ten days.[16]

The next experiment of this type was carried out at Sheffield in England during World War II; the volunteers were conscientious objectors to military service. The basic diet included a number of foods such as milk, dehydrated meat, potatoes, and carrots, which would all have contributed vitamin C if they had not been cooked in special ways. The milk was aerated for thirty minutes at 70°C with one part per million of added copper. Dried potato strips were boiled in large volumes of water, left to stand in the water for ninety minutes, then mashed, and kept hot for thirty minutes before being served. It was calculated that the daily intake of vitamin C was less than 1.0 mg and probably less than 0.5 mg. The levels of other vitamins and of iron were all satisfactory.[17]

After a period in which they received 50 mg supplementary ascorbic acid per day, ten of the volunteers received no more of the vitamin for a test period of 26–38 weeks. Ten others received either 10 mg or 70 mg per day. Placebos (dummy supplements) were used so that, until deficiency symptoms appeared, neither the subjects nor the examining clinicians knew to which group they belonged. The results were then very similar to those already recorded for Crandon's experiment on himself. It took between four and eleven weeks for the plasma levels of vitamin C to fall almost to the limit of detection, but no serious consequences were seen for a considerable period. After seventeen weeks, the subject whose plasma level had fallen fastest showed some hyperkeratotic follicles on his upper arm; four weeks later, six of the ten were showing them, and after twenty weeks all were doing so, with hemorrhages in six of them.[18] (Although the hyperkeratotic follicles were unexpected at the time of these two experiments, a French description of scurvy cases at sea in 1802 had reported, together with all the usual signs, that "the whole of the skin presented at the root of the hair small round spots of the colour of wine lees.")[19]

It was only after thirty weeks without vitamin C that changes began to be seen in the gums. By the thirty-sixth week, nine out of the ten were showing gross changes: The gums became purplish, swollen, and spongy, with areas of necrosis and bleeding. The authors of the final report also commented on things they did *not* see. There were no significant weight changes, nor any indication of edema or anemia; neither were there changes in white cell counts nor in apparent susceptibility to infections such as colds. Wounds

[16] Ibid., 362.     [17] Bartley, Krebs, & O'Brien (1953) 6, 56–67.     [18] Ibid., 8–9, 90–109.
[19] Pinkerton (1812), 891.

inflicted in the period from thirteen to twenty-six weeks into the experiment all healed normally; those made after this did not. Subjects also complained repeatedly of pain and stiffness in their joints.[20]

In the twenty-sixth week, a routine chest x-ray of one subject revealed an abscess in one of the vertebrae which was interpreted as an active tubercular lesion. When the x-ray taken at the beginning of the trial was reexamined, a slight shadow could be made out in the same position, indicating that the abscess was already in existence. He was immediately dosed with ascorbic acid and given conservative treatment in hospital. The tuberculous process healed, and three years later there was no evidence of any active process. It was thought interesting that this subject should also have been 'the one to develop obvious scurvy most quickly; and it seemed likely (though not, of course, proven) that the development of tuberculosis was precipitated by the deprivation of the vitamin. Three weeks later, the one woman in the group (who had the same family name, and was of similar age to the one discovered to have tuberculosis, and so may well have been his wife) also asked to receive a vitamin C supplement. She had begun to show scurvy at a rate of development similar to that of the men.[21]

In the thirty-sixth week of the experiment, the first "special incident" (to use the language of the report) occurred. One of the group, a twenty-two-year-old student, the day after performing an agility test that involved heavy physical exercise, woke up in severe pain and breathing with difficulty. His blood pressure was very low, and he appeared to be critically ill. He was immediately taken to hospital and given 1,000 mg ascorbic acid by injection. He made an uninterrupted recovery. It was considered probable that this was a cardiac attack brought on by scorbutic hemorrhage. This subject was one of the most severely affected at the time.[22]

Two and one-half weeks later, another subject, who had shown relatively few signs of deficiency "woke during the night with a constrictive pain in the chest which was intensified by deep breathing." Listening to the heart beat with a stethoscope, the physician heard a systolic murmur; the electrocardiogram also showed some changes. The diagnosis was uncertain but seemed consistent with a local scorbutic hemorrhage in the heart. The subject was given large doses of ascorbic acid, and within twenty-four hours the pain and systolic murmur had disappeared.[23]

In view of these "incidents," the remainder of the group were then each given a daily supplement of 10 mg ascorbic acid. All six showed distinct improvement after two weeks; after eight weeks their skin appeared normal, except for a slight brown color remaining where there had been hemorrhages. Their gums were completely normal after ten to fourteen weeks. The seven who received 10 mg ascorbic acid from the beginning also developed

---

[20] Bartley, Krebs, & O'Brien (1953), 9–11, 44–5.    [21] Ibid., 84–5.    [22] Ibid., 10, 80.
[23] Ibid., 10, 87–8.

no signs of deficiency during the trial, although the levels of vitamin in their blood plasma and white cells both fell almost as severely as in the "zero ascorbic acid" group.[24]

Before we leave the Sheffield study, one other point must be addressed. Their basal diet included "plum jam . . . given to meet any possible criticism that factors included under the term vitamin P were omitted."[25] Szent-Györgyi's group in Hungary, after it was proven that his "hexuronic acid" was antiscorbutic, came to believe that lemon juice also contained a second factor that was necessary for capillary walls to retain their normal strength and permeability, and was essential for guinea pigs.[26] They called it vitamin P ("P" for permeability). A number of papers appeared giving results that seemed to support the general claim, but disagreeing as to which chemical factor was active, and some of the studies could not be replicated later.[27] By 1939, Glen King (Szent-Györgyi's old rival), in a review article, drew together "further evidence that vitamin P does not exist, at least as an essential factor for guinea pigs."[28] This has remained the general opinion.

The third study of experimental scurvy to be discussed was carried out over twenty years later in the United States. Four male volunteers, who were all prisoners, consumed for 100 days a liquid, purified diet based on casein, sucrose, starch, oils, and added supplements of minerals, vitamins (other than C), and the amino acid cystine. This mixture contained absolutely *no* ascorbic acid. The subjects were required to walk some ten miles a day, and they kept approximately constant weight on their 3,000-calorie diet.[29]

The observations were very similar to those seen in the other studies except that signs of deficiency appeared earlier – skin changes in 8 to 13 weeks and gum changes in 11 to 19 weeks. The authors suggested that this might have resulted from the more complete removal of ascorbic acid from the diet.[30] After 100 days, the subjects were given doses of 6.5–34.5 mg ascorbic acid per day. Even the subject receiving only 6.5 mg lost all signs of scurvy.[31]

## Recommended allowances of vitamin C

With increasing interest in nutrition and with so much new information becoming available, attempts began to be made in the later 1930s to draw up recommendations as to the quantity of each mineral and vitamin required in the daily diet. The League of Nations (the predecessor of the United Nations Organization) appointed a committee to draw up a set of international standards.[32] They had been asked to define "the principles of nutrition best

[24] Ibid., 13–14.   [25] Ibid., 6.   [26] Rusznyak & Szent-Györgyi (1936), 27; Bensáth, Rusznyák, & Szent-Györgyi, (1936), 798.   [27] Scarborough (1945), 271–2.   [28] King (1939), 401. [29] Hodges et al. (1969), 536–7.   [30] Ibid., 546.   [31] Baker et al. (1969), 558.   [32] Technical Commission on Nutrition, League of Nations (1938), 461.

suited to ensure the fullest development and the maintenance of the organism." With respect to vitamin C, they concluded "The adult's requirement is no doubt covered by about 30 milligrammes daily, which has been shown to be a curative dose for adults suffering from scurvy. There is evidence that the requirement of vitamin C is increased in, and following, febrile conditions." [33] (In some reports of this period, quantities of vitamin C were expressed in IU, i.e, international units; 1 IU was originally defined as the activity of 100 mg freshly squeezed lemon juice, then redefined as 0.05 mg ascorbic acid.)[34] Two papers published in Britain in this period concluded that intakes of 15–20 mg were also adequate, although, of course, they carried a smaller margin of safety.[35]

These standards were to become a factor in some important decisions that had to be made in Britain from 1939 on, with the outbreak of World War II. Because of the attacks on shipping and of priority going to military materials, space for imports of food had to be reduced as much as possible.[36] Imported citrus fruit had been providing a significant proportion of the vitamin C in the British diet. "Would it reduce the fitness and productivity of the people if these imports were entirely cut out?" Drummond, who had actually coined the term "vitamin" in general, and the term "vitamin C" in particular, was made of Chief Nutritional Adviser to the Government. He gave it as his opinion, that it would do no harm, *provided* that home production of potatoes was expanded and their consumption encouraged. It was also decided that "concentrated orange juice" (tested for its activity) would be made available as a free ration for pregnant women and children under two years of age.[36] Underlying this policy was the calculation that the ordinary pattern of the British diet would still provide at least 20 mg vitamin C for adults, and that this would be sufficient.

Undoubtedly there was some increase in the incidence of scurvy as the war progressed. In the hospitals of Edinburgh and Glasgow combined the average number of cases treated per year, prior to 1940, was under 50; this increased to 110 in 1941–42.[37] What was seen was typically "bachelor" scurvy, mostly in men over sixty-five years old. It appeared that these individuals did little cooking, and, when fruit became scarce, their low intakes of potatoes and vegetables became critical. One of the cases resulted from the patient's having been meticulous in following a diet prescribed for a gastric ulcer. Such cases had been reported previously in the 1920s and 1930s, both in Britain and the United States, when physicians had recommended fiber-free diets based on rice, milk, eggs, and white meats, without either fruit, vegetables, or a vitamin supplement.[38] Presumably, there would have been many more cases if the "doctor's orders" had been followed more conscientiously!

[33] Ibid., 475.      [34] Coward (1935), 710.      [35] Kellie & Zilva (1939), 163; Fox (1941), 313.
[36] Hammond (1954), 147–9.      [37] McMillan & Inglis (1944), 235.      [38] Martin (1931), 293.

Several studies were made of the status of the general population. Plasma concentrations of vitamin C were often low, but vitamin supplements for both children and adults seemed to have no effect on growth, incidence of sickness, or productivity.[39] In one large residential training school for boys in southern Scotland, the food was kept hot for many hours between cooking and meal times, resulting in great loss of vitamin C: The intake was estimated to be from 10 to 15 mg per day. In this instance, sixty boys who received supplements of 50 mg of ascorbic acid per day subsequently did have a rather better health record than those not receiving the supplement.[40] There was a high incidence of bleeding gums among servicemen, but this sign did not seem related to a marginal deficiency because vitamin C supplements were not found to reduce the incidence, whereas direct treatment was effective.[41]

In Norway, after the German occupation in 1940, there was a sharp decline in supplies of fruit, meat, milk, eggs, and fats. However, the population made up for this loss of calories by doubling their consumption both of potatoes and also of other roots and vegetables. The net effect was that the calculated average intake of vitamin C actually increased, and studies of vitamin C status confirmed that there was no problem of deficiency in the population.[42]

When the United States entered the war in 1941, the U. S. National Research Council (NRC) had just issued the first edition of their Recommended Dietary Allowances, which included 75 mg vitamin C for an adult man.[43] The U. S. Army endeavored to provide diets for their men that met the national standards. When large numbers of U. S. troops were stationed in Britain prior to the invasion of Europe, there was the ironic situation of two allied armies working together, one with apparently 2½ times the vitamin C requirement of the other and being supplied with grapefruit and other items rich in vitamin C, which the other army had been without for four years and were apparently none the worse for the lack of. It was, of course, a measure of progress that here were large armies in the field, and, in contrast to the experience of previous centuries, the discussions on their provisioning focused on how large a margin of safety was required, rather than on how best to deal with a devastating epidemic of scurvy.

The reasoning behind the NRC's higher recommendation was elaborated only in later editions of their publication. In the general introducton to the 1953 edition, it was stated that: "the recommendations are not requirements, since they represent, not merely minimal needs of average persons, but nutrient levels selected to cover individual variations in a substantial majority of the population and . . . to provide for increased needs in times

[39] Bransby, Hunter, Magee, Milligan, & Rodgers (1944), 78; Craig, Lewis, & Woodman (1944), 455–7.    [40] Glazebrook & Thomson (1942), 5, 13–15.    [41] Stamm, MacRae, & Yudkin (1944), 241.    [42] Hansen (1947), 264–6.    [43] National Research Council (1941), 5.

of stress. . . ."[44] In relation to ascorbic acid, they said that the levels recommended were some seven times the amounts required to protect against the gross signs of scurvy, because there was "evidence that such intakes may not be satisfactory for the preservation of optimal health through long periods of time. . . ."[45] One of the studies cited describes experiments with guinea pigs in which those that received 0.8 mg ascorbic acid per day grew as well as those receiving 5.0 mg per day, and showed no obvious sign of deficiency. Yet, when they were given a dose of diphtheria toxin, their teeth were severely injured, whereas the teeth of those receiving the higher level of the vitamin remained normal.[46] Another paper describes a study of mild gingivitis (inflammation of the gums) in Canadian servicemen. As in the earlier British study, vitamin supplements proved of no value in clearing up the condition, but when the condition had been corrected by local treatment, men who were then given 75 mg ascorbic acid per day did not have such an early recurrence as those receiving only 10 mg.[47] A later review of a number of studies indicated that about 30 mg per day was necessary for the maintenance of healthy gums.[48]

Another argument found in the papers cited in the 1953 report was that all animals that made their own ascorbic acid had levels in their tissues that were substantially higher than those found in guinea pigs receiving only the amounts needed to avoid survy.[49] It was argued from this that the higher levels were the "natural" ones. The NRC committee members believed that an intake of 75 mg resulted in tissue levels in humans similar to those in the "synthesizing" species.[44]

In 1974, the NRC issued a new set of recommendations in which the allowance of vitamin C for adults was reduced to 45 mg. The argument in favor of this reduction was presented very succinctly: "Studies of ascorbic acid turnover . . . in the adult human male indicate that an intake of 30 mg/day is sufficient to replenish the quantity of ascorbic acid metabolized daily. An intake of 45 mg/day will maintain an adequate body pool of 1500 mg."[50] This information was obtained from the repletion stage of the experiment carried out in the United States on four human volunteers which was already referred to.[31] When the repletion began, the subjects each received also a small dose of ascorbic acid labeled with a radioactive isotope of carbon. There was reason to believe that this would be handled in the body exactly like ordinary ascorbic acid and that a fraction would be incorporated into the body's store (or pool). Thus, by measuring the proportion of the ascorbic acid appearing in the urine in subsequent weeks and by measuring the proportion of the ascorbic acid that was radioactive, it was possible to estimate the size of the body stores and its rate of turnover. It

[44] National Research Council (1953), 1–2.    [45] Ibid., 19–20.    [46] King, Musulin, & Swanson (1940), 1071.    [47] Linghorne & McIntosh (1946), 108–17.    [48] Goldsmith (1961), 233.
[49] Lowry (1952), 431–48.    [50] National Research Council (1974), 63–4.

appeared "that on a high intake of ascorbic acid only a limited quantity of the ingested vitamin is equilibrated with the body ascorbate pool."[51]

Following this, further studies with radiolabeled ascorbic acid were undertaken, and the first results were also recalculated, making allowance for the variability between subjects; on this basis, and estimating that only 85% of the ingested vitamin was absorbed into the bloodstream, the next edition of the NRC booklet, published in 1980, raised the recommendation for vitamin C to 60 mg.[52] The British, Canadian, and United Nations (FAO/ WHO) allowances had remained at 30 mg.[53]

In the postwar period, the scale of manufacture of ascorbic acid in the United States increased from 17 tons in 1940 to about 3,000 tons in 1960, and in 1985 the total market was 16,000 tons. In the same period, the bulk price fell from $100 to as low as $6 per kilogram, despite the general tenfold decline in the purchasing power of the dollar with continuing inflation. In 1975, even the retail customer could buy a kilogram of the vitamin for $10.[54] At that price, a year's supply of the full RDA of 60 mg per day for an individual, which amounted to 22 g, would have cost no more than 22 cents, a sum which would have been earned in less than five minutes, even by an unskilled worker. The consumption of the synthetic vitamin in 1983 corresponded to nearly 200 mg per day per head of the entire U. S. population.

## Ascorbic acid in food processing

During World War II, there was increasing use of vitamin "pills" or other forms of supplements by the public, which continued into the postwar period; we shall return to this topic later in the chapter. The other immediate use for ascorbic acid was by food manufacturers to fortify (or enrich) their products. For example, black currants were a rich source of vitamin C, and the public had been educated to think of black currant juice as healthful, because of its vitamin content, as well as flavorful. However, when black currants were shipped in bulk for the manufacture of juice they had to have a preservative added, which resulted in almost complete loss of the vitamin. When the juice was prepared, synthetic ascorbic acid could be added, and the final product was still flavorful and could genuinely be promoted as a rich source of the vitamin.[55] Other "fruit" drinks were also fortified. Dehydrated potatoes, prepared as granules or flakes for "instant" reconstitution into mashed potatoes, had the same problem of loss of vitamin C. And, as we have seen, potatoes have served for some social groups as their major source of the vitamin. Again it was possible to develop a procedure for fortifying the dried products quite cheaply with ascorbic acid.[56]

[51] Baker et al. (1969), 557.    [52] National Research Council (1980), 75–6.    [53] Truswell (1976), 8.    [54] Anonymous (1984), 62; Pauling (1976), 160.    [55] Bauernfeind & Pinkert (1970), 223–32.    [56] Hadziyev & Steele (1970), 99–100; Bauernfeind (1982), 436–8.

In this way, the food industry became familiar with the use of ascorbic acid. At the same time, many other chemicals that had previously been used as food additives were being restricted by government orders because of suspicions that they might be harmful if consumed regularly over many years. It was natural, therefore, that studies should have been made of the possible value of ascorbic acid as an additive for improving the keeping quality or physical character of foods, and even of wines and beer.[57]

One industry that relied heavily on the use of additives was large-scale bread-making. It had been traditional knowledge that for a loaf to rise well and keep its own texture after leaving the oven, the wheat flour should be allowed to age for several months after the grain had been milled, and that the mixture of the dough with yeast should be allowed to "ripen" for some three hours before baking.[58] Then, finally the dough was placed in an oven. As it became warmer, the fermentation of the carbohydrates intensified and bubbles of carbon dioxide gas formed; when the temperature in the dough rose further, the wheat gluten "set" so that the bubbles did not collapse when the loaf cooled again. In order for bread to be mass-produced more economically, there was a strong incentive to shorten the time required for the early stages. Research showed that molecules of the protein, gluten, in the presence of oxygen, gradually formed cross-linkages that increased its sticky properties. It was found that these changes could be reproduced by adding a small quantity of an oxidizing agent to the flour, and about 10 parts per million of potassium bromate had commonly been used since the 1920s. Second, it was discovered in the 1960s that dough could be "ripened" without the three-hour delay if it were mixed (or beaten) very vigorously. However, the level of "improver" (chemical additive) needed to be increased if it was to do its work in a shorter period, and by this time, the tendency of government regulation was to enforce reductions, rather than to allow higher levels of chemicals in foods.[59]

As far back as 1935, it had been found that ascorbic acid was as effective an improver as potassium bromate. At the time this was of no practical significance, because ascorbic acid was then a rare chemical, but was of theoretical interest because it was a reducing rather than an oxidizing agent. By 1960, it was inexpensive and one of the few chemicals not under suspicion of toxicity. Further research indicated that it was first oxidized in the dough to dehydroascorbic acid which then participated in the oxidation of the protein. In the 1970s, most of the bread in Britain was made with the addition to the bread flour of 30 ppm (parts per million) of both potassium bromate and ascorbic acid. In Britain alone, it has been estimated that over 60 tons per year of ascorbic acid were being used for this purpose; some other countries have used it at higher concentrations. In another development, high-energy mixing could be avoided via the addition of an amino

[57] Bauernfeind & Pinkert (1970) 277–87.     [58] Chamberlain (1981), 89.     [59] Ibid., 90–101.

acid, but ascorbic acid was still required at 30–50 ppm. Unfortunately, none of the vitamin activity remained in the final loaf.[59]

In the late 1940s, ascorbic acid was also found to have possible uses in meat processing. Dipping fresh meat in a dilute solution of the chemical before placing it in a chilled display cabinet delayed by one day the change from a fresh red appearance to a staler brown. This use was prohibited in some countries as being "deceptive to the public," though it was claimed that the same result could be obtained by feeding animals a high level of ascorbic acid before their slaughter.[60] It continued to be used in fresh (un-cured) sausages, and has been of special interest as an additive in cured products.

The traditional "curing" of meat to bacon, ham, etc., involves their being pickled with a solution of salt and potassium nitrite (or potassium nitrate, which is then converted to the nitrite in the pickling bath). The fully cured meats could be stored with little risk of infection by the highly pathogenic organisms of the *Botulinus* family, even without refrigeration. The meats also developed an attractive, characteristic pink color, which resulted from a complex reaction between the nitrite and the muscle protein to form nitro-sylmyoglobin.[61] Concern over the safety of this type of processing came from the discovery that nitrite could also react with another class of com-pounds, secondary amines, to form nitrosamines, which could be carcino-genic at very low concentration.[62] Pressure was therefore applied on the food industry to find ways of curing meat with lower levels of nitrite. Ascorbic acid was found to be a useful additive in the development of an attractive color in "cooked cured meats" of lower nitrite content. It did not appear to have any synergistic effect with nitrite in protection against mi-crobial attack, but this property may be less important wth the advent of modern refrigeration of food both in retail displays and in homes.[63]

## *The megavitamin concept*

In 1966, Irwin Stone, an industrial chemist, put forward a rather startling concept. It was that humans and other primates were the victims of a genetic disease or an "inborn error of metabolism," i.e., failure to synthesize ascor-bic acid, which could be fully corrected only by supplying the amounts that were produced by the livers of animals, such as rats, which did not have this genetic defect. He calculated that, for an average man, the amount needed would be in the range of 1,800–4,000 mg, to be provided in a series of smaller doses throughout a day. Therefore, in studies in which researchers had been investigating the possible effects of an increased vitamin C intake on resistance to infection, with doses in the range of 100–200 mg per day,

[60] Ranken (1981), 107–8.     [61] Ibid., 107–9.     [62] Crosby & Sawyer (1976), 7.     [63] Ranken (1981), 112–21.

they had on this basis, still been using only about one-tenth of the "true" natural level.[64]

These calculations were based on earlier experiments with rats. In one study, it had been estimated that young rats produced in their liver 0.2 mg per hour per 100 g body weight. If a man weighing 70 kg (154 lb) were to produce ascorbic acid at the same rate (per 100 g body weight), the amount produced in twenty-four hours would certainly be approximately 4,000 mg (i.e., 4 g). However, these calculations were later criticized on two grounds: The first was that the data had been obtained under artificial conditions, and that the normal rat synthesized less. The second was that the nonsynthesizing species had developed mechanisms for using ascorbic acid more economically.[65]

In the following year (1967), Williams and Deason published a paper arguing that humans probably had great individual differences in their needs for vitamin C, with some requiring twenty times as much as others. These investigators argued that the Food and Drug Administration in the United States, and the medical profession generally, by thinking always in terms of the average person, "are overlooking and failing to develop a set of *major weapons* against disease." [66] The actual data presented in Williams and Deason's paper referred to the variability in individual growth rates within groups of guinea pigs, each of which was receiving a different level of ascorbic acid. From this it was concluded that a small proportion of these animals had an exceptionally *low* requirement for the vitamin.[67]

Roger Williams was in his seventies in 1967, but he had been well known for the discovery of the vitamin pantothenic acid, and had served twenty years earlier as a member of the Food and Nutrition Board, which is appointed by the National Research Council in the United States, and oversees the preparation of the Recommended Dietary Allowances. He was now to be joined by an eminent scientist with even more prestigious credentials. Linus Pauling was one of the very few recipients of two Nobel Prizes, the first for Chemistry in 1954, the second for Peace in 1963, and of almost every kind of honor given to a scholar of the first rank, including the Davey Medal of the Royal Society in England, the Pasteur Medal in France, and the National Medal of Science in the United States.[68]

The first paper by Pauling that was directly relevant to the present subject, appeared in 1968 under the title "Orthomolecular Psychiatry," which he defined as "the treatment of mental disease by the provision of the optimum molecular environment for the mind, especially the optimum concentrations of substances normally present in the human body." [69] He thought it probable that some people had a deficiency in the system that allowed suitable molecules to be transferred from the bloodstream into the

---

[64] Stone (1966), 133–4.    [65] Ginter (1979), 126.    [66] Williams & Deason (1967), 1641.
[67] Ibid., 1640.    [68] Press (1979), 5, 3865.    [69] Pauling (1968), 265.

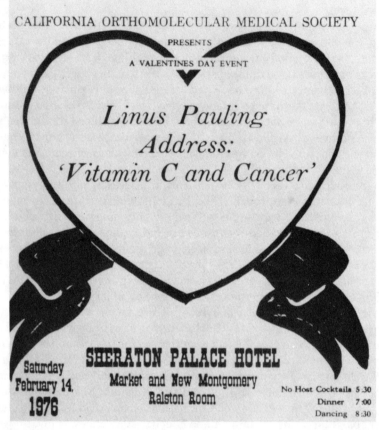

A poster illustrating the popular interest in the use of ascorbic acid as a megavitamin in the 1970s. (Author's collection.)

cerebrospinal fluid. With such a defect, an individual could have a vitamin or other nutrient deficiency in the brain without its being apparent in other tissues; furthermore, such a deficiency could possibly be countered by increasing the level of the nutrient in the blood so as to compensate for the inefficient transfer mechanism.[70] He also pointed out that other investigators had found the level of vitamin C, even in the circulating blood of schizophrenics, to be lower than that in normal subjects. "It is my opinion, from the study of the literature, that many schizophrenics have an increased metabolism of ascorbic acid, presumably genetic in origin, and that the ingestion of massive amounts of ascorbic acid has some value in treating mental disease."[71] This kind of treatment has since been termed "megavitamin therapy"; "mega" derives from the Greek and means "very large."

[70] Ibid., 270.    [71] Ibid., 269.

In 1970, Pauling argued that a consumption of some 2,000 mg ascorbic acid per day (as had been recommended by Stone on the basis of a comparison with the rate of its synthesis by rats) was not necessarily "unnatural," but rather, it could have been the normal consumption of humanity's ancestors at the time when the gene for its synthesis was lost – assuming they were living largely on green food supplemented with a little meat. He calculated, for the 110 raw natural plant foods listed in a table of food values, the quantity of vitamin C present in the weight of each that would supply 2,500 Kilocalories (i.e., the average daily energy requirement of humans who are not doing heavy work). The average from all these values was 2,300 mg. He suggested that this was an independent confirmation of Stone's estimate, although he accepted the idea that some other mutations that had occurred since the loss of synthesizing capacity, had probably resulted in a more efficient utilization of the vitamin.[72]

In the same year, Pauling also published the first edition of a bestseller book, *Vitamin C and the Common Cold*. In 1976 he published an expanded version, in which he said: "There is a continually increasing body of evidence that the optimum intake of vitamin C decreases both the morbidity and mortality with heart disease, cerebrovascular disease, and cancer, as well as infectious diseases in general." He also declared: "It is now my opinion that for most people the improvement in health associated with the ingestion of the optimum amount of ascorbic acid is such as to lead to an increase in life expectancy that . . . probably lies in the range twelve to eighteen years." [73] In 1979, he published *Cancer and Vitamin C* jointly with a Scottish surgeon, Ewan Cameron. In this they argued that the true optimal intake lay between 3,200 and 12,000 mg per day, and instanced that goats, of the same body weight as humans, had been found to synthesize 13,000 mg per day. They also said that "there is now little doubt that both the incidence and the outcome of cancer are closely related to the intake of this important substance." [74] In 1984, he himself was taking 12,000 mg per day, and increased this to 40,000 mg whenever he sensed that he was catching a cold.[75]

As Pauling himself acknowledged, the medical profession, and scientists in general, responded to his claims with considerable skepticism. For example, the low level of ascorbic acid in the blood of schizophrenics was attributed to their poor diet rather than to abnormal metabolism.[76] In connection with the argument of an evolutionary genetic disease, the logic was to be disputed. Even if the gorilla's daily feed included a particular quantity of vitamin C, it also included particular quantities of many other nutrients, and there was no reason to suppose that every one of these corresponded, in some miraculous way, to the exact optimum.[77] Another comment was that

---

[72] Pauling (1970), 1647–8.    [73] Pauling (1976), 2.    [74] Cameron & Pauling (1979), 107.
[75] Anonymous (1985), 6–7.    [76] McDonald (1958), 368.    [77] Jukes (1974), 1950; Hughes (1977), 121.

this evolutionary guessing game is a double-edged sword, for one might argue a quite different view, that our ancestors never did ingest such large amounts of vitamin C, that these amounts are more harmful then beneficial, and that this accounts for the success of the mutation which prevented manufacture of vitamin C. Such games . . . solve nothing. . . . Theory alone can never by itself provide answers to questions of benefit and toxicity. The answer must come from research designed to answer the specific questions at hand.[78]

With regard to the common cold, there had been, at the very least, twenty published experiments by 1979. Overall, the results suggested that the number of colds suffered by subjects on a high intake (i.e., 1,000–2,000 mg vitamin C) was not greatly reduced, but that their average duration and the average days of sickness for all reasons were shorter by about 30%.[79] Within the data there were also unexplained differences from one study to another, even when both were carried out by the same group. We shall consider just two studies carried out in Canada, which set out to use the conditions specified by Pauling, i.e., at least 1,000 mg per day normally, increased to 4,000 mg if a cold was coming on. It was his claim that, given in this way "protection against the common cold . . . becomes nearly complete."[80]

These two studies were "randomized double-blind trials." "Randomized" refers to the fact that whether a particular subject was assigned to the treatment or "control" (nontreated) group was not at the discretion of those running the study, but rather was determined by a prearranged order of appearance, to the particular treatment coded as A, B, etc. "Double-blind" means that neither the participating subjects nor the people collecting the data knew to which group they belonged. This was achieved by having tablets made up of lactose and citric acid which imitated the appearance of the vitamin C tablets and had a similar flavoring. The vitamin tablets were made from a mixture of sodium ascorbate and ascorbic acid, to mask the characteristic taste of the free acid alone. People who were not going to participate in the study as subjects were used to verify that it was not possible to distinguish the placebo from the active vitamin.[81] The two types of tablets were then given to a third party to be labeled A or B, so that those running the trial would also not know which was the active vitamin until all the results had been tabulated and the conclusions reached as to which group performed better. Only then was the code broken.[82]

One thousand volunteers, all of whom had said that they usually experienced at least one cold in the period from January to March, were recruited. The study covered this period in 1972. Nearly 200 subjects dropped out of the trial for some reason, usually loss of interest, but in almost exactly the same proportion from the two treatment groups, leaving just over 400 in

[78] Vander (1981), 104.     [79] Pauling (1976), 182; Briggs (1984), 4–6.     [80] Ibid., 47.     [81] Anderson, Reid & Beaton (1972), 503.     [82] Ibid., 504.

each. The results can be summarized as follows (asterisks are explained in the text):[83]

| | Gp. I (ascorbic acid) | Gp. II (placebo) | Gp. I value as % of Gp. II value |
|---|---|---|---|
| Episodes of illness/100 subjects | 138 | 148 | 93% |
| Total days with symptoms/ 100 subjects | 525 | 602 | 87% |
| Days confined to house/100 subjects | 130 | 187 | 70%** |
| Percentage of subjects ill at some time during trial | 74 | 82 | 90%* |

Even if the ascorbic acid had no effect, we would expect still some differences in the results for the two groups, simply because one could not be certain that the subjects in the two groups would be identical in their behavior. However, it was possible to work out the probability that a particular difference – or a greater one – would occur just by chance. In principle, the methods employed are comparable to those used in determining the chance that when a coin is tossed in the air, it will repeatedly land with the same face up, when there is really an equal chance for "heads" or "tails" in any single throw. There is a 50% chance that the second throw will be the same as the first, a 25% chance for three in a row, 12.5% for four, 6.25% for five, 3.12% for six, and so on. The convention in biological studies is not to consider a difference between the mean (average) values for two groups to be "statistically significant" unless the probability of so large a difference occurring just by chance is less than 5%. Thus, in the example of coin tossing, one would judge the bias to be "significant at the 5% level" only if the coin fell the same way six times in a row when tested.

Returning to the Canadian results, the difference in the "percentage of subjects ill at the same time" was greater than could have occurred by chance with a 5% probability, and the asterisk (*) against this row is the conventional symbol used to express this. The proportional difference in "days confined to house" was greater (i.e., 70%), and statistical analysis indicated that there was less than a 1 in 1,000 probability of its occurring just by chance (hence two asterisks, **).[83] In both groups, over 90% of the illness was of the "nose, throat, chest" type.

In a study carried out in the United States, there was reason to believe that

[83] Ibid., 505–7.

many of the subjects had, from the taste of the supplements, correctly guessed whether they were receiving the vitamin or the placebo. Further, it seemed that, among these subjects, those who guessed that they were receiving the vitamin had fewer days in which they considered themselves sick, whereas among the subjects that had not identified their supplement, there was no such effect. This indicated that subjects tended to feel less ill if they believed they were receiving treatment that they had some faith in.[84] In the Canadian study, the subjects were questioned, but there was no evidence that they had been able to identify which treatment they had been receiving. The researchers, who said that they had not expected to find any such response, could therefore only conclude that the ascorbic acid had in fact had an effect in reducing illness. On the other hand, the effect was not nearly as great as Pauling had predicted.

A second study was then carried out by the same group in Toronto, which was designed to test different levels of vitamin C, and to compare the value of a continuing supplement with one taken only when a cold was beginning. It was difficult to draw conclusions from the results. Two "placebo" groups, each of nearly 300 people, were used, with their "treatments" differing only in how many tablets they were to take, but their mean "days of symptoms" were 540 and 416 per 100 subjects, respectively, which was a significant difference. The six different groups receiving vitamin C all gave intermediate values, though lower than for the average of the two placebo groups.[85] Another pair of well-controlled trials carried out in Scotland also gave inconsistent results, with the first indicating a significant and substantial advantage from vitamin C, and the second showing no difference. Also, in the second trial, an additional group that had received isoascorbic acid (a chemical very similar to vitamin C, and also an antioxidant but with only one-thirtieth the vitamin activity) did show an improved health record.[86]

There has been much debate about the results of these and similar trials. It seems undoubtedly to be the case that some people are helped by large doses of vitamin C, but that not everyone is. It has been pointed out that volunteers for experiments tend to have a more than average interest in health and may not therefore be representative of the whole population. However, similar results have been obtained with unselected groups, such as servicemen or children in boarding schools. An example of the latter was a study made in Arizona at a boarding school for Navajo Indian children. With 320 subjects in each group, those that had received 1 or 2 g vitamin C per day (according to whether they were less or more than ten years old) for fourteen weeks had, on average, about 30% fewer days of illness than those that had received a placebo.[87]

As mentioned already, in 1979, Pauling, in collaboration with Cameron,

---

[84] Lewis et al. (1975), 510.    [85] Anderson, Suranyi, & Beaton (1974), 32–5.    [86] Charleston & Clegg (1972), 1402; Clegg & McDonald (1975), 974–5.    [87] Coulehan et al. (1974), 7–8.

published *Cancer and Vitamin C*. The first claim made by the authors was that patients with advanced, untreatable cancers had a greatly increased life expectancy and felt less ill if given very high doses (roughly 10,000 mg per day) of vitamin C. Cameron, the surgeon, said that he did not feel justified in carrying out a randomized, double-blind trial because he was convinced of the value of the vitamin for his patients, and it would therefore be unethical to withhold it from those who would be serving as controls. Instead they used "historical controls," i.e., the records of past patients whose condition appeared from the documentation to have matched that of Cameron's subjects at the point at which he began dosing with vitamin C. From this comparison, it was concluded that only 12% of the 1,000 controls survived for 100 days, and the corresponding value for the 100 subjects was 53%, with 16% surviving for as long as 400 days. The difference was similar, whatever the type of cancer being watched.[88] Very comparable results to those of Cameron and Pauling were later reported from a Japanese study, but again there was no strict randomization to "placebo" or "vitamin" treatment.[89]

A randomized, double-blind trial was carried out in the United States at the Mayo Clinic. After 56 days, 50% of the "vitamin" group and 40% of the "controls" were still surviving but by 100 days there were 19% of survivors in each group. Of the vitamin group, 63% reported some improvement in symptoms after the trial began, as did 58% of the controls. It was concluded that the differences were no greater than could have been expected to occur by chance, and that megadoses of vitamin C could not be recommended for such patients.[90] The authors pointed out that their patients had all previously received either irradiation or chemotherapy, which would have had a suppressing effect on their immune systems. In a subsequent trial at the Mayo Clinic, 100 patients with cancer originating in the colon or rectum, and who had not been given chemotherapy, received either 10,000 mg vitamin C or a placebo each day until there was an objective progression of the disease. This had occurred in 50% of those receiving vitamin C after approximately three months, and in the controls after four months. The difference was not statistically significant, but the study clearly showed no advantage from the use of ascorbic acid in this way.[91]

Many other scientists have explored mechanisms by which ascorbic acid might possibly inhibit the development of different kinds of cancer. One idea was that having ascorbic acid in the urine, as a result of a high, "saturating" intake, might reduce the incidence of bladder cancer. The reasoning behind this was that some chemicals excreted by the kidney could then become carcinogenic in the bladder as a result of reaction with oxygen. This might be prevented by the presence of ascorbic acid, which itself acts as an

---

[88] Cameron & Pauling (1979), 133–9.     [89] Murata, Morishige, & Yamaguchi (1982), 107–12.     [90] Creagan et al. (1979), 688–9.     [91] Moertel et al. (1985), 140–1.

"oygen scavenger" and might thus greatly reduce the oxidation of the potential carcinogens.[92]

Most work has been done on the possible effects of ascorbic acid in reducing the formation of nitrosamines. This has already been referred to in connection with the concern over the formation of these carcinogens during the traditional "curing" of meat with potassium nitrite. Nitrates are present in drinking water and in many vegetables, and can be reduced to nitrites in the mouth as well as the gut. Various amines are present in foods, and several workers demonstrated that nitrosamines could be formed from reaction of the two compounds in the gastrointestinal tract.[93] However, ascorbic acid reacted even more readily with nitrites, so that it might be expected to reduce nitrosamine formation. This has been demonstrated under some conditions;[94] however, with some amines the reverse happened, and nitrosamine production actually increased.[95]

Several papers have reported that cigarette smokers had lower levels of ascorbic acid in their blood than did nonsmokers with a similar intake of the vitamin. It was thought that chemicals absorbed into the bloodstream from the smoke in some way reduced the availability of the vitamin. It was concluded that, whatever the mechanism might be, it would be prudent for smokers to have a higher intake of vitamin C to compensate for this effect.[96] (It would, of course, be even more prudent to give up smoking.) Papers were also published indicating the value of a high ascorbic acid intake for subjects with asthma, but, as with so many claims for this vitamin, other studies failed to confirm such an effect.[97] Yet other investigators proposed that general nervous stress, or the "rat race," of modern life was sufficient to increase the requirement for the vitamin.[98]

While one group of investigators was focusing on the possible benefits to be derived from consuming up to 10,000 mg ascorbic acid per day, another group was concerned with possible deleterious effects of the practice. Because humans can metabolize ascorbic acid to oxalic acid, it was thought that the latter compound might be excreted in the urine at levels high enough to cause oxalate stones to form in the kidneys. Taking 1,000 mg per day was found to result in a doubling of the level of oxalic acid in the urine. However, still higher levels caused no further increase, perhaps because the enzymatic mechanism was already saturated.[99] Whether or not stones are formed also depends on other factors such as the pH (degree of acidity) of the urine, so that it does not necessarily follow that the risk would be increased by the higher intake of the vitamin, and as yet, no evidence has been published showing that such a complication can develop from the practice.[100]

[92] Schlegel (1975), 434–5.    [93] Oshima & Bartsch (1981), 216–19.    [94] Ibid., 219–21; Kim, Tannenbaum, & Wishnok (1982), 581–3.    [95] Hughes (1981a), 27–8.    [96] Pelletier (1975), 160–6; Stone (1972), 172–7.    [97] Irwin & Hutchins (1976), 845; Basu & Schorah (1982), 111.    [98] Lewin (1976), 141–2.    [99] Hughes, Dutton, & Truswell (1981), 277–9.
[100] Hanck (1982), 229–33.

The one commonly reported, short-term problem resulting from the ingestion of megadoses of vitamin C was diarrhea.[101] This was to be expected when the absorptive capacity of the small intestine was exceeded. The excess, reaching the large bowel, presumably stimulated fermentation there. The same result is seen when people with a limited capacity to digest lactose (milk sugar) eat products containing milk. Another effect of increasing vitamin C intake was that the absorption of some metal ions from foods was found to be increased. In the case of iron, this was thought to be beneficial because iron-deficiency anemia was a common condition.[102] On the other hand, it was also reported that the absorption of mercury, which is a toxic element, could be increased.[103] The availability of other metal ions, including copper and cadmium (another toxic element), was reduced.[104] Irwin Stone has summarized the evidence supporting the use of high levels of ascorbic acid for improving resistance to poisoning from lead and other heavy metals in the industrial environment.[105]

Because of the extent of the controversy and the conflicting results, it was to be expected that there would be no general agreement as to either the desirability or the safety of a continued intake of vitamin C at megadose levels.[106] Nevertheless, very large numbers of people have adopted the practice of taking supplementary vitamin C, usually in the form of pills, even though their intake of the vitamin from the foods that they eat exceeds the RDA.

In one survey of approximately 3,000 adults, chosen at random from an area in northern California in 1974, nearly 900 took such pills regularly and another 600 took them occasionally. Of those using supplements, some 250 took 1,000 mg or more per day. There was a strong tendency for the highest intakes to be taken by those with most education and the highest income. No difference was seen between men and women.[107] Interestingly, there was a statistically significant association between the amount of vitamin C consumed and "mean days in bed" per year, *but* it was in a different direction from that expected: Those who took *most*, spent *more*, that is, 8.0 days were spent in bed by the high-dose group whereas 3.1 days were spent in bed by the low-dose group.[108] Of course, it is always dangerous to assume a simple cause-and-effect from such a correlation. For example, we cannot conclude from these data that taking vitamin C made people ill. There are many alternative possibilities, one of which would be that people with chronic health problems were more likely to try to improve their general state by purchasing dietary supplements; another possibility might be that people who spent more time worrying about their health would also be more likely both to buy possible "health protectors" *and* to coddle themselves by staying in bed when they had a minor infection of some kind.

[101] Ibid., 236; Pauling (1976), 107–9.     [102] Solomons & Viteri (1982), 553–7.     [103] Hallberg (1981), 51–7; Hughes (1981a), 52.     [104] Solomons & Viteri (1982), 559–60, 566.     [105] Stone (1972), 152–6.     [106] Hughes (1981a), 47–53.     [107] Shapiro et al. (1983), 773–4.     [108] Ibid., 775.

Some further data are to be found in another study carried out, for quite a different purpose, in southern California in 1976. Out of a group of fifty nonvegetarian adults, twelve (i.e., 24%) took vitamin C supplements which contained approximately 400 mg on average.[109] From the data in the previous paper, one can imagine that such an "average" is, in no sense, a *typical* intake, but rather the result of a few taking megadoses of 1,000 mg or more and the remainder taking about 100 mg. A national survey carried out in the United States in 1971–4 obtained data for 20,000 people; 21% of these reported that they took vitamin or mineral supplements regularly, and another 11% took them occasionally.[110] On the assumption that the great majority of these supplements would have included ascorbic acid, it would seem then that in one country alone (with a population of some 250 million), at least 50 million on any particular day in the late 1970s were eating some of the crystals, the first few milligrams of which were isolated by Albert Szent-Györgyi in 1928. Meanwhile, Szent-Györgyi himself was still working actively in his laboratory, seeking further discoveries.

[109] Calkins et al. (1984), 901.     [110] Shapiro et al. (1983), 776.

# 10

---

## *Retrospect*

The intention in the preceding chapters was to present findings as they appeared at the time. The purpose of this final chapter is to reexamine some of the more important recorded observations in the light of modern knowledge and to consider to what extent they can now be explained. In general, references to primary sources will not be repeated if they have already been given in earlier chapters. Nor will the megavitamin concept be reconsidered here, for it is too recent for any attempt at retrospective evaluation.

### *Classical scurvy and vitamin C*

The first point is that modern analyses confirm that the traditional sailor's diet on long voyages was almost totally lacking in vitamin C. Wheat flour, salted meat, oatmeal, dried peas, cheese, and butter all give essentially zero values;[1] therefore, it is not difficult to understand why scurvy should have appeared after twelve to sixteen weeks at sea. The wonder is that anyone on board, restricted to these supplies, should have escaped it.

But was the disease that developed on the old expeditions simply the result of a deficiency of vitamin C? Certainly the experiments carried out in this century demonstrated that eating an otherwise good diet, except for the omission of ascorbic acid, resulted, after a depletion period of several months, in characteristic signs described also in the earliest outbreaks – weakness, stiffness of the limbs, spots on the legs, and changes in the gums. But some of the old accounts also refer to other signs, one of which was edema, or what one early writer called "the wet scurvy, with hydropic tumefaction of the limbs, that pits under the fingers as if a man had altogether the dropsie."[2] This condition was seen particularly in ships returning from the East Indies and is now considered to have been beriberi.[3] Edema is

---

[1] Adams (1975), 4–174.    [2] Moyle (1702), 250–1.    [3] Creighton (1891), 593; Keevil (1957–8) 1: 100–1; Grmek (1966), 507.

a feature of "wet beriberi," now known to result from a deficiency of the B vitamin thiamine (also called vitamin $B_1$, or aneurin, in the older literature).[4] This compound, although present in all grains, is at a particularly low level in polished rice, which may have replaced wheat flour in the victualing of some European ships returning from the Far East.

Night blindness (nyctalopia) was another condition seen occasionally in scorbutic sailors. As mentioned in Chapter 5, the fact that the condition also occurred independently of scurvy made some observers believe that it was only a coincidence when they appeared together. It is now known that night blindness is one of the first signs of mild vitamin A deficiency.[5] Green food such as cabbage is a good source of both vitamin C and vitamin A (or, more precisely, its precursor, carotene). Sailors receiving butter and cheese in their rations would be obtaining vitamin A, but not C. On the other hand, those receiving potatoes or lemons would be receiving vitamin C but not A from these sources. With a diet deficient in both vitamins, depletion of A to the point of overt deficiency symptoms would normally take longer than the depletion of vitamin C, if the previous diet had been fairly rich in both factors. In contrast the bad effects of eating polar bear liver (described in Chapter 6) are now explained by its containing vitamin A at levels high enough to be toxic.

The association of rickets with infantile scurvy has also been discussed in Chapter 7. Rickets is now known to be associated usually with a lack of vitamin D, which is found in the fatty portion of milk, eggs, and livers, but is usually obtained in greater quantity from irradiation of the skin in sunlight.[6] Infants kept indoors *and* fed on evaporated or condensed products made from skimmed milk (i.e., with most of the fat removed) and starchy gruels would be expected to become deficient in both vitamins C and D, as many obviously did. There were some superficial similarities in the changes in the appearance of the bones in the two diseases, though they were quite different when studied microscopically,[7] and, as we saw before, one disease could be treated and corrected while the other remained.

Anemia has also been a common finding in cases of scurvy since procedures for measuring it were developed in the middle of the nineteenth century.[8] There are two main types of nutritional anemia. In the first, the red blood cells are, on average, microcytic (smaller than normal); this condition commonly results from a deficiency of iron in the diet and/or from hemorrhages.[9] The loss of blood could, of course, be external or internal. Because scurvy in an advanced form can result in characteristic hemorrhages around the long bones, this alone might cause anemia in a subject whose iron status is marginal. Lind said of some postmortem examinations: "The quantity of

---

[4] Goodhart & Shils (1980), 686–7.    [5] Ibid., 142–3.    [6] Ibid., 693–6.    [7] Follis (1958), 361–403.    [8] Cox (1968), 635; Reuler, Broudy, & Cooney (1985), 806.    [9] Goodhart & Shils (1980), 339–46.

effused stagnating blood was sometimes amazing: . . . almost a fourth part of this vital fluid had escaped from its vessels."[10]

The second type of nutritional anemia is classified as megaloblastic or macrocytic (large-celled). This condition can result from a deficiency of either of two B vitamins, folic acid or cobalamin (vitamin $B_{12}$).[11] For most people the greater part of their folic acid intake is derived from green vegetables. In studies of scurvy cases in recent years, where the blood picture has been examined in detail, megaloblastic anemia has been a common finding, and, in some cases, dosing with ascorbic acid has corrected this.[12] On the other hand, the subjects have typically been old men who lived alone and did minimal cooking, and thus ate little in the way of green vegetables or any other good source of folic acid. Also in some cases, dosing the anemic, scorbutic patient with folic acid stimulated the production of red blood cells, whereas dosing with ascorbic acid did not.[13] In the controlled studies of vitamin C depletion there has been no evidence of anemia developing. It has been suggested that the association of scurvy with this type of anemia may result from an ascorbic acid deficiency, making the utilization of an already marginal intake of folic acid even less efficient.[14]

In summary, the diets with which scurvy has been associated are clearly likely to be relatively deficient in a number of nutrients. Nevertheless, all of the evidence points to lack of ascorbic acid as primarily responsible for the characteristic signs of the disease. Can vitamin P, Szent-Györgyi's second factor, be ignored? There is certainly no evidence that guinea pigs require it when they have a good intake of ascorbic acid, nor that it will lengthen their survival when they are given a diet completely lacking vitamin C. However, there is good evidence that, in the intermediate situation, when they are receiving only marginal vitamin C, flavonoid compounds of the type found in orange peel do help to maintain levels of the vitamin in the tissues.[15] Possibly these compounds help to reduce losses of the vitamin by acting as general antioxidants.

## Antiscorbutic foods

A great number of foods were recommended as supplements to the sailor's diet in the period 1740–90, when the disease was such a serious problem. Many were suggested on the ground that their traditional diet was difficult to digest. Freshly baked bread, oatmeal, rice, cocoa, sugar, and molasses were all repeatedly recommended, but analyses have showed them to be devoid of vitamin C. Nor do analyses of the ingredients used to make

---

[10] Lind (1772), 496.   [11] Goodhart & Shils (1980), 252–5.   [12] Chazan & Mistilis (1963), 357.   [13] Will & Murdoch (1960), 502–4.   [14] Cox (1968), 650–1.   [15] Ambrose & De Eds (1949), 316; Hughes & Jones (1971), 551; Wilson, Price-Jones, & Hughes (1976), 661.

"portable soup," that is, dried animal offals, suggest that it would have had any intrinsic preventive value. It was indirectly of importance, as Cook himself stated, because it made a more palatable base for serving up green vegetables.

In general, analyses do confirm the opinion of writers such as Bachstrom and Trotter, who extolled the benefits of salads and "recent" (fresh) vegetables in "imparting a 'something' to the body (and) fortifying it against disease." [16] This is confirmed in Tables 10.1 and 10.2. Not only green leafy material, but also roots and tubers such as potatoes, turnips, and yams are healthful in this regard. However, these are all bulky to transport (at least 80% of their weight is water), and they cannot be stored indefinitely. Of the provisions that sailors could take with them, onions, which Lind had recommended, were a good source of the vitamin, and were also appreciated as a flavoring for other foods. Onions, when boiled, lose a large proportion of their vitamin C, but, because in the eighteenth century they were stored individually by the sailors themselves, they were presumably sliced and eaten raw.[17] The point often made in the 1700s, that *dried* leaves or herbs had lost their potency, has also been confirmed; to conserve their potency the drying must be carried out under special conditions that have been developed only since 1930.[18] Dried potatoes would have lost much of their vitamin content, but not necessarily all; how much would depend on the nature of the drying process and on the length and conditions of storage before they were reconstituted, cooked, and eaten.

Analyses also confirm that, among the fruits, the acid ones are generally the most potent. We shall return later to the controversy surrounding the quality of the "lemon juice" and "lime juice" issued to armies and navies. It is interesting that apples are relatively low: A medium-sized apple has been estimated to contain 6–8 mg of ascorbic acid, as compared with 60–100 mg in an orange. However, two apples per day, supplying about 12 mg, would still be expected to protect an adult from scurvy, even if the rest of the diet supplied absolutely none. And Trotter, in saying that apples in great quantity were curative and made a beneficial change from acid fruit, was almost certainly correct.[19] Berries, such as cloudberries, were prized as antiscorbutics in northern Europe, as were rose hips.[20]

However, it can be misleading to examine only the levels (i.e., concentrations) of the vitamin in different foods in order to assess their relative historical importance in the prevention of scurvy. For example, potatoes are by no means as rich in ascorbic acid as some fruits and vegetables, but they have been a cheap staple food eaten in quantity day after day, and were available during the winter when fruits and vegetables were scarce. Thus,

[16] Trotter (1804), 424.     [17] Norris (1983), 335.     [18] Hess (1918), 942; Delf & Skelton (1918), 462.     [19] Trotter (1786), 110–12; Trotter (1804), 421.     [20] Nordenskiöld (1881), 44, 480; Nicolaysen (1980), 303–5.

Table 10.1. Typical values for the vitamin C content of common items in European and North American diets

| | Weight of item (g) | Ascorbic acid (mg) | | Weight of item (g) | Ascorbic acid (mg) |
|---|---|---|---|---|---|
| *Vegetables* | | | *Fruit* | | |
| Broccoli (boiled), 1 cup | 155 | 140 | Strawberries, 1 cup | 150 | 88 |
| Cabbage (boiled), 1 cup | 170 | 40–50 | Orange (2½ in. in diameter) | 180 | 66 |
| Potato (baked in skin) | 200 | 30 | Banana (with peel) | 175 | 12 |
| Potato (boiled & reheated) | 200 | 5–15 | Apple (3 in. in diameter) | 180 | 7 |
| Green peas (sold frozen, then boiled), 1 cup | 160 | 20 | *Animal products* | | |
| Tomato (raw) | 100 | 20 | Liver (beef or lamb, cooked) | 85 | 15–30 |
| Carrots (boiled), 1 cup | 155 | 6 | Cow's milk (pasteurized) or yogurt, 1 cup | 250 | 2 |
| Lettuce (chopped), 1 cup | 55 | 4 | Butter, cheese, eggs, well-cooked meat or fish | All negligible or zero | |
| Bread, flour, margarine, chocolate, dried peas, or beans | All negligible or zero | | | | |

*Note:* One ounce is equivalent to approximately 28 grams (g).

Table 10.2. *Analytical values for some of the sailors' traditional antiscorbutics*

| | Ascorbic acid (mg/100 g or /100 ml for liquids) | | Ascorbic acid (mg/100 g or /100 ml for liquids) |
|---|---|---|---|
| Cloudberries | 80 | Cabbage, fresh | 45–60 |
| Cranberries | 5–10 | Sauerkraut (stored 1 month) | 10–15 |
| Gooseberries, fresh | 60–65 | Onions, fresh | 10 |
| Gooseberries, preserved (as recommended by Lind) | 0 | Onions, pickled | 0 |
| Apple cider (fresh, unpasteurized) | 4–5 | Lemon juice, fresh | 45 |
| Scurvy grass (leaves and buds) | 200 | Lime juice, fresh | 30 |
| Spruce pine needles | 65–200 | Orange juice, fresh | 48 |
| Spruce (leaves and young shoots) | 30–270 | Rob of oranges (juice concentrated ten fold to Lind's directions), fresh | 240 |
| Spruce (fresh aqueous infusion) | 14–100 | Rob of oranges as described above, after 28 days of storage | 60[a] |
| Spruce (fermented aqueous infusion) | <0.5 | Wine (French varieties) | <0.5 |
| Freshly sprouted barley seed | 30–100 | Miscellaneous foods (sugar, molasses, fresh bread, rice, vinegar, coffee, portable soup) | All negligible or zero |
| Malt, dried and powdered | 10 | | |
| Wort, made with boiling water | 0.1 | | |

[a] As pointed out by R. E. Hughes (1975, p. 347), who did the experiment, this value corresponds to only 13% of the vitamin originally present in the juice that was evaporated down.

they are considered to have been the key factor in keeping the population of northern Europe free from scurvy since 1800, at least when crop yields were normal. In Great Britain, for example, the mean daily intake of vitamin C from potatoes (even allowing for 50% loss in cooking) was at least 17 mg in working-class households over the whole period from 1909 to 1949.[21] This represents some 40% of the total intake of the vitamin in the average household.

People with "average" diets would still have avoided scurvy even if their potatoes had lacked vitamin C; however, for some groups potatoes have been, and continue to be, the only food keeping them out of the danger zone. The first such group includes men on pensions, who live alone on a low income, doing little cooking and feeling that fruit is a frivolous luxury. If they cook potatoes once a day, they are protected, whereas if they try to subsist with bread as their sole staple, they can become deficient. The second group includes men doing heavy physical labor, who have a hearty appetite and a disdain for what they consider to be "fancy" ideas about nutrition, but who (in Britain at least) are always ready to enjoy a meal of bacon, fried eggs, and chips (French fries). Finally, there are many young men in large cities who live in lodgings without cooking facilities and eat at "fast food" outlets or hamburger joints where French fries would be about the *only* food containing vitamin C. It has been estimated that a single serving of potatoes contributes 5–40 mg of vitamin C, depending on the season and how they are cooked.[22]

## Germinated seeds and malt

All mature, dry seeds are almost or entirely devoid of vitamin C. This is the case for all kinds of grain (wheat, rice, corn, etc.), as well as for legumes (peas and beans), and, of course, for flours made from them. However, with germination, the synthesis of ascorbic acid begins almost immediately;[23] thus germinated seeds could have been beneficial on board ship. We have seen that the Dutch tried to establish "gardens" on their East Indies fleet in order to grow ordinary plants, but that they found it impracticable. In 1798, an article appeared in the *Gentleman's Magazine* whose main point was that scurvy was caused by excessive salt. But the author also recommended sprouted beans as an antiscorbutic.[24] Shipley, writing in 1929, said that their value was "the common knowledge of every naval surgeon in the latter half of the eighteenth century."[25] However, I have not found references to the value of "sprouting" in any of the ten or so eighteenth-century treatises dealing with the prevention of scurvy. A retired naval surgeon, writing in 1807 on the diseases encountered by sailors, said in relation to the prevention of scurvy that

[21] National Food Survey Committee (1951), 4, 51–2.    [22] Adams (1975), 129–30.    [23] Lugg & Weller (1943), 13.    [24] Sherwen (1798), 192–5.    [25] Shipley (1929), 8.

. . . there is a plan . . . recommended by a Mr. Young of the Navy . . . highly deserving of attention. . . . Any kind of . . . seeds brought under the malting or vegetating process are converted into the state of a growing plant . . . and if eaten in this state, [after] separating and rejecting the husks . . . cannot fail to supply precisely what is wanted . . . [which is] fresh vegetable chyle.[26]

He cites no examples of its actual use in the Navy, and the fact that the idea is referred to as a "plan" suggests that it had still to be tested.

As we saw in Chapter 8, the antiscorbutic property of sprouted beans was confirmed in early experiments with guinea pigs, and was then made use of in Russia during World War II. Chemical analyses added further confirmation, as in the following experiment: Peas and beans were soaked and spread out on wet cotton wool in an environment maintained at approximately 70°F. After two days they had already begun to sprout, and analysis of the "seeds + sprouts" at this stage gave values of 35–40 mg vitamin C per 100 g starting material. After five days, the values had risen to 60–100 mg;[23] 300–500 g of lemons would have to be squeezed to obtain the same quantity of ascorbic acid from the juice.

Experiments with barley have given values in the region of 30 mg per 100 g starting material (i.e., rather lower than with beans). MacBride was correct, therefore, in believing that sprouted (i.e., malted) barley had antiscorbutic properties, although his reasoning, i.e., that this material would be useful because it supplied "fixed air" (carbon dioxide), was wrong. The doubts arise in connection with the value of malt after it has been dried and stored on board ship as a powder. When dried, bean sprouts, as well as malt, were found to have lost their protective value for guinea pigs.[27] We have seen many old reports in which wort made from dried malt was found to be inactive at sea, and modern analyses have confirmed its very low ascorbic acid content.[28] The use of malt soup, made by heating up malt extract with a certain amount of milk, was found by Hess and Fish (as we saw in Chapter 7) to be associated with a high incidence of infantile scurvy. However, Gerstenberger, another American pediatrician, later reported good results when one particular batch of malt extract was given to scorbutic infants, suggesting that it was in fact antiscorbutic.[29] He speculated that the batch might have been made from barley that had been allowed to sprout for a longer period than usual, and thus developed greater activity; possibly it was also more freshly made than other batches had been.

Beer also has repeatedly been recommended as an antiscorbutic. However, the word "beer" is applied to beverages made by a variety of processes. At one extreme is "Kaffir beer," which was "largely used in South Africa to arrest scurvy in prisons and mines." [30] A small quantity of millet grain was germinated by being steeped for 48 hours; it was then dried in the sun for a

[26] Curtis (1807), 41–2.    [27] Chick & Hume (1917), 169; Fürst (1912), 129.    [28] Trotter (1792), 189–90; Norris (1983), 335.    [29] Gerstenberger (1921), 324–5.    [30] Dyke (1918), 515.

day, and within the next 24 hours was mixed with boiled water, and a little yeast was added. After 36–48 hours, it was poured through a coarse strainer, and the turbid fluid was then usually drunk on the same day.[30] The dried sprouts were never prepared in bulk, nor were they stored before the beer was made; in addition, the wort was not boiled after the hot water was added; finally, it was drunk in large quantities, almost immediately after the fermentation period. Thus one can appreciate how it could have actually been an effective antiscorbutic.

At the other extreme is the commercial type of beer that has been mass-produced since 1850, using "high-dried, kilned malt," and stored to maturity before being sold. This type of beer has not been found to have antiscorbutic activity.[31] Whether beer that was made from malted barley that had received a milder drying was ever a reliable antiscorbutic is debatable. Most of the naval surgeons in the eighteenth century thought of beer, along with wine or any fermented liquors or even fermented oatmeal, as being antiscorbutic.[31] Beer taken on a voyage remained "good" only for the first six to ten weeks; therefore, it was to be expected that the period during which beer was available would coincide with freedom from scurvy, even if it and the rest of the diet were entirely free of vitamin C, because the sailors could have been living on their reserves. There is no reason to believe that fermentation with yeasts or any other type of microorganism leads to the synthesis of the vitamin; on the contrary, it is more likely to hasten its destruction.[32]

Another drink prized by sailors was "spruce-beer." The name may have led to some misconceptions. It originates from the anglicization of the German *"sprossen-bier,"* which is beer made from *sprossen* (or sprouts), the green leaf buds of fir trees, and which has been used as a beverage by sailors in the Baltic Sea at least since the sixteenth century.[33] This kind of decoction can have a significant ascorbic acid content. Thus, in one investigation, extracts made from leaves of the kind of tree thought to have been used by the Canadian Indians who showed their remedy to Cartier yielded some 200 mg vitamin C per 100 g of leaves.[34] Hughes made an infusion of spruce leaves (which contained 55 mg vitamin C per 100 g); when fresh, it contained 14 mg/100 ml, but after fermentation the vitamin content had virtually all disappeared.[35] Lind wrote:

Although the pines and firs . . . differ from each other in their size and outward form, . . . they seem all to have analogous medicinal virtues, and great efficacy in this disease. The shrub spruce . . . affords a balsam superior to most turpentines. . . . A simple decoction of the tops, cones, leaves, or even bark and wood of these trees, is antiscorbutic: but it becomes much more so when fermented, as in making spruce beer; where the molasses contributes. . . .[36]

---

[31] Smith (1918), 814.    [32] Hughes (1975), 349.    [33] De Veer (1876), 114–15.    [34] Rousseau (1953), 128–9.    [35] Hughes (1975), 348.    [36] Stewart & Guthrie (1953), 166.

As we have seen, modern analyses do not confirm Lind's belief in the beneficial effect of fermentation. The reference to "turpentines" (resins) may relate to Bishop Berkeley's claims in the 1740s that tarwater (an aqueous extract of tar that had been prepared by distilling the wood of pine or fir trees) was a cure for scurvy as well as for many other diseases.[37]

Spruce beer was one of the items said by La Pérouse (after his circumnavigation in the 1780s) to be "not sufficient for the actual cure of scurvy, but . . . [to] certainly retard its progress."[38] Beer brewed with the addition of dried spruce leaves, or flavored with "essence of spruce" continued to be regarded as an important precautionary measure to ward off scurvy as late as the 1850s, when ships were searching in the Arctic for Sir John Franklin's expedition. To quote from Mrs. Smith: "The essential element, of course, from the point of view of scurvy, was the freshness of the vegetable ingredient, and, as has happened in the history of other antiscorbutics, the belief in the value of the drink persisted after the elimination of the element on which that value depended."[39]

Cider (fermented apple juice), another drink recommended as an antiscorbutic in the eighteenth century, did seem to show some activity in Lind's classic experiment. In Britain, ordinary commercial cider nowadays contains little or no vitamin C, but it has been argued that the low levels result from changes in its manufacture, and that stronger, traditional cider made without pasteurization may contain 40–50 mg per liter.[40] In Lind's experiment, the men who drank just over one liter of cider per day showed a little improvement, which would be consistent with their receiving, say, 5 mg of the vitamin per day – or some 10% of the amount that has been found in the analysis of fresh, top-quality cider. Lind said that it was "inclinable to be pricked" (turning vinegary), so that it probably had lost much of its original activity.

## Meat, fish, and Eskimo diets

One of the problems for nineteenth-century students of scurvy who believed in the special properties of fresh vegetables was that Eskimos normally remained free from scurvy, although they had no access to fruits and vegetables. In Chapter 6, we have already considered some of the debates on this subject that took place in the period 1860–1900. The modern dietitian has a similar problem with the Eskimo diet. Conventional teaching dictates that a good diet consists of a balance of items from the different food groups – cereals, fruits and vegetables, meat or fish, and dairy products. Yet here is an ethnic group whose traditional diet came almost entirely from one group – meat and fish.[41] This has to be generally true, even though the

---

[37] Chance (1942), 458, 460–1; Clerk of the California (1968), 2, 12.    [38] La Pérouse (1807), 3, 398.    [39] Smith (1918), 813.    [40] French (1982), 64–5.    [41] Draper & Bell (1972), 14.

environments in which individual Eskimo groups lived differed widely as regards the availability of fish and game and the growth of vegetation in the summers. Some writers have cited examples of Eskimo groups that were able to gather berries at certain times of the year and to store them in seal oil,[42] and of others who killed caribou that had been living on lichens, and who had a special liking for the vegetable material in their rumen (first stomach).[43]

However, there seems no reason to explain the Eskimo freedom from scurvy in terms of possible occasional sources of vegetable food. Most animals, as we have seen, synthesize their own ascorbic acid, and it is distributed throughout their tissues; however, its concentration in animal tissues is lower than in some vegetable foods and is relatively easily destroyed by cooking. But if a population eats large amounts of meat in a raw, or only lightly cooked state, there is no reason to anticipate a deficiency of the vitamin.

In both Western and Asian cultures, meat has become, for many people, little more than a rather expensive garnish or flavoring, for a diet in which most of the calories are derived from grains, sugar, and vegetable oils. Moreover, it is so thoroughly cooked – partly to develop flavors, partly to prevent food poisoning – that its contribution of ascorbic acid to the diet is negligible, and not even listed in most food tables. But in the Eskimo culture, the quantities of meat and fish eaten are of a different order; moreover, the cooking, if any, is so mild that the vitamin C contributed is considerable, even though the average concentration is relatively low. Some analyses are summarized in Table 10.3. Eskimos have been reported to eat the livers of both seals and caribou raw, and even a few ounces of such organ meat would satisfy a day's requirement for the vitamin.[44,45] An adult male would generally require something like 2 lb (900 g) of ordinary meat to satisfy his need for calories, assuming that it had 30% fat content. If he were eating leaner meat, that quantity would have to be doubled. The traditional Eskimo custom was also to eat their meat or fish raw, or, if it was lightly warmed (rather than even brought to a boil), then to drink the liquor in which the meat had been steeped. It was often difficult for them to cook because of a shortage of fuel. Seal oil, although serving as a source of light when burned, was not much better than a candle for cooking.[43] This restriction, of course, resulted in a better yield of ascorbic acid, so that the basic meat diet could be expected to have provided them with some 15–20 mg vitamin C per day – enough to ward off scurvy. The occasional meal of liver or whale skin would provide them with a further supplement. It is interesting that whale skin was prized by the Eskimos long before its high ascorbic acid content was discovered.[46]

---

[42] Ibid., 15.    [43] Jenness (1922), 97–8.    [44] Ibid., 100.    [45] Høygaard & Rasmussen (1939), 943; Hoppner et al. (1978), 258; Geraci & Smith (1979), 137.    [46] Bertelsen (1911), 538–9.

Table 10.3. *Analytical values for the vitamin C content of items in traditional Eskimo diets*[45]

|  | Ascorbic acid (mg/100 g) | |
|---|---|---|
|  | Raw | Lightly boiled |
| Seal flesh | 0.5–3 | 0.5–2.5 |
| Seal liver | 18–35 | 14–30 |
| Whale skin (narwhal) | 18 | n.d.[a] |
| Whale skin (Beluga) | 35 | n.d. |
| Blubber (Beluga) | 5 | n.d. |
| Animal flesh, raw | | |
| (caribou, musk ox, polar bear) | 0.8–1.8 | 0.5 |
| Fish flesh (cod, char) | 0.5–2 | n.d. |
| Cod roe | 44 | n.d. |
| Bird flesh, raw | 1–2 | 0.3–1 |
| Licorice root | 21 | 4 |
| Mountain sorrel | 36 | 5 |
| Angelica | 14 | – |

[a] I.e., "not determined."

Stefansson argued repeatedly from his long experience in the Arctic that it was perfectly possible for people of European stock to live for long periods on a traditional and entirely carnivorous Eskimo diet. He, in fact, was enthusiastic about the texture and tastiness of frozen raw fish that was just beginning to melt in the warmth of an igloo. He believed that many explorers in the Arctic had developed scurvy just because they would not follow the Eskimos and place trust in their instinct and experience.[47] Because of the skepticism that greeted his writings, he and a colleague volunteered to subsist on nothing but meat, under medical supervision in New York, for one year starting in February of 1928. They each consumed between 100 and 140 g protein per day, with the remaining calories coming from fat. Both men remained in good general health and gave no indication of incipient scurvy. It was, of course, too early for vitamin C analyses of either their diet or their own blood.[48] Stefansson recalled that he was amused at the doctors' certainty that he was attempting something extremely dangerous, and at his having to sign a statement relieving them of any responsibility for the outcome.[49]

It has been estimated that a traditional Eskimo diet, even without any plant material, would typically contain 40 mg vitamin C.[50] Unfortunately, the arrival of people from other cultures in their territories, along with the opportunities for trading with them, has resulted in nutritional problems

[47] Stefansson (1918), 1717–18; Stefansson (1946), 16–17.    [48] Lieb (1929), 21.    [49] Stefansson (1946), 60–1.    [50] Høygaard & Rasmussen (1939), 943.

among the Eskimos and some concern as to the vitamin C status of mothers and their infants, even though there is no longer any risk of outright famine in a particularly harsh season.[51]

## The eighteenth-century controversy over lemon juice

Herbert Spencer, the Victorian philosopher and sociologist, cited a number of instances of Government inefficiency in order to support the argument, in one of his books, that further state intervention in social matters was, in general, ineffectual and undesirable. He said that of all the examples that he used, the most striking was the treatment of the scurvy problem in the British Navy over the forty years from 1757 to 1797. It was an "amazing perversity of officialism" that over all this period the Admiralty had not adopted a procedure "after a chief medical officer of the Government had given conclusive evidence of its worth." [52] No one seems to have disagreed with Spencer.

We have already discussed the events of this period in Chapters 3 and 4 in terms of what was known at the time. Do they look different from a modern perspective? Some of the modern analyses of citrus products are set out in Table 10.2. Hughes has provided valuable analyses of a "rob of oranges" prepared according to Lind's directions. Evaporating 800 ml juice down to one-tenth of this volume resulted in the loss of one-half of the vitamin C. When the rob was stored for a month at room temperature, less than one-seventh of the original vitamin was still present.[53] Presumably, the loss of the vitamin would have continued with longer storage. Yet, the rob would probably only have *begun* to be used as a treatment for sailors showing incipient scurvy some three months after the beginning of a voyage, and it could not always be prepared immediately before a voyage began. In practice, it might be a year or more between its production and the need for it.

It would appear therefore that the advice given to the Admiralty that "rob of lemons or oranges" was *not* an effective antiscorbutic in practice was correct. Because this was the procedure that Lind had recommended, Spencer was wrong in thinking it obvious that the Admiralty should have adopted it. Further, he was wrong in describing Lind as a chief medical officer of the Government, with the implication that he was one of the group responsible for advising the administrators. In fact, as we saw earlier, it was the physicians of the Sick and Hurt Board who had that responsibility, and the administrative admirals would certainly have been censurable if they had not taken the advice of their professional experts. As we have seen in Chapter 4, in the 1780s this was to the effect that the rob did not work, that unconcentrated juice was unlikely to be that much superior, and that the testimony from Captain Cook and others was in favor of carrying malt or

[51] Nares (1878), 2, 183; Clow, Laberge, & Scrives (1975), 625–6; Draper (1977), 310.
[52] Spencer (1879), 162–3.     [53] Hughes (1975), 347.

any type of easily fermentable materials. Spencer's charge leaves the impression that the Admiralty had shown "inertia and torpor" in the face of the serious scurvy problem. Again this hardly stands up to scrutiny. Part of the difficulty was that the Admiralty gave captains of expeditions so many materials to try out (from carrot marmalade to soda water) that it was almost impossible to ascribe the good health of the crews to one particular cause. As we have seen, the reports from Cook's expeditions actually confused the matter rather than clarifying it.

The question remaining in my mind is, why was not more done to develop and try out different methods of preserving large quantities of oranges and lemons on long voyages? Thomas Trotter seems to have been the only person with ideas on the subject. Because the rob was believed to have lost its activity during the heating used to concentrate the juice, he tried "concentrating it by freezing [and removing the ice] to one-eighth of its bulk" and concluded from the response of a scorbutic patient that it "retains all the virtues of the fruit in its recent state." [54] Unfortunately, as we saw in Chapter 4, he then went further and recommended actual crystallized citric acid, which he found to be antiscorbutic whereas others did not. Other people applied their minds instead to discovering entirely novel preventives. And yet we know from correspondence between Nelson's fleet and their agents in Sicily that lemons were being shipped in brine as far as Russia.

We also know that what was assumed to be impossible for the sailors was standard practice for the officers. To quote again from Lind's last work: "Officers . . . who make use of oranges and lemons . . . [might] reserve the peels to be put into the spirits served to the men." [55] Could it be that, subconsciously, this provision for the officers reflected the idea that their needs differed from those of their men? There are many instances of officers' giving some of their special supplies for the use of the sick, and of this being regarded as a suitable act of charity. Perhaps in some way a sick sailor was also considered to be in a delicate state more comparable to that of an officer whose duties characteristically involved the brain work of navigation and organization. The physical labor of the ordinary sailor was thought to promote (and even to require) the digestion of coarser food. Even Thomas Trotter, who had so strongly advocated that ships carry lemon juice, did not want sailors to have it to take for long periods: "It cures scurvy and preserves human life, but at the same time it weakens the digestive powers, consumes fat, and lessens muscular vigour." [56]

## The nineteenth-century controversy over lime juice

The 1800s began with nothing but praise for the potency of lemon juice. There were repeated urgings from medical officers at the chief ports in

[54] Trotter (1795), 58.    [55] Lloyd (1965), 43.    [56] Trotter (1804), 74, 77; Nagy (1980), 14–17.

Britain, who continued to see cases of scurvy in the crews of merchant ships, that the Government should enforce the same issue of lemon juice in these ships as in the Royal Navy.

Now that the experience of nearly half a century has established the infallible efficacy of lemon-juice in preventing scurvy on the longest voyages . . . and when lemon-juice is so cheap . . . it may well excite surprise that . . . no regulation has been made for compelling our merchant ships to take a supply of it. . . . Every year [the appearance of scurvy cases] teaches us a lesson of humility by showing how slow we still are . . . in giving effect to discoveries most important to the well-being of our fellow men.[57]

This was a difficult problem for Governments that believed, in principle, in laissez-faire economics. In fact, a series of regulations were enacted, although they were not always followed and needed several revisions to ensure some control over the use of adulterated juice and over the size of the issue.[58]

As the century progressed, it no longer seemed quite so evident that citrus juices were universally effective – perhaps partly because "successes" were no longer newsworthy whereas a failure was. Even in 1824, an editorial in a British medical journal stated that "it has long been known to many intelligent observers that . . . lemon juice is by no means an infallible cure for scurvy . . . notwithstanding the evidence of Sir Gilbert Blane, so positively advanced to the contrary."[59] The article described an outbreak of scurvy that occurred "despite large quantities of lemon juice plentifully administered," in the crew of a naval ship sailing from Trincomalee (in Sri Lanka) to the Cape of Good Hope, where they recovered. Specimens of the juice were analyzed in London and were found to be good.[59] As we have seen in Chapter 5, there were many later complaints that lemon juice or lime juice purchased in the Indian subcontinent was of little value, and this was attributed to deliberate adulteration by wily merchants. If the analysts in London were using acidity as their indicator of quality, they could, of course, have been deceived by the use of acid adulterants. In 1848, an arctic expedition had to return early because of scurvy and, in this instance, samples of their lemon juice were found to have only one-tenth of the normal acidity. From then on special care was taken over the quality of the juice taken on such voyages.[60]

With the development of steam engines and the provision of a more varied diet on ships, the value of antiscorbutics was not being put to the test so regularly. More critical conditions were encountered on military campaigns and polar expeditions. As we noted earlier, the comments on the value of the lemon or lime juices issued to the British Army in the Crimean War were equivocal. They referred to "differences of opinion" and seemed

---

[57] Budd (1842), 634.    [58] Lloyd & Coulter (1963), 4, 114–15.    [59] Anonymous (1824), 232.    [60] Smith (1919), 101.

to make excuses for its lack of effect rather than to endorse its value. By then, the terms "lemon juice" and "lime juice" were being used indiscriminately for the same product.

Public attention was drawn to the questionable value of lime juice with the early return of the Nares Arctic expedition in 1876 as a result of scurvy. What happened was described at length in Chapter 6. On their return, the remaining juice was checked by analysts and was reported to meet normal standards. Similar failures of lime juice to protect the men in other expeditions then led to the development of entirely new theories as to the cause of the disease, though lime juice continued to be a compulsory issue in British ships. To use a phrase from Hirsch, "the reality of facts well authenticated began to be doubted altogether." [61] Thus, Captain Scott, in planning his expedition at the beginning of the present century, was advised that there was no such thing as an antiscorbutic and that his party would be at risk of scurvy from bad meat or an unpredictable acidosis. A warning was even given that lime juice could have an adverse effect because of its acidity.[62]

Some order was restored to the field by the development of guinea pig assays, as described in Chapter 8. Most relevant here was the finding in 1918 that samples of the lime juice issued to the armed services were of extremely low potency and that even fresh lime juice had only one-third to one-fifth the value of fresh lemon juice. Investigation showed no evidence of any kind of adulteration on the part of the manufacturers. Alice Henderson Smith, of the Lister Institute, then searched old Admiralty records in order to find out whether there had been any clear break in practice between the time when "lime juice" had worked and the time when it ceased to do so. Her conclusion was that this corresponded to their changeover from the use of Mediterranean lemons to West Indian limes for the preparation of their standard issue of juice in the 1860s.[63]

Lloyd has implied that the change was another example of the Admiralty's short-sighted economy and indifference to the sailor's needs;[64] it could also be construed as their giving in to the lobbying of British planters in the West Indies on the lookout for a new market. On the other hand, it can equally be argued that it was a wise decision, when Mediterranean lemon juice was in short supply, to establish a source of supply in an area firmly under British control where the time of harvest and every stage of preparation could be supervised. With limes being *more* acidic than lemons (and acidity having always been regarded as an indicator of quality), they could be expected to be *more* antiscorbutic, and certainly many of the older writers had referred appreciatively to the value of limes.[65] Finally, when the changeover began, limes were actually more expensive than lemons.[63]

[61] Hirsch (1885) 2, 514.     [62] Bullmore (1900), 873; Wright (1904), 87.     [63] Smith (1919), 102, 206–8.     [64] Lloyd (1961), 131.     [65] Hulme (1768), 67–8; Lind (1772), 522; Evans (1878), 14; Lloyd & Coulter (1961), 132, 134.

That there had been a change of fruit used was itself not very obvious because of the confusion over terminology. In Arabic-speaking countries the sweet lime is called a *limoon*. The German for lime is *Limone*, which is also Italian for lemon. Even the systematic Linnean terminology was not very helpful. Lemons (now *Citrus limonum*) were called by Chick *Citrus medica*, var. *limonum* and sour limes, *Citrus medica*, var. *acida*.[66] The latter, now *Citrus aurantifolia* (Swingle) are variously known as West Indian, Key, Kagzi, Mexican, or Galego limes.[67]

Modern analyses of sour lime juice have given values ranging from 23 to 49 mg ascorbic acid per 100 g, with an average of approximately 30 mg. The corresponding values for lemon juice are 31–61 mg, with an average of 45 mg per 100 g.[68] In other words, lime juice was found to have about two-thirds the vitamin C value of lemon juice. How then are we left? *Yes*, the new analyses do confirm that limes have a generally lower vitamin C content than lemons. But, *no*, they do not provide a confirmation, or explanation, of the three- to fivefold difference found for the fresh juices in the 1917 guinea pig assays. Could it be that the vitamin level in fruit from the particular variety of trees that provided the juice was especially low, or that in limes it breaks down more rapidly after harvest than in lemons? It was noted in the 1918 paper that, for the "fresh lime juice" treatment, the fruit was about four weeks in transit from the West Indies (because of the War), and that the expressed juice was then refrigerated and up to two months old when given to the guinea pigs. A threefold difference was, however, obtained again in another study after the War.[69]

Whether or not commercial lime juice must inevitably be so much poorer than commercial lemon juice remains to be determined. However, it seems almost certain, despite the relatively favorable, modern analyses of fresh lime juice, and the repeated endorsement of the value of fresh limes in the eighteenth century, that commercial lime juice in the period 1860–1920 was of very little value. Further, defective material was produced by reputable manufacturers under repeated inspection. The "wily merchants of the East" may have been unfairly suspected of adulteration. Possibly much of the vitamin was lost in the long period (apparently it could last a month) when the juice was held in settling tanks, to allow the decanting of a clear liquid.[70] We do not know what the tanks or vats were made of, but there is reason to think that any pumping of the juices from one container to another would have been done with copper tubing.[71] There was, of course, no knowledge at that time of the potential destructive effect of metals on the antiscorbutic value of materials.

It is sometimes stated in introductory comments to a paper on vitamin C

[66] Chick, Hume, Skelton, & Smith (1918), 736.     [67] Hodgson (1967) 1, 573–8.
[68] Munsell et al. (1949), 160; Munsell et al. (1950), 44; Garg & Ram (1973), 38; Calvarano & Gallino (1975), 289; Nelson & Tressler (1980), 163, 173.     [69] Davey (1921), 102.     [70] Smith (1919), 101.     [71] Parkes (1830), 249.

or scurvy that "the juice of the West Indian sour lime contains no vitamin C." [72] This is clearly untrue and one more myth obscuring the real complexity of the subject.

## Unexplained cures

This chapter would present a simpler, and perhaps more pleasing, story if it dealt only with those of the earlier observations that can now be explained in terms of modern analyses. However, it would not be honest; we must force ourselves also to consider the still unexplained records.

First we have Lind's description of his disappointments with the experiments at Haslar Hospital, designed to test the value of different antiscorbutic treatments. His "negative controls" (men restricted to a diet essentially of bread and butter with floury gruels or puddings and no meat, fruit, or vegetables) always recovered from scurvy as quickly as those receiving supplements of vegetable juices.[73] We know that there were disciplinary problems at Haslar, as one might expect with many of the men having been "pressed" into service, and having a chance, now that they were back on English soil, of escaping to their families.[74] The conditions must therefore have been rather like those of a prison, and those kept on a restricted experimental diet must have felt that a further arbitrary punishment was being imposed on them. There was no such thing as "informed consent" or per diem compensation, and one can well imagine that the men would make every effort to bribe their attendants to bring in lemons or other "comforts." It was probably fairly easy for this to happen, for example, on night shifts, when there was no danger of a physician's discovering what was going on. Lind, as Director of the large hospital, must have had so many other responsibilities that he could not have supervised the trials as closely as he had done as a junior surgeon in H.M.S. *Salisbury*. Strangely enough, in one modern study, two (out of eleven) scorbutic patients also improved while remaining in a hospital ward and receiving a scorbutic diet: Their skin changes cleared up and their blood picture became almost normal, despite there being no detectable ascorbic acid in their blood plasma.[75]

It is even more difficult to suggest explanations for some of the cures reported to have occurred at sea. For example, we have Paterson's description in 1795 of his repeated successes in curing severely scorbutic men in British naval ships, using a mixture of vinegar and potassium nitrate. There seems no doubt that his descriptions do refer to the cure of scurvy: gums healing, lips becoming more flexible, and skin growing again over ulcers.[76] There seem to be only three possibilities. The first is that the men really did recover when transferred to the sick bay, but that it came from an attendant there providing, or selling, something like lemon juice from a store un-

[72] Kark (1953), 280.     [73] Lind (1772), 538–9.     [74] Rolleston (1915), 183.     [75] Vilter, Woolford, & Spies (1946), 619–20.     [76] Paterson (1795), 16.

known to Paterson. But it would have had to be a very large store because 180 cases were treated on board the ship in a period of twenty-one months. The regular sick bay diet might also have included an unrecognized antiscorbutic, though Paterson said that it was the ordinary sick fare and consisted of barley, peas, portable soup, salop, and wine.[77] Second, he might not have been telling the truth as to their recovery. But, if there really were many seriously ill and they did *not* recover, this would have been known to the captain, who could then have been expected to denounce Paterson to the Admiralty when the book appeared. Alternatively, the sailors were not really so ill, or Paterson knowingly gave them something else, and pretended that the niter had been responsible for the cure. But why would someone stake his reputation on proposing a remedy which he knew would fail when tested by others? Or was he fooling himself, just because he believed so strongly in the "oxygenating" theory behind the remedy, and wanted the fame of discovery? Yet we know that he had letters from two other surgeons who confirmed the efficacy of the treatment from their own experience, and that two more surgeons were to say similar things in the 1830s.[78]

The last possibility, of course, is that the men really did recover without any additional treatment. If so, was it a "placebo" effect? We cannot point to any modern, well-controlled experiment in which a mixture of vinegar and potassium nitrate was tested and failed. Trotter did refer in 1804 to treatment with niter alone having failed in the hands of several surgeons,[79] but this does not necessarily prove that the five claims of positive results were wrong. We are really forced to make a choice: Either we believe so strongly in our concept of scurvy that we will reject any observations that disagree with it, or we must keep an open mind on the matter. The later claims made for the curative value of potassium salts generally, as described in Chapter 5, and the cures reported by Trotter himself with crystalline citric acid, leave us in the same dilemma. It seems inherent in human nature that we find it difficult to keep something in mind which is out of harmony with our generalizations on the subject. It requires a positive effort therefore to remember that there are reported observations that have not always been repeatable and do not fit our present ideas as to the nature of scurvy and, in particular, to know that some of them came from James Lind, whose judgment and objective evaluation is so highly esteemed.

## Dietary factors inducing scurvy

So far, the only scorbutic factor considered in this chapter has been a lack of vitamin C in the diet. But some others also deserve consideration. Jones and Hughes drew attention recently to the eighteenth-century paper suggesting

---

[77] Ibid., 19, 23.   [78] Cameron (1830), 751–2; Henderson (1839), 15.   [79] Trotter (1804), 402n.

that "the use of copper cooking vessels in the Navy is one of the principal causes of the sea scurvy."[80] The original author, as we saw in Chapter 3, envisaged scurvy as being straightforward copper poisoning from verdigris dissolved in the fat or "slush" being eaten by the men on board. Now, of course, the destructive effect of even very low levels of copper salts on ascorbic acid has been discovered. An experiment in which cabbage was cooked in a copper pot resulted in an average loss of 65% of the vitamin after twenty to thirty minutes, whereas cabbage cooked in an iron pot showed only an 18% loss.[81] Captain Cook, who was so keen to encourage the use of freshly gathered green foods, said that they were boiled with "portable soup" to make them more palatable.[82] The level of ascorbic acid in naval rations at sea was, at best, extremely low anyway, but the extra loss in cooking, when green vegetables were available, must certainly have added to the problem. The moral that this story illustrates is that an observation may be correct, but that what appears at the time to be the "obvious" explanation can still be entirely wrong.

The next possible scorbutic factor is also related to the ships' coppers. Cook, in his report to Pringle (reproduced in Chapter 4), said that he believed that "slush," the fat rising to the top of the coppers when meat was being boiled in them, was productive of scurvy, and he forbade his men to use it.[83] Several naval surgeons and captains were to say essentially the same thing in the next seventy years.[84] This in itself is, of course, no proof of the correctness of the idea because we could collect even more quotations for the antiscorbutic value of sugar, which no one today would believe.

An observation that may possibly tie in with the excessive use of fat is that there are several examples of ships' cooks being the first to die of scurvy on voyages.[85] Obviously they had the best opportunity of selecting their own diet items, forbidden or not, and the point has often been made that human beings do not always know (or act as if they know) what is good for them. However, there are also instances where cooks escaped the scurvy suffered by others.[86] Trotter suggested that eating excessive fat led to obesity, and that it was obesity which, in turn, made people more susceptible to scurvy.[87] Yet, as De Lisle pointed out in 1877, the Eskimos, who remained largely free from scurvy despite their harsh conditions, ate a diet that was very high in fat.[88]

Sir James Watt has argued that the "slush" might have been particularly harmful because the contact with copper and the boiling in the presence of oxygen would have led to "oxidative rancidity," particularly in pork fat.[89] A

---

[80] Travis (1762), 1.  [81] Jones & Hughes (1976), 81.  [82] Cook (1776), 403.  [83] Ibid., 405.
[84] Trotter (1795), 53–4; Gillespie (1798), 2; Henderson (1839), 5; Clowes (1899), 4, 148; Lamb (1984), 4, 1471–2, 1481.  [85] La Pérouse (1807), 3, 119; C. R. Markham (1881), 148; Beaglehole (1961) 2, 185n, 186n.  [86] Smith (1919), 202.  [87] Trotter (1795), 54.  [88] De Lisle (1877), 302.  [89] Watt (1979), 77; Watt (1981), 58–9; Watt (1982), 41.

fat is said to be "rancid" whenever it has developed an unpleasant flavor. There are two types of chemical reaction that can cause this. With butter fat, the only reaction is *hydrolysis,* which fat undergoes in any case when it is eaten and digested. Rancid butter is unattractive but harmless. The second type of reaction is *oxidation,* which can happen only to fats of the type classified as "unsaturated." Even such oxidized fats are not directly toxic to animals.[90] However, there is circumstantial evidence that links their consumption with diarrhea and malabsorption conditions in humans,[91] and Watt's argument was that these conditions have, in turn, repeatedly been associated with scurvy – the stress of one reducing resistance to the other. Even more recently, another scientist has argued that rancid fat predisposed seafarers to scurvy,[92] on the basis of work suggesting that vitamin C and vitamin E may act together in the detoxification of rancid fat.[93] These arguments are suggestive, but the history of ideas about scurvy has shown the danger of treating an attractive theory as anything more than a hypothesis in the absence of direct proof.

## Factors other than diet

Lind and many of his contemporaries believed that damp, cold weather at sea was productive of scurvy. As we saw in Chapter 3, he thought that this was explained by "a stoppage of perspiration" under those conditions. In Holland, the cold and damp of winter were thought to have the same effect, though we would now think that the seasonal lack of fresh vegetables was a sufficient explanation. Lind's example of a surprisingly early appearance of scurvy on a voyage in late spring also seems to be fully explained now by the previous stay in their home port in England having been at the season of scarcity of fresh fruit and vegetables, so that the sailors' reserves of vitamin C were likely to have been depleted. That cold, wet weather had any direct effect also seemed inconsistent with later observations of scurvy outbreaks in the dry season in Africa and India and in the hot, dry conditions of the California gold fields.

Another belief of the early travelers was that idleness was conducive to the disease. Hawkins said that as long as he could get his men to dance on deck every day, he knew that they were not going to go down with the scurvy; and the leaders of the early French expeditions in Canada believed that the only safeguard was to keep happy and active. We now suspect that these observers were reversing cause and effect. As has been pointed out, there is evidence both from the old outbreaks and from modern experiments that the first effects of vitamin C depletion are fatigue and lassitude, continuing for as long as six weeks before any more objective signs appear.[94]

---

[90] Frazer (1962), 48–51.    [91] Klipstein & Corcino (1974), 1194.    [92] Reid (1983), 167–8.    [93] Packer, Slater, & Wilson (1979), 738.    [94] Hughes (1981b), 79–80.

Therefore, being unwilling or unable to dance may have been the first symptom of scurvy. In other words, one could say that it was a diagnostic test of trouble ahead, without it following that the dancing itself had any preventive value. Once again, we probably have an example of a completely correct observation from an earlier period, although the apparently obvious conclusions drawn from it at the time now seem quite mistaken.

Linked with physical inactivity is melancholy. This, of course, was the very first factor to be associated with scurvy in the sixteenth- and seventeenth-century medical writings discussed in Chapter 2. Bishop Berkeley, a much-admired philosopher in his time, obviously felt that this was a penalty likely to be inflicted on the thinker: "Many . . . scorbutic ailments . . . afflict the people of condition [upper classes] in these islands, often rendering them, on the whole, much more unhappy than those whom poverty and labour have ranked in the lowest of life." [95] In the same vein is the remark of an early eighteenth-century missionary in South Carolina, to the effect that scurvy was particularly difficult to cure "in those whose business requires a sedentary life as the clergy's does." [96]

The idea survived into the nineteenth century. The captains of Arctic expeditions, when scurvy had appeared, tried every means to rouse their men from lassitude so that they would "keep a rapid circulation," and, when recording a death from scurvy, a typical note was that "he hastened his own end by want of common energy." [97] However, like many others before and since, the Arctic explorer Nansen and his companion spent a whole winter in a small hut in almost complete inactivity. He commented afterward that their freedom from scurvy was an illustration of how fallacious it was to think that it could be brought on by idleness. [98]

Another factor associated with lassitude as a cause of scurvy has been the failure to maintain a discipline conducive to good hygiene – washing regularly, keeping living quarters clean, maintaining fresh air through ventilation, and so on. Cook placed as much emphasis on this as on the use of dietary antiscorbutics in long voyages. It is understandable that some of these precautions would reduce infectious disease, and that this might in some indirect way prevent any increased drain on their reserves of vitamin C. On the other hand, we know that some native communities lived in what seemed like squalor to Western observers, yet remained free from scurvy. We also know that men who were forced to overwinter in the Arctic or Antarctic without preparation, and had no soap or change of clothing, and lived on meat and frozen blood, emerged filthy and stinking, but with no trace of scorbutic taint. Lind, too, pointed out that in the ships of his day the carpenters had to spend long periods working near the bottom of the ship, in the vapors rising from putrid bilge-water, but their health record was no worse than that of sailors who worked mostly up on deck.

[95] Chance (1942), 460–1.    [96] Dufy (1953), 11.    [97] Back (1838), 172–3, 187; Belcher (1995), 2, 89–91.    [98] Nansen (1897), *II*, 402–3.

Finally, there is the opposite factor of overexertion as a possible cause of scurvy. Certainly, once someone has the disease, any physical effort may be sufficient to cause a fatal heart attack from the bursting of a blood vessel. On several voyages, men were described as dying from the effort of getting out of their hammocks.[99] This is understandable in a disease where the basic defect is a failure to synthesize connective tissue of normal strength.

The issue that is not so clear-cut is whether or not heavy, stressful exertion actually makes a person more likely to develop scurvy on a marginal diet, or to develop it more rapidly on a completely deficient diet. It is difficult to find instances where the degree of exertion was the only major difference in two otherwise comparable groups. Thus, those said to have remained healthiest through the winter in the early French expeditions to Canada were the hunters, who were also, presumably, having the lion's share of the fresh meat that they obtained. Again, people may be inactive because they are suffering from another disabling, stressful condition.

Norris has recently drawn together evidence relevant to "heavy exertion as an exacerbating influence on scurvy,"[100] and instances the 1875–6 Arctic expedition, in which some men went down with the disease after only three weeks of dragging heavy sledges. At the time, the sudden exertion after a period of relative inactivity seemed the obvious cause, rather than dietary depletion, because they had been taking lime juice until they left the ship. Now that we know that the lime juice they had used as their principal antiscorbutic for the previous eight months was probably almost inactive, it seems quite possible that they had already approached the condition of marginal scurvy.

Norris has also compared the time taken for signs of the disease to appear in the different depletion experiments carried out from 1940 on (and discussed in Chapter 9). The difficulties in making such comparisons come both from not knowing the state of ascorbic acid reserves of different individuals before the depletion period began, and from the uncertainty as to whether all the depletion diets were really entirely devoid of ascorbic acid. Even 1 or 2 mg per day might have delayed depletion significantly. Thus Norris has associated the fact that the men in the 1960 experiment took more exercise (walking 10 miles per day) than those in the earlier experiments with the observation that they showed deficiency signs sooner. On the other hand, the scientists in charge of that experiment associated the more rapid depletion with their having devised a diet entirely free from ascorbic acid, whereas the earlier diets had still probably contained traces of it.

The experience of Scott's Antarctic expeditions has also been contrasted with that of sedentary experimental subjects, and the tentative conclusion has been drawn that the heavy exertion in the sledging expeditions did

---

[99] Walter (1748), 145; Murray (1838–9), 294.     [100] Norris (1983), 325–38.

speed depletion.[101] I have been left with an open mind on this point. In Scott's final Polar group they were out for 150 days and subsisting on a scorbutic diet, and at the beginning were probably far from saturated with vitamin C from their previous diet. Yet there is no positive evidence that any of them were showing specific signs of scurvy at any time, even though they had subjected themselves to exceptional exertion and had sustained a terrible disappointment.

Evans's death, following what was thought not to have been a very serious concussion, *could* have been due to brain hemorrhage as a result of marginal deficiency. Oates's bad leg *could* also have been a symptom of scurvy, but equally it *could* be explained by a combination of frostbite and his old wound. Wilson, the surgeon in the party, wrote his diary for the first 120 days, and made no mention of signs of scurvy. Nor did Scott, even at the end, when he was trying to set down the reasons for their being unable to complete the return journey. There was no inducement for him to avoid doing so, because the disease was not regarded by him and his colleagues as something that could always be avoided, but rather as an unpredictable Act of God. The other surgeon, Atkinson, who had already diagnosed and treated scurvy, and who actually saw the frozen bodies the next spring, attributed their deaths to lack of food, weakness, and frostbite, and *not* to scurvy.

This is not to deny that lack of the vitamin must have had a weakening effect on the party. But it does seem that even these terrible conditions did not elicit the classical signs of the disease as seen after only a short period of sledging in the 1875 expedition. On the other hand, as described in Chapter 5, the relatively short siege of Paris in 1870 "provoked an explosion of scurvy," with cases occurring even among people who did not have to endure fatigue and cold. It seems only reasonable that heavy exertion should exacerbate a deficiency condition but, as Norris says: "Only a specific experiment under properly controlled conditions could establish the proposition conclusively." [101]

There have been many suggestions that other kinds of stress – including burns, surgical operations, radiation, and chemical toxins – all deplete the body of ascorbic acid, and so increase the requirement for the vitamin. Stone, who has argued the case, gives a substantial body of references.[102] But this remains controversial. Kark has said that "our generation inclines to the belief that stress stimulates adrenocortical activity [activity of the portion of the adrenal or suprarenal gland that secretes corticosteroids] and the opinion has been expressed that this glandular excitation destroys or consumes vitamin C," but he concludes that there is no good evidence for this from direct experiments. Also, sufferers from Cushing's disease, caused by a severe overactivity of the adrenal cortex, are not more than usually prone to

---

[101] Ibid., 338.    [102] Stone (1972), 152–85.

scurvy, which is not what one would expect if their requirement for vitamin C were increased.[103]

## *Are some people immune?*

It has been suggested that some people may be immune from scurvy, because of the evidence that on most expeditions there were some who remained healthy while others were going down with the disease. Cartier has been cited as a particular example because virtually the whole of his crew were sick. Anson was another example of an apparently exempt commander. Of course, the captain and officers of an expedition always had their own special supplies, so that it is not unexpected that they should have had a different, and usually better, record as regards the deficiency diseases. Nevertheless, it would, as has been suggested recently, be of great interest to follow up any indication that a particular individual was truly a synthesizer of ascorbic acid.[104]

Investigators have also been puzzled as to how certain cultural groups apparently continue to avoid scurvy when they do not seem to have an adequate supply of antiscorbutics available to them. The first such group was the Eskimos, but, as we have already seen, their traditional carnivorous diet does supply vitamin C, and they are subject to scurvy when they are able to buy other kinds of food.

It has also been suggested that the nomadic tribes living in the deserts of North Africa may be able to synthesize ascorbic acid because they appear to survive without scurvy on diets consisting primarily of cooked meat and containing no more than 2 mg vitamin C per day, by one calculation.[105] However, they, too, can suffer severely from scurvy when they are unable to carry on their accustomed life and have to live on purchased or donated foods.[106] Normally, they are only in completely arid areas when moving from one oasis to another. At an oasis, where they can graze their flock, they may be able to gather dates and citrus fruit, to supplement the meat and milk from their flocks. Arabs commonly value the fresh organ meats from a carcass even more highly than the muscles, and these are also generally considerably higher in vitamin C content. Not all the Bedouin groups drink fresh milk, but those that do are said to be the best protected from the disease.[107]

It was noted in Chapter 7 that one reason for the reluctance to identify Barlow's disease as the infantile form of scurvy was that it was apparently unknown in Russia even though adult scurvy was an endemic problem. At that time, breast-feeding was universal in Russia. Modern studies have shown that the level of vitamin C in breast milk is influenced by the level in the mother's blood plasma.[108] Nevertheless, the level in the milk can be as

---

[103] Kark (1953), 291.    [104] Cummings (1981), 298.    [105] Lewin (1976), 174–5.    [106] Fauré (1943), 271; Moulin (1959), 312, 314.    [107] May (1967), 145.    [108] Yüceðglu (1949), 149.

much as seven times as high as that in the maternal plasma, and this seems to explain the general immunity of breast-fed infants.[109] But how are lactating women able to supply this quantity? One study found no explanation for the good vitamin C status of Indian women who apparently had little of the vitamin in their diet and continued to secrete a larger quantity in their breast milk.[110]

Another puzzling group are the Bantu infants studied in Johannesburg. There is considerable malnutrition among these children after they are weaned early onto a cereal-based pap, but scurvy is extremely rare. Out of 9,000 hospital admissions, only 4 cases were seen. In routine checkups, x-rays of the femur showed no abnormality and their plasma levels of vitamin C were actually higher, on average, than those of artificially fed infants in the United States.[111] If there were biosynthesis by the infants, it would have had to be limited to that period of their life because the disease is seen regularly in Bantu men in the same urban community, though it is much more rare among the women.[112] Possibly the infants are given, from time to time, fruit which the women did not mention to their questioners because they thought it unimportant, or likely to be disapproved of. Wild fruits can be very rich in vitamin C; one, from a tree of the sweet almond family, has so much that a piece the size of a single grape (1.4 g) contains 100 mg.[113]

The very great majority of recorded cases of scurvy have occurred in men. This has usually been attributed to their having made up the old expeditions that had such limited dietaries, and, in modern times, to their lack of interest in cooking for themselves. But could there also be a true difference in the requirements of the two sexes, that is, one greater than the proportional difference in body size and total food requirement? It seems unlikely. The only female volunteer in the depletion experiments considered in Chapter 9 began to show signs of deficiency at a similar time to that of her male colleagues; also many of those that developed scurvy during the siege of Paris were women.

## Scurvy since World War II

In some other countries, infantile scurvy became an increasing public health problem in the period 1945–65. It was of particular concern in Canada.[114] As in the outbreaks studied at the beginning of the century, the problem was confined to babies that had not been breast-fed to any significant extent, and whose substitute foods contained little vitamin C. Evaporated cow's milk was the commonest alternative food. It was thought that no more than

[109] Salmenpera (1984), 1052.      [110] Rajalakshmi, Deodhar, & Ramakrishnan (1965), 379–81.      [111] Andersson, Walker, & Falcke (1956), 101–3      [112] Grusin & Kincaid-Smith (1954), 323.      [113] Nicol (1958); Brand et al. (1982), 873.      [114] Grewar (1958), 679.

10% of babies were being breast-fed, and that the shorter period that women now spent in hospital after childbirth reduced the opportunity to educate the mother in the proper alternative feeding of her baby.[115] There seemed no need to postulate any explanation for the increased incidence of disease other than there were more infants receiving an inadequate intake of the vitamin. Orange juice was available free of charge, but most physicians were uncertain as to its stability and were recommending multivitamin preparations instead.[116]

A nationwide study organized in 1961 by the Canadian Pediatric Society brought out one finding in striking contrast to that of the similar study which had been carried out in the United States in 1898 (see Chapter 7). At that time the problem had been largely confined to the better off, well-regulated households. Now the parents were typically from small communities and had less than average education and income.[117] The explanation proposed for the Canadian finding was that the artificial feeding of infants had by then spread through all the social classes, but that many of the mothers with scorbutic infants neither knew of the need for vitamin C in an infant's diet nor went to obtain regular advice from a health center or private pediatrician. It was concluded that the simplest preventive measure would be for "evaporated milk" to be fortified with ascorbic acid, and for cans of sweetened condensed milk to be labeled "unsuitable for infant feeding."

The experience in Australia was very similar to that in Canada. The disease appeared to be on the increase, and the parents were again typically of the lower socioeconomic groups. There was also the problem that many of the mothers were recent immigrants who did not understand English. There was a significant tendency, seen also in the Canadian studies, for the affected child to have come late in the family. The mothers, it was thought, did not attend Infant Welfare Centers as frequently as they had done with their earlier children. The recommendations were again that free orange juice be made available and that evaporated milk be fortified.[118]

A report of four cases of infantile scurvy seen at a clinic in Malaysia within a short period was accompanied by the suggestion that the rarity with which the disease was reported from the Tropics could be partly due to the lack of medical services to rural and poor urban populations.[119] Traditionally in Malaysia a woman who could not breast-feed her baby would seek out someone else to wet-nurse it. Now it was becoming common for mothers to use artificial feeding. Sweetened condensed milk was the cheapest form of milk available and had been given to all four of the cases studied. Manufacturers were encouraging, rather than discouraging, its use, and the incidence of the disease was expected to increase.

---

[115] Whelan et al. (1958), 179.    [116] Severs, Williams, & Davis (1961), 218.    [117] Demers et al. (1965), 574–5.    [118] Turner, Pitt, & Thomson (1959), 245–6.    [119] MacLean & Kamath (1970), 206.

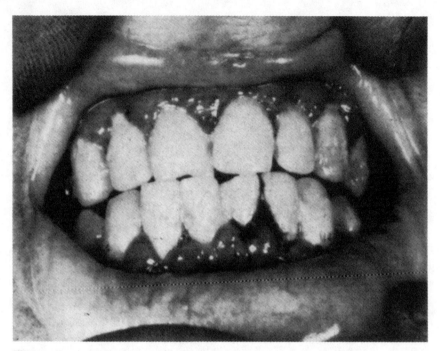

The swollen gums and hypertrophied papillae of a woman who developed scurvy on a fad diet in the 1960s. (From *Journal of the American Medical Association 199*: 794, 1967; copyright 1967, American Medical Association.)

Among adults in Western countries cases have continued to be reported from time to time, usually among widowers living alone and unaccustomed to cooking.[120] A new class of case appeared in the United States as a result of eating a Zen macrobiotic diet.[121] The patient, a woman thirty-eight years old, had used the most extreme form of the diet and eaten nothing but brown rice sprinkled with sesame seeds for the previous eight months. She had all the classical signs of scurvy as well as generalized malnutrition, but was still unwilling to change her diet because of her faith in the "macrobiotic philosophy." Finally her family persuaded her to receive an intramuscular injection of ascorbic acid. She responded rapidly and then agreed to change to a more normal diet. In another bizarre case, a nine-year-old girl developed both skin and mouth changes after living on nothing but tuna fish sandwiches (without lettuce) and iced tea (without lemon) for many months.[122]

[120] Anonymous (1983), 152; Reuler, Broudy, & Cooney (1985), 805–7.    [121] Sherlock & Rothschild (1967), 131–2.    [122] Ellis, Vanderveen, & Rasmussen (1984), 1212.

## Factors impeding progress in the nineteenth century

A solution to the practical problem of preventing scurvy seemed to have been worked out by 1800, and yet there continued to be outbreaks in the second half of the ensuing century. It was not just that there was a practical preventive available in the form of lemon juice; the modern concept of the disease, that is to say its being due to a simple dietary deficiency, was also clearly spelled out in the first half of the century. Elliotson's lecture on the subject, published in 1831, has already been referred to at the beginning of Chapter 5. He described scurvy as "a purely chemical disease . . . [in which] each part of the system is ready to perform all its functions, but one of the external things necessary for its doing so is taken away." [123]

Ten years later, George Budd, at another of the London teaching hospitals, made the same analysis of scurvy as being a deficiency disease. He also seems to have been the first to explain Lind's experience of the early appearance of scurvy in ships sailing from England in the spring, in terms of the depletion of the sailors' reserves of the antiscorbutic element during the preceding winter, rather than in Lind's terms of cold, wet weather being the inducing factor. [124] In addition, Budd said that scurvy was only one of a number of diseases due to specific dietary deficiencies; another was rickets and a third, which we would now describe as vitamin A deficiency, was "characterised by a peculiar ulceration of the cornea." [125]

As two authors have pointed out, Budd was a prophet. [126] But, in regard just to scurvy, it would be wrong – and another writer has documented the point – to think that his idea was unorthodox. [127] Nevertheless, it is true that there is surprisingly little reference to the antiscorbutic factor in most of the general works on food and dietetics that appeared in the next fifty years, [128] and the concept of deficiency diseases was almost lost to view by the end of the nineteenth century. Let us consider some factors that could be responsible for this.

First there was the development of methods of chemical analysis for carbon and nitrogen, and Liebig's division of food components into protein, the nitrogenous fraction which was "truly nutritive," and the other organic compounds which were merely "respiratory" and a source of calories. Analyses for these two elements, combined with determinations of the digestibility of different foods, provided two generations of researchers with a full-time occupation; and other qualities of foods that were not yet measurable came to be forgotten. Thus, even as late as 1902, the U. S. Department of Agriculture, in its well-meant studies aimed at showing the poor how to eat more cheaply, was making its calculations just in these terms. As a consequence it classed green vegetables and fruit as expensive sources of both

---

[123] Elliotson (1831), 653.     [124] Budd (1840), 67.     [125] Budd (1842), 632.     [126] Harris (1935), 8; Hughes (1973), 132.     [127] Carter (1977), 121–2.     [128] Hughes (1973), 133–4.

protein and energy, with special value only in providing laxative bulk.[129] It acknowledged that a more varied diet was pleasing to the aesthetic sense but warned that ". . . indulgence in luxuries simply pleases the palate without properly nourishing the body."[130]

Another factor reducing interest in the deficiency disease concept may have been the discovery of the alkaloids by French scientists and their work on the analogy between morbid causes and poisons.[131] Also there was the incidental observation that dogs, found so useful in research on other nutrients, failed to develop scurvy when they were kept on what would be a scorbutic diet for humans.[132] As we have seen, it was only in this century, through the chance use by Holst and Frölich of guinea pigs, one of the few animal species that do require the antiscorbutic factor, that real progress began to be made.

Several scholars have argued that it was the success of the "germ theory of disease" that caused the study of scurvy to be diverted in unprofitable directions.[133] One writer has said: "As a result of the tremendous influence of these positive agents, the bacteria and their products, it was difficult to think in terms of negative causes of disease."[134] To quote from another essay: "The germ theory of disease proved vastly more successful than any previous medical concept. . . . With the emphasis . . . on sanitation. . . from 1870 onward there was a new success . . . which created a temptation to believe that microorganisms might be responsible for all diseases.[135] On the other hand, a third writer has suggested that the development of the germ theory, rather than being an obstacle to the study of scurvy, acted as a challenge by providing a new standard for the theoretical understanding of disease. Viewing it only as an obstacle "seems to reflect a serious lack of historical perspective."[136] Certainly, it was work that began as a study of beriberi from the perspective of its being an infectious disease that led the microbiologists and pathologists to the evidence of its being a deficiency condition. The work of bacteriologists also demonstrated the great value of using a variety of animal models, and it was this that led to the Norwegian production of experimental scurvy in guinea pigs.

My own feeling is that it was the repeated failure of lime juice after 1860 that was most important in leading investigators to doubt the whole structure of experience and conclusions about scurvy that had been built up in the previous two hundred years. The very kernel of the old school of thought was that lemon juice was virtually a specific for the disease, yet now (given the confusion between lemons and limes, and ignorance of the losses in processing and storage) it was found to be almost useless. In this situation the investigator was induced to look at the whole subject anew, rejecting

---

[129] Milner (1902), 397, 405–6.    [130] Ibid., 388.    [131] Lesch (1984), 137–44.    [132] Budd (1842), 743.    [133] Stewart (1953), 408.    [134] Follis (1960), 307.    [135] Ihde & Becker (1971), 16.    [136] Carter (1977), 136.

earlier knowledge which now seemed unreliable, and accepting only the first-hand experience and ways of thought of his own generation. For people like Jackson and Koettlitz, whose experience in the Arctic had been that those who ate fresh meat remained healthy, whereas those who ate preserved meat developed scurvy (even though they took lime juice), it is understandable that they should have come to believe that it was caused by ptomaine poisoning.

Another factor that may have weakened confidence in the deficiency concept was that the specific claims as to the identity of the antiscorbutic factor – first that it was citric acid and then potassium – did not stand up to examination. The "diminished alkalinity" theory, which came next, is understandable as a hypothesis. But, like the potassium theory, it obviously did not explain why foods lost value as a result of drying or processing. Nor did studies of the blood in cases of scurvy support it. The fact that it continued to be put forward for so long, and to receive support in England, seems to have been due entirely to the eminence and contentiousness of one individual, Sir Almroth Wright. The "nuisance value" of the theory was that it persuaded some people that the disease had been explained and therefore no longer needed investigation. There was, in any case, the continued difficulty that the human disease occurred only sporadically, and usually in remote positions where there was no facility or preparation for a systematic study.

## General conclusions

The negative contribution of Sir Almroth Wright, just referred to, prompts the generalization that the contributions of men already eminent for another piece of work have, when it comes to scurvy, been rather uniformly of this character. The basis for this conclusion is set out in Table 10.4. In most instances the theory advanced was related in some way to the work for which the man had become famous. In contrast, the people such as Bachstrom, Lind, Elliotson, Budd, and Holst, who made contributions and drew conclusions that we now consider well founded, seem equally consistently to have escaped the usual marks of general recognition and appreciation. Perhaps success in one field, and the subsequent respect in which their opinions are held, tend to give the eminent over-confidence in proposing theories in other fields which they have not really had time to study in depth, in the way that they had in their original work.

Certainly, theories are beguiling things, and human nature finds it difficult to admit to *not* having an explanation for a phenomenon. As a consequence, we have seen how discovery after discovery in chemistry led to successive explanations of scurvy: "acid and alkali," carbon dioxide, oxygen, citric acid, potassium, and ptomaines. As Trotter admitted in 1795: "It is a difficult, if not dangerous attempt to reconcile appearances in the living

Table 10.4. *Views of the most eminent men appearing in the history of scurvy*

| Subject and positions attained | Work primarily responsible for eminence | Theory of scurvy | Present view of the theory |
|---|---|---|---|
| Sir John Pringle (1707–87) President of the Royal Society; Copley medalist | Association of typhus with poor hygiene; introduction of hygienic reform in the Army | A result of putrefaction, correctable by foods fermenting to yield carbon dioxide | Wrong |
| Sir Robert Christison (1797–1882) President, British Medical Association; physician to Queen Victoria | Pioneer in forensic toxicology | Due to protein deficiency | Wrong |
| Jean-Antoine Villemin (1827–92) Member of the Academy of Medicine, Paris | Experimental proof that tuberculosis was an infectious disease | Caused by a contagious miasm | Wrong |
| William A. Hammond (1828–1900) U. S. Surgeon-General | Administrative reforms during the Civil War | Due to a deficiency of potassium and/or iron | Wrong |
| Lord Lister (1827–1912) President of the Royal Society; surgeon to Queen Victoria | Introduction of antiseptic procedures into surgery | A result of ptomaine intoxication | Wrong |
| Sir Almroth Wright (1861–1947) Royal Society medalist | Development of antityphoid inoculation and of immunology generally | Due to the blood's being insufficiently alkaline | Wrong |

body, to the laws of chemical affinity. In the fond attachment to this be-witching study, amidst the enthusiasm of enquiry, we may be sometimes betrayed into imaginary facts and fallacious conclusions." [137]

As emphasized already, the whole subject was put on a different footing once it was discovered that the guinea pig could serve as an animal model. The use of animals in medical research is a controversial and distressing subject, but in the present instance it is difficult to imagine how vitamin C could have been identified without the use of guinea pigs. The justification for all the animal experiments with ascorbic acid carried out since that period is more open to argument, now that the means of both preventing and curing scurvy are readily at hand.

Certainly, the work of the chemists in discovering the structure of vitamin C and in developing cheap ways of synthesizing it seems an unmixed blessing. It was possible, of course, because of the basic studies in organic chemistry already carried out without relation to any particular medical application. It still seems extraordinary how quickly the structure of Szent-Györgyi's crystals was worked out in the early 1930s, on the basis of a relatively small number of observed properties. It is perhaps an ironic consequence that ascorbic acid – and other synthetic vitamins – are now being used in large quantities mainly by those who can already afford a well-balanced diet, rather than by those who cannot.

McCord has argued that scurvy should be classed as an "occupational disease," perhaps even as history's foremost occupational disease. For the work forces of sailors from 1500 to 1800 he has accumulated records of two million deaths.[138] He says:

"One of the warped notions running through early scurvy history is the belief that only a few nations were subject to it, chiefly the English, Spaniards, Portuguese and Russians . . . these people have furnished the best records. . . . While scurvy is ever the mark of ignorance . . . it is also the mark of national boldness. . . . they suffered more because they risked more." [139]

To quote from McCord again: "The British navy appears to be the greatest contributor of occupational scurvy, but this appearance may be deceptive. No other nation has so well recorded its epidemics and catastrophes." [138] Furthermore, the people who put these problems on record were also actively trying to understand and overcome them. I think particularly of Thomas Trotter's being in trouble with his admiral for trying to hold up the sailing of a ship until it had received a full issue of vegetables; and, despite his dignified position as Physician to the Fleet, thinking it "no disgrace" to go around the markets of Portsmouth himself, collecting up salads for his sailors.[140] His theories about the mode of action of vegetables now seem almost ridiculous, but his sincerity and good heart are above question.

---

[137] Trotter (1795), 33.     [138] McCord (1959), 316.     [139] McCord (1971), 307.     [140] Trotter (1804), 73–4.

Undoubtedly there was the same dedication in the laboratory work removed from actual suffering, for example, that of Harriette Chick and her colleagues during World War I, with their very careful assays – all of whose results have stood the test of time.

I will end with a loose translation of a passage in Mahé's scholarly monograph, written in the 1870s after the experience of the siege of Paris:

From this long enumeration of the facts relating to the reign of scurvy . . . I would like the reader to remember the following points. . . . In preceding centuries it was in full view, today it is more in the shadows but it is still scurvy, an intimate and profound change in the organism which weakens the force of life even when it does not extinguish it. . . . It is a result of bad conditions of existence for which we are responsible because of our ignorance and even more because of our foolhardy improvidence. . . . Scurvy has too often saddened, paralysed and brought to nothing the greatest enterprises of men both at sea and on land. . . . But it would be childish just to have traced such a sombre aspect of human history. We must now go on to penetrate further into the secret of the causes or conditions which engender the disease, for we must never forget that *to know is to anticipate and to prevent.*[141]

Mahé's prophecy was certainly correct. Let us honor and remember all the men and women who contributed to the spectacular advances of the first thirty-five years of this century.

[141] Mahé (1880), 80–1.

# References

Acerra, M.-M. (1981). Le scorbut: la peste du marin. *L'Histoire*, no. 36: 74–5.

Ackerknecht, E. H. (1982). *A Short History of Medicine*. Baltimore, MD: Johns Hopkins University Press.

Adams, C. F. (1975). *Nutritive Value of American Foods in Common Units*. Washington, DC: U.S. Department of Agriculture.

Adams, F., trans. (1884). *The Seven Books of Paulus Aegineta*. 3 vols. London: Sydenham Society.

Addington, A. (1753). *An Essay on the Sea Scurvy wherein is Proposed an Easy Method of Curing that Distemper at Sea*. Reading: Mickelwright.

Admiralty Committee on Scurvy (1877). *Report on the Cause of the Outbreak of Scurvy in the Recent Arctic Expedition. Parliamentary Papers LVI*: 557–1137. London: H. M. Stationery Office.

Aldridge, J. (1847). On the comparative nutritive and pecuniary values of various kinds of cooked food. *Proc. R. Dublin Soc.* 1846–7 (no. 18): 123–52.

Aldridge, J. (1862). Potash in scurvy. *Lancet ii*: 268.

Alvarez, W. (1924). Intestinal autointoxication. *Physiol. Rev. 4*: 352–93.

Ambrose, A. M., & De Eds, F. (1949). The value of rutin and quercetin in scurvy. *J. Nutr. 38*: 305–17.

Ancell, H. (1843). Liebig, his chemistry and reviewers. Part X. *Lancet i*: 605–71.

Andel, M. A. van (1927). Der Skorbut als niederlandische Volkskrankheit. *Arch. Gesch. Med. 19*: 82–91.

Anderson, A. (1847). On the recent differences of opinion as to the cause of scurvy. *Monthly J. Med. Sci. 8*: 176–81.

Anderson, T. W., Reid, D. B. W., & Beaton, G. H. (1972). Vitamin C and the common cold: a double-blind trial. *Can. Med. Assoc. J. 107*: 503–8.

Anderson, T. W., Suranyi, G., & Beaton, G. H. (1974). The effect on winter illness of large doses of vitamin C. *Can. Med. Assoc. J. 111*: 31–6.

Andersson, M., Walker, A. R. P., & Falcke, H. C. (1956). An investigation of the rarity of infantile scurvy among the South African Bantu. *Br. J. Nutr. 10*: 101–5.

Anonymous (1824). Lemon juice in scurvy. *Medico-Chirurg. Rev. [n.s.] 1*: 232.

Anonymous (1847). John Oliver Curran, M. B. *Dublin Q. J. Med. Sci. [N.S.] 4*: 500–11.

Anonymous (1848). Analytical and critical review on the pathology and treatment of scurvy. *Br. Foreign Medico-Chirurg. Rev. ii*: 439–74.

Anonymous (1983). Scurvy in an old man. *Nutr. Rev. 41*: 152–4.

Anonymous (1984). Chemical profile: ascorbic acid. *Chemical Marketing Reporter*. January 2: 62.

Anonymous (1985). Coldbusters. *Delicious.* New Hope Publications, New Hope, PA. February: 6–7.

Arber, E., ed. (1879). Prince's Chronological History of New England. In: *An English Garner,* vol. 2. London: Arber.

Armitage, A. B. (1905). *Two Years in the Antarctic.* London: Arnold.

Armstrong, A. (1857). *A Personal Narrative of the Discovery of the Northwest Passage.* London: Hurst & Blackett.

Armstrong, A. (1858). *Observations on Naval Hygiene and Scurvy.* London: Churchill.

Aschoff L., & Koch, W. (1919). *Skorbut, Eine pathologisch-anatomische Studie.* Jena, E. Germany: Fischer.

Atkinson, E. L. (1915). The British Antarctic Expedition, 1910–1913. *J. R. Naval Med. Serv.* 1: 1–14.

Ausset, E. (1902). La maladie de Barlow, est-elle une forme spéciale de rachitisme ou du scorbut infantile? *Bull. Soc. Pédiatrie (Paris)* 4: 320–38.

Aykroyd, W. R. (1974). *The Conquest of Famine.* London: Chatto & Windus.

Bachstrom, J. F. (1734). *Observationes circa scorbutum.* Reprinted in *De Scorbuto Liber* (1766). Venice: Pezzana.

Back, G. (1838). *Narrative of an Expedition in H.M.S.* Terror . . . *1836–7.* London: J. Murray.

Badenoch, J. (1776). Observations on the use of wort in the cure of scurvy at sea. *Med. Obs. Inquiries Soc. Physicians (London)* 5: 61–72.

Baker, E. M., Hodges, R. F., Hood, J., Sauberlich, H. E., & March, S. C. (1969). Metabolism of ascorbic-1-$^{14}$C in experimental human scurvy. *Am. J. Clin. Nutr.* 22: 549–58.

Baly, W. (1843). On the prevention of scurvy in prisoners, pauper lunatic asylums etc. *London Med. Gaz. [n.s.]* 1: 699–703.

Banks, J. (1896). *Journal during Captain Cook's First Voyage. 1768–71.* London: MacMillan.

Barlow, H., & Barlow, A., ed. (1965). *Sir Thomas Barlow, Bt. 1845–1945.* London: Dawsons.

Barlow, T. (1883). On cases described as 'acute rickets' which are probably a combination of scurvy and rickets, the scurvy being an essential, and the rickets a variable, element. *Med. Chir. Trans. (London)* 66: 159–220.

Barnes, G. R., & Owen, J. H. (1938). *The Private Papers of John, Earl of Sandwich,* vol. 4, 1781–2. London: Navy Records Society.

Barnes, R. E., & Hume, E. M. (1919). A comparison between the antiscorbutic properties of fresh, heated and dried cow's milk. *Lancet ii:* 323–4.

Barrett, J. (1849). Observations on scurvy in Bath and its neighbourhood in the spring of 1847. *Provincial Med. J.* 148–53; 173–7; 211–13.

Bartenstein, L. (1905). Beitrage zur Frage des Kunstlichen Morbus Barlow bei Tieren. *Jahrb. Kinderheilk.* 61: 6–35.

Bartley, W., Krebs, H. A., & O'Brien, J. R. P. (1953). *Vitamin C Requirement of Human Adults.* Medical Research Council Special Report Series, no. 280. London: H. M. Stationery Office.

Barton, J. K. (1897). The value of sterilised milk. *Br. Med. J.* i: 14.

Basu, T. K., & Schorah, C. J. (1982). *Vitamin C in Health and Disease.* London: Croom Helm.

Baudens, L. (1862). *On Military and Camp Hospitals and the Health of Troops in the Field.* (F. B. Hough, trans.). New York: Bailliere Bros.

Bauernfeind, J. C. (1982). Ascorbic acid technology in agricultural, pharmaceutical, food and industrial applications. In: *Ascorbic Acid: Chemistry, Metabolism, and Uses* (P. A. Leib & B. M. Tolbert, eds.), pp. 395–497. Washington, DC: American Chemical Society.

Bauernfeind, J. C., & Pinkert, D. M. (1970). Food processing with added ascorbic acid. *Adv. Food Res.* 18: 219–315.

Beaglehole, J. C., ed. (1955). *The Journals of Captain James Cook I. The Voyage of the Endeavour.* Cambridge: Hakluyt Society.

Beaglehole, J. C., ed. (1961). *The Journals of Captain James Cook II: The Voyage of the Resolution and Adventure.* Cambridge: Hakluyt Society.

Beaglehole, J. C. (1974). *The Life of Captain James Cook.* London: Hakluyt Society.

Beddoes, T. (1793). *Observations on the Nature and Cure of Calculus, Sea Scurvy etc.* London: Murray.

Beke, C. T., ed. (1853). *A True Description of Three Voyages by the North-East Towards Cathay and China: 1594, 1595, 1596.* London: Hakluyt Society.

Belcher, E. (1855). *The Last of the Arctic Voyages.* 2 vols. London: Lovell Reeve.

Bellot, J. R. (1855). *Memoirs.* London: Hurst & Blackett.

Bennett, G. (1832). The porphyra nautica, or sea scurvy. *London Med. Gaz.* 10: 573–4.

Bensáth, A., Rusznyák, S., & Szent-Györgyi, A. (1936). Vitamin nature of flavones. *Nature* 138: 798.

Berncastle, J. (1842). Potatoes as a preventative of sea-scurvy. *Lancet ii:* 892–3.

Bertelsen, A. (1911). Animalske antiscorbutica i Grønland, *Hospitalstidende (Copenhagen)* 54: 537–44.

Berthenson, L. (1892). Zur Statistik und Aetiologie des Scorbuts. *Dtsch. Arch. f. Klin. Med.* 49: 127–55.

Bestermann, T. ed. (1956). *Voltaire's Correspondence,* vols. 20 & 23. Geneva: Institut et Musée Voltaire.

Biggar, H. P. (1901). *Early Trading Companies of New France.* Toronto: University of Toronto Library.

Biggar, H. P. (1924). *The Voyages of Jacques Cartier.* Ottawa: Acland.

Birdwood, G., ed. (1893). *The Register of Letters etc. of the Governors and Company of Merchants Trading into the East Indies. 1600–1619.* London: Quaritch. Reprint, 1965.

Bisset, C. (1755). *A Treatise on the Scurvy.* London: Dodsley.

Black, P. (1876). *Scurvy in High Latitudes: an Attempt to Explain the Cause of the 'Medical Failure' of the Arctic Expedition of 1875–6.* London: Smith, Elders & Co.

Blane, G. (1813). Observations on the comparative prevalence, mortality and treatment of different diseases. *Med. Chirurg. Trans.* 4: 89–141.

Blane, G. (1819). *Elements of Medical Logic.* London: Underwood.

Bolle, C. (1902–3). Zur Therapie der Barlow'schen Krankheit. *Z. f. die Gesamte Physikalische Therapie (Leipzig)* 6: 354–6.

Bostock, J., & Riley, T. H., trans. (1856). *The Natural History of Pliny,* book 25, chap. 6, lect. 3. London: Bohn.

Boussingault, J. B. (1845). *Rural Economy in Its Relations with Chemistry, Physics and Meterology.* London: Bailliere.

Boxer, C. R., ed. (1959). *The Tragic History of the Sea.* Cambridge: Hakluyt Society.

Boycott, A. E. (1917). Discussion on beriberi and scurvy. *Trans. Soc. Trop. Med. Hyg.* 10: 179.

Brand, J. C., Cherikoff, V., Lee, A., & Truswell, A. S. (1982). An outstanding food source of vitamin C. *Lancet ii:* 873.

Bransby, E. R., Hunter, J. W., Magee, H. E., Milligan, E. H. M., & Rodgers, T. S. (1944). The influence of supplements of vitamins on growth, health and physical fitness. *Br. Med. J. i:* 77–8.

Breeden, J. O. (1975). *Joseph Jones, M.D., Scientist of the Old South.* Lexington, KY: University Press of Kentucky.

Briggs, M. (1984). Vitamin C and infectious disease. In: *Recent Vitamin Research* (M. H. Briggs, ed.), pp. 39–81. Boca Raton, FL: CRC Press.

Brock, A. J. (1929). *Greek Medicine.* London: Dent.

Brown, T. M. (1968). *The Mechanical Philosophy and the "Animal Oeconomy": A Study in the Development of English Physiology in the Seventeenth and Early Eighteenth Century.* Ph.D. Dissertation, Princeton University.

Bruff, J. G. (1949). *Gold Rush.* New York: Columbia University Press.

Bryson, A. (1850). On the respective value of lime juice, citric acid and nitrate of potash in the treatment of scurvy. *Med. Times Gaz. (London)* 21: 212–14, 435–6.

Buchan, W. (1769). *Domestic Medicine.* Edinburgh: Balfour, Auld & Smellie.

Budd, G. (1840). Scurvy. In: *The Library of Medicine. Practical Medicine* (A. Tweedie, ed.), vol. 5: 58–95. London: Whittaker.

Budd, G. (1842). Disorders resulting from defective nutriment. *London Med. Gaz.* 2: 632–6, 712–16, 743–9, 906–15.

Buffum, E. G. (1850). *Six Months in the Gold Mines.* Philadelphia, PA: Lea & Blanchard.

Bullmore, C. (1900). Beri-beri. *Lancet ii:* 873–5.

Buño, W. (July–Dec., 1953). Escorbuto durante la exploracion y conquista de América. *Arch. Ibero-Amer. de Historia de la Medicina* 5: 576–83.

Burnett, W. (1854–5). Reports made to the Board of Admiralty and the Board of Trade on the subject of preparing lemon-juice to render it efficacious and anti-scorbutic. *Med. Times Gaz. (London)* 30: 635–6.

Burney, J. (1975). *With Captain James Cook in the Antarctic and Pacific.* Canberra: National Library of Australia.

Buzzard, T. (1866). Scorbutus. In: *A System of Medicine* (J. R. Reynolds, ed.), pp. 731–55. London: Macmillan.

Calkins, B. M., Whittaker, D. J., Rider, A. A., & Turjman, N. (1984). Diet, nutrition intake, and metabolism in populations at high and low risk for colon cancer. Nutrient intake. *Am. J. Clin. Nutr.* 40: 896–905.

Calvarano, M., & Gallino, M. (1975). Contributo allo studio del limao Galego (*Citrus aurantifolia* Sw.) coltivato in Brasile. *Essenze Derivati Agrumari* 45: 279–91.

Cameron, C. (1830). Nitre, a remedy for scurvy. *London Med. Gaz.* 5: 751–2.

Cameron, E., & Pauling, L. (1979). *Cancer and Vitamin C.* Menlo Park, CA: Linus Pauling Institute of Science and Medicine.

Campbell, H. J. (1896). The advantages and disadvantages of the use of sterilized milk for infant feeding. *Br. Med. J. ii:* 623–6.

Campbell, M. E. D., & Chick, H. (1919). The antiscorbutic and growth promoting value of canned vegetables. *Lancet ii:* 320–2.

Carpenter, K. J., ed. (1981). *Pellagra: Benchmark Papers in the History of Biochemistry.* Stroudsburg, PA: Hutchinson Ross.

Carpenter, K. J. (1984). Biological Assays. In: *Methods of Vitamin Assay,* (J. Augustin, ed.), pp. 17–34. New York: Wiley.

Carter, K. C. (1977). The germ theory, beriberi, and the deficiency theory of disease. *Med. Hist.* 21: 119–36.

Castiglioni, A. (1958). *A History of Medicine.* 2nd ed. New York: Knopf.

Cell, G. T. ed., (1982). *Newfoundland Discovered: English Attempts at Colonisation, 1610–1630.* London: Hakluyt Society.

Chamberlain, N. (1981). The use of ascorbic acid in breadmaking. In: *Vitamin C (Ascorbic Acid).* (J. N. Counsell & D. H. Hornig, eds.), pp. 87–104. London: Applied Science Publishers.

Chance, B. (1942). Bishop Berkeley and his use of tar-water. *Ann. Med. Hist. [ser. 3]* 4: 453–67.

Charleston, S. S., & Clegg, K. M. (1972). Ascorbic acid and the common cold. *Lancet i:* 1401–2.

Chatterjee, I. B., Majumder, A. K., Nandi, B. K., & Subramanian, N. (1975). Synthesis and some major functions of vitamin C in animals. *Ann. N. Y. Acad. Sci.* 258: 24–47.

Chazan, J. A., & Mistilis, J. P. (1963). The patho-physiology of scurvy. A report of seven cases. *Am. J. Med.* 34: 350–8.

Cheadle, W. B. (1878). Three cases of scurvy supervening on rickets in young children. *Lancet ii:* 685–7.

Cheadle, W. B. (1882). Osteal or periosteal cachexia and scurvy. *Lancet ii:* 48–9.

Chick, H. (1953). Early investigations of scurvy and the anti-scorbutic vitamin. *Proc. Nutr. Soc.* 12: 210–18.

Chick, H., & Dalyell, E. J. (1920). Eine Skorbutepidemie unter Kindern im Alter von 6 Bis 14 Jahren. *Z. f. Kinderh.* 26: 257–69.

Chick, H. & Delf, E. M. (1919). The anti-scorbutic value of dry and germinated seeds. *Biochem. J.* 13: 199–218.

Chick, H., & Hume, E. M. (1917). The distribution among foodstuffs of the substances required for the prevention of beriberi and scurvy. *Trans. Soc. Trop. Med. Hyg.* 10: 141–78.

Chick, H., Hume, M., & MacFarlane, M. (1971). *War on Disease: A History of the Lister Institute.* London: Deutsch.

Chick, H., Hume, E. M., & Skelton, R. F. (1918). The anti-scorbutic value of cow's milk. *Biochem. J.* 12: 131–53.

Chick, H., Hume, E. M., Skelton, R. F., & Smith, A. H. (1918). The relative content of the antiscorbutic principle in limes and lemons. *Lancet ii:* 735–8.

Chick, H., & Rhodes, M. (1918). An investigation of the antiscorbutic value of the raw juices of root vegetables, with a view to their adoption as an adjunct to the dietary of infants. *Lancet ii:* 774–5.

Christison, R. (1847a). Account of an epidemic of scurvy which prevailed in the general prison at Perth in 1846. *Monthly J. Med. Sci.* 7: 873–91.

Christison, R. (1847b). Account of scurvy as it has lately appeared in Edinburgh, and of an epidemic of it among railway labourers in the surrounding country. *Monthly J. Med. Sci.* 8: 1–22.

Churchill, J. (1704). *A Collection of Voyages and Travels,* vol. 2, London: Awnsham & Churchill.

Clark, J. (1773). *Observations on the Diseases in Long Voyages to Hot Countries.* London: Wilson & Nicol.

Clark, R. W. (1983). *Benjamin Franklin. A Biography.* New York: Random House.

Clegg, K. M., & McDonald, J. M. (1975). L-ascorbic acid and D-isoascorbic acid in a common cold survey. *Am. J. Clin. Nutr.* 28: 973–6.

Clemetson, C. A. B. (1980). Histamine and ascorbic acid in human blood. *J. Nutr.* 110: 662–8.

Clerk of the California, The (1968). *An Account of a Voyage for the Discovery of the North-West Passage (1749).* New York: Johnson Reprint Corp.

Clow, A., & Clow, N. L. (1952). *The Chemical Revolution.* London: Batchworth Press.

Clow, C. L., Laberge, C., & Scrives, C. R. (1975). Neonatal hypertyrosinemia and evidence for deficiency of ascorbic acid in Arctic and sub-Arctic people. *Can. Med. Assoc. J.* 113: 624–6.

Clowes, W. L., ed. (1899). *The Royal Navy. A History,* vol. 4. Boston, MA: Little, Brown.

Coale, E. (1842). Notes on the scurvy, as it appeared on board the U.S. Frigate Columbia in her cruise around the world, 1838–40. *Am. J. Med. Sci. [n.s.]* 3: 68–77.

Cockburn, A. (1845). Biographical sketch of the late Dr. Thomas Trotter, Physician to the British Fleet. *Edinburgh Med. Surg. J.* 64: 430–41.

Cockburn, W. (1736). *Sea Diseases.* 3rd ed. London: Strahan.

Cohen, B., & Mendel, L. B. (1918). Experimental scurvy of the guinea pig in relation to the diet. *J. Biol. Chem.* 35: 425–53.

Cohen, J. M., ed. (1969). *The Four Voyages of Christopher Columbus.* London: Penguin.

Colan, T. (1883). Discussion on the etiology of scurvy. *Lancet i:* 363–5, 406–8.

Colly, M. (1956). Le scorbut chez les enfants de l'Aumône Générale et de la Charité de Lyon aux XVIe et XVIIIe siècles. *Cahiers Lyonnais d'Hist. Méd.* 1:33–40.

Commission on Milk Standards (1912). Report of the Commission on Milk Standards appointed by the New York Milk Commission. *Public Health Rep.* 27: 673–700.

Comrie, J. D. (1920). Scurvy in North Russia. *Edinburgh Med. J.* 24: 207–15.

Comstock, D. A. (1982). *Gold Diggers and Camp Followers.* Grass Valley, CA: Comstock Bonanza Press.

Connell, S. J. B., & Zilva, S. S. (1924). The reducing properties of antiscorbutic preparations. *Biochem. J.* 18: 638–40.

Cook, J., ed. (1679). *Select Observations on English Bodies by John Hall.* 2nd ed. London: Shirley. [Reprinted in Joseph (1964).]

Cook, J. (1776). The method taken for preserving the health of the crew of His Majesty's ship the Resolution during her late voyage round the world. *Philos. Trans. R. Soc.* 66: 402–6.

Coplans, M. (1904). On the etiology of scurvy. *Trans. Epidemiol. Soc. (London):* 79–94.

Corlette, C. E. (1900). An explanation of the cause of infantile scurvy with suggestions as to its prevention. *Br. Med. J. ii:* 573–5.

Corney, B., ed. (1855). *The Voyage of Sir Henry Middleton to Bantam and the Maluca Islands.* London: Hakluyt Society.

Coulehan, J. L., Reisinger, K. S., Rogers, K. D., & Bradley, D. W. (1974). Vitamin C prophylaxis in a boarding school. *N. Engl. J. Med.* 290: 6–10.

Counsell, J. N., & Hornig, D. M., eds. (1981). *Vitamin C (Ascorbic Acid).* London: Applied Science Publishers.

Coward, K. H. (1935). The biological standardisation of vitamins. *Nutr. Abstr. Rev.* 4: 705–14.

Cox, E. V. (1968). The anemia of scurvy. *Vitam. Horm.* 26: 635–52.

Craig, A. A., Lewis, F. J. W., & Woodman, D. (1944). Survey of vitamin C levels in wartime in pregnant women. *Br. Med. J. i:* 455–7.

Crandon, J. H., Lund, C. C., & Dill, D. B. (1940). Human experimental scurvy. *N. Engl. J. Med.* 223: 353–69.

Creagan, E. T., Moertl, C. G., et al. (1979). Failure of high-dose vitamin C (ascorbic acid) therapy to benefit patients with advanced cancer. *N. Engl. J. Med.* 301: 687–90.

Creighton, C. (1891). *A History of Epidemics in Britain,* vol. I. Cambridge University Press.

Crooke, W., ed. (1909). *A New Account of East India and Persia Being Nine Years' Travels, 1672–81 by John Fryer.* London: Hakluyt Society.

Crosby, N. T., & Sawyer, R. (1976). N-nitrosamines: a review of chemical and biological properties and their estimation in foodstuffs. *Adv. Food Res.* 22: 1–71.

Cummings, M. (1981). Can some people synthesize ascorbic acid? *Am. J. Clin. Nutr.* 34: 297–8.

Curran, J. O. (1847). Observations on scurvy as it has lately appeared throughout Ireland, and in several parts of Great Britain. *Dublin Q. J. Med. Sci. [n.s.]* 4: 83–130.

Curtis, C. (1807). *An Account of the Diseases of India.* Edinburgh: Laing.

Dalton, W. (1842). The potato in sea-scurvy. *Lancet ii:* 789.

Davey, A. J. (1921). Determination of the minimum doses of some fresh citrus juices which will protect a guinea-pig from scurvy. *Biochem. J.* 15: 83–103.

Davis, K. G., & Johnson, A. M. (1963). *Northern Quebec and Labrador Journals and Correspondence, 1819–35.* London: Hudson's Bay Record Society.

Debus, A. G. (1977). *The Chemical Philosophy: Paracelsian Science and Medicine in the Sixteenth and Seventeenth Centuries,* vol. 2. New York: Science History Publications.

De Hullu, J. (1913). Ziekten en dokters op de schepen der Oost-Indische Compagnie. *Bijdr. Taal-, Land-, en Volkenkunde Ned.-Indië,* 67: 245–72.

Delacoste, J., trans. (1715). *Boerhaave's Aphorisms Concerning the Knowledge and Cure of Diseases.* London: Cowse & Innys.

Delf, E. M., & Skelton, R. F. (1918). The effect of drying on the antiscorbutic and growth promoting properties of cabbage. *Biochem. J.* 12: 448–63.

De Lisle, F. I. (1877). Scurvy; its cause, its prevention and its antidotes. *Med. Times Gaz. (London) ii:* 301–3.

Delpech, A. (1871). Le scorbut dans le siège de Paris. *Ann. d'Hyg. Publ. (Paris) [n.s.]* 35: 297–359.

Demers, P., Fraser, D., et al. (1965). An epidemiological study of infantile scurvy in Canada: 1961–63. *Can. Med. Assoc. J.* 93: 573–6.

De Mertans, C. (1778). Observations on the scurvy. *Philos. Trans. R. Soc.* 68: 661–80.

De Veer, G. (1876). *Journal of the Three Voyages of William Barents to the Arctic Regions.* London: Hakluyt Society.

De Villiers, J. A. J., ed. (1906). *The East and West Indian Mirror.* London: Hakluyt Society.

*D. N. B.* [Dictionary of National Biography] (1893). London: Oxford University Press.

Dobson, M. (1779). *A Medical Commentary on Fixed Air.* London: Cadell.

Dolman, C. E. (1973). Joseph Lister. In: *Dictionary of Scientific Biography* (C. C. Gillispie, ed.), vol. 18: 399–413.

Donno, E. S. (1976). *An Elizabethan in 1582. The Diary of Richard Madox, Fellow of All Souls.* London: Hakluyt Society.

Donovan, A. L. (1975). *Philosophical Chemistry and the Scottish Enlightenment.* Edinburgh: University Press.

Draper, H. H. (1977). The aboriginal Eskimo diet in modern perspective. *Am. Anthropol. 79:* 309–16.

Draper, H. H., & Bell, R. R. (1972). The changing Eskimo diet. *Illinois Res. 14* (4): 14–15.

Drinkwater, J. (1786). *A History of the Late Siege of Gibraltar.* 2nd ed. London: Spilsbury.

Drummond, J. C. (1919). Note on the role of the anti-scorbutic factor in nutrition. *Biochem. J. 13:* 77–80.

Drummond, J. C. (1920). The nomenclature of the so-called accessory food factors (vitamins). *Biochem. J. 14:* 660.

Drummond, J. C., & Wilbraham, A. (1935). William Stark, M.D.: an eighteenth century experiment in nutrition. *Lancet ii:* 459–62.

Dubos, R., & Dubos, J. (1952). *The White Plague. Tuberculosis, Man and Society.* Boston, MA: Little, Brown.

Dudley, S. F. (1953a). James Lind: laudatory address. *Proc. Nutr. Soc. 12:* 202–9.

Dudley, S. F. (1953b). The Lind tradition in the Royal Naval Medical Service. In: *Lind's Treatise on Scurvy.* (C. P. Stewart & D. Guthrie, eds.), pp. 369–86. Edinburgh: University Press.

Dudley, S. F. et al. (1953). Lind bicentenary symposium. *Proc. Nutr. Soc. 12:* 201–344.

Dufrenoy, J., Dufrenoy, M. L. & Rousseau, J. (1954). Les plantes antiscorbutiques. *Rev. horticole,* no. 2197: 993–5.

Dufy, J. (1953). *Epidemics in Colonial America.* Baton Rouge, LA: Louisiana State University Press.

Dulieu, L. (1984). Pierre Chirac et les maladies des équipages des vaisseaux. *Rev. Hist. Sci. 37:* 66–70.

Dunmore, J., ed. (1981). *The Expedition of the St. Jean-Baptiste to the Pacific 1769–1770.* London: Hakluyt Society.

Dyke, H. W. (1918). An outbreak of scurvy in the South African native labour corps. *Lancet ii:* 513–15.

Echthius, J. (1541). De Scorbuto, vel Scorbutica passione Epitome. In: *De Scorbuto Tractatus* (D. Sennertus, ed.) (1654), pp. 181–6. Frankfurt: Mevius & Schumacher.

Edinburgh Board of Health (1848). Instructions respecting the prevention and treatment of cholera. *Lancet ii:* 484–5.

Editorial (1847). Observations on scurvy. *Lancet ii:* 312–13.

Elliotson, J. (1831). Clinical lecture. *Lancet i:* 649–55.

Ellis, C. N., Vanderveen, E. E., & Rasmussen, J. E. (1984). Scurvy. A case caused by peculiar dietary habits. *Arch. Dermatol. 120:* 1212–4.

*Encyclopaedia Brittanica* (1771). Scurvy. vol. 3: 106–10. Edinburgh: Bell & MacFarquar.

*Encyclopaedia Brittanica,* 3rd ed. (1797). Brewing. vol. 3: 543–50. Edinburgh: Bell & MacFarquar.

Erdman, J. W., & Klein, B. P. (1982). Harvesting, processing and cooking influences on vitamin C in foods. In: *Ascorbic Acid: Chemistry, Metabolism and Uses* (P. A. Seib & B. M. Tolbert, eds.), pp. 499–532. Washington, DC: American Chemical Society.

Estes, J. W. (1982). Naval medicine in the age of sail: the voyage of the *New York* 1802–1803. *Bull. Hist. Med. 56:* 238–53.

Evans, E. R. G. R. (1921). *South with Scott.* London: Collins.

Faber, H. K. (1920). Sodium citrate and scurvy. *Proc. Soc. Exp. Biol. Med. 17:* 140–1.

Faulkner, A. (1887). The efficacy of salicylic acid in the treatment of scurvy. *Ind. Med. Gaz. 22:* 198–200.

Fauré, R. M. (1943). Sur quelque cas de scorbut observés dans le Sahara Central. *Arch. Inst. Pasteur d'Algérie 21:* 270–2.

Ferguson, C. D. (1948). *California Gold Fields.* Cleveland, OH: Williams.

Fernandez de Ybarra, A. M. (1907). The letter of Dr. Diego Alvarez Chanca, dated 1494, relating to the second voyage of Columbus to America. *Smithsonian Misc. Publ. 48:* 428–57.

Fisher, M., & Fisher, J. (1957). *Shackleton.* London: Barrie.

Follis, R. H., Jr. (1958). *Deficiency Disease.* Springfield, IL: Charles C. Thomas.

Follis, R. H. (1960). Cellular pathology and the development of the deficiency disease concept. *Bull. Hist. Med. 34:* 291–317.

Foltz, J. M. (1848). Report on scorbutus, as it appeared on board the United States squadron blockading the posts in the Gulf of Mexico in the summer of 1846. *Am. J. Med. Sci. [n.s.] 15:* 38–57.

Forry, S. (1841). On the endemic influences of the United States. *Am. J. Med. Sci. [n.s.] 2:* 293–327.

Forry, S. (1842). On scorbutus, which prevailed in the United States Army at Council Bluffs and St. Peters. *Am. J. Med. Sci. [n.s.] 3:* 77–84.

Foster, W., ed. (1897). *Letters Received by the East India Company from Its Servants in the East,* vol. 2 (1613–15). London: Sampson, Low, Marston.

Foster, W. (1910). *The English Factories in India (1630–33).* Oxford: Clarenden Press.

Foster, W., ed. (1928). *A supplementary Calendar of Documents in the India Office relating to India or to the Home Affairs of the East India Company (1600–1640).* London: H. M. Stationery Office.

Foster, W., ed. (1934). *The Voyage of Thomas Best to the East Indies (1612–1614).* London: Hakluyt Society.

Foster, W., ed. (1940). *The Voyages of Sir James Lancaster to Brazil and the East Indies (1591–1603).* London: Hakluyt Society.

Fox, F. W. (1941). Experimental human scurvy. *Br. Med. J. i:* 311–13.

Frazer, A. C. (1962). The possible role of dietary factors in the aetiology and pathogenesis of sprue, coeliac disease and idiopathic steatorrhea. *Proc. Nutr. Soc. 21:* 42–52.

Freeman, R. G. (1898). Should all milk used for infant feeding be heated for the purpose of killing germs. *Arch. Pediatr. 15:* 509–14.

French, R. K. (1982). *The History and Virtues of Cyder.* New York: St. Martin's Press.

Friedman, M., & Rosenman, R. H. (1959). Association of specific overt behaviour patterns with blood and cardiovascular findings. *J. Am. Med. Assoc. 169:* 1286–96.

Friedman, M., Thoresen, C. E., et al. (1982). Feasibility of altering type A behaviour after myocardial infarction. *Circulation 66:* 83–92.

Frölich, T. (1912). Experimentelle Untersuchingen uber den infantilen Skorbut. *Z. f. Hyg. 72:* 155–82.

Fruitnight, J. H. (1894). Infantile scurvy, especially its differential diagnosis. *Arch. Pediatr. 11:* 486–96, 573–84.

Funk, C. (1912). The etiology of deficiency diseases. *J. State Med. 20:* 341–68.

Funk, C. (1913). The nitrogenous constituents of lime-juice. *Biochem. J. 7:* 81–6.

Fürst, V. (1912). Weitere Beitrage zur Ätiologie des experimentellen Skorbuts des Meerschweinchens. *Z. f. Hyg. 72:* 121–54.

Gallagher, R. E. (1964). *Byron's Journal of his Circumnavigation (1764–1766).* Cambridge: Hakluyt Society.

Garg, R. C., & Ram, H. B. (1973). Effect of waxing on the storage behaviour of kagzi limes. *Prog. Horticult. 4* (3/4): 35–44.

Garrod, A. B. (1848). On the nature, cause and prevention of scurvy. *Monthly J. Med. Sci. (London, Edinburgh) 8:* 457.

Geiger, V., & Bryarly, W. (1950). *Trail to California, Overland Journal* (D. M. Potter, ed.). New Haven, CT: Yale University Press.

Geraci, J. R., & Smith, T. G. (1979). Vitamin C in the diet of Inuit hunters from Holman, Northwest Territories. *Arctic 32:* 135–9.

Gerstenberger, H. J. (1921). Malt soup extract as an antiscorbutic. *Am. J. Dis. Child. 21:* 316–26.

Gibbs, F. W. (1965). *Joseph Priestley: Adventurer in Science and Champion of Truth.* London: Nelson.

Gihon, A. L. (1871). *Practical Suggestions in Naval Hygiene.* Washington, DC: Government Printing Office.

Gillespie, L. (1785). Observations on the putrid ulcer. *London Med. J. 6:* 373–400.

Gillespie, L. (1798). *Advice to the Commanders and Officers of His Majesty's Fleet Serving in the West Indies.* London: Cuthell.

Ginter, E. (1979). Chronic marginal vitamin C deficiency: biochemistry and pathophysiology. *World Rev. Nutr. Diet. 33:* 104–41.

Gittings, J. C. (1923). Infantile scurvy. *Arch. Pediatr. 40:* 508–18.

Glauber, J. R. (1659). *La consolation des navigants.* Paris: Jolly.

Glazebrook, A. J., & Thomson, S. (1942). The administration of vitamin C in a large institution and its effect on general health and resistance to infection. *J. Hyg. (Cambridge) 42:* 1–19.

Glisson, F. (1651). *A Treatise of the Rickets Being a Disease Common to Children.* London: Peter Cole.

Goldsmith, G. A. (1961). Human requirements for vitamin C and its use in clinical medicine. *Ann. N. Y. Acad. Sci. 92:* 230–45.

Goodhart, R. S., & Shils, M. E. (1980). *Modern Nutrition in Health and Disease.* Philadelphia, PA: Lea & Febiger.

Grant, J. O. (1863). Remarks on the disease termed "black leg" as observed amongst the Ottawa lumbermen. *Med. Times Gaz. (London),* 669.

Grant, W. L., ed. (1907). *Voyages of Samuel de Champlain 1604–1618.* New York: Scribner.

Gray, A., ed. (1887). *The Voyage of Francois Pyrard.* London: Hakluyt Society.

Greely, A. W. (1886). *Three Years of Arctic Service,* 2 vols. New York: Charles Scribner's Sons.

Greene, T. W. N. (1883). The influence of diet on scurvy. *Lancet i:* 714.

Greenlee, W. B., ed. (1958). *The Voyage of Pedro Alvares Cabral to Brazil and India.* London: Hakluyt Society.

Grenet, A. L. Z. (1871). Le scorbut au fort de Bicêtre. *Ann. d'Hyg. (Paris) [n.s.] 35:* 278–84.

Grewar, D. (1958). Infantile scurvy in Manitoba. *Can. Med. Assoc. J. 78:* 675–80.

Griffith, J. P. C., Jennings, C. G., & Morse, J. L. (1898). The American Pediatric Society's collective investigation on infantile scurvy in North America. *Arch. Pediatr. 15:* 481–508.

Grmek, M. D. (1966). Les origines d'une maladie d'autrefois: le scorbut des marins. *Bull. Inst. Océanographique.* Numéro special 2: 505–23.

Grusin, H., & Kincaid-Smith, P. S. (1954). Scurvy in adult Africans. *Am. J. Clin. Nutr. 2:* 323–35.

Guerra, F. (1950). Hispanic-American contributions to the history of scurvy. *Centaurus 1:* 12–23.

Guerlac, H. (1957). Joseph Black and fixed air. *Isis 48:* 124–51, 433–56.

Guggenheim, K. Y. (1981). *Nutrition and Nutritional Diseases: The Evolution of Concepts.* Lexington, MA: D. C. Heath.

Gupta, S. D., Chaudhuri, C. R., & Chatterjee, I. B. (1972). Incapability of L-ascorbic acid synthesis by insects. *Arch. Biochem. Biophys. 152:* 889–90.

Guthrie, D., & Meiklejohn, A. P. (1953). James Lind and some of his contemporaries. In: *Lind's Treatise on Scurvy* (C. P. Stewart & D. Guthrie, eds.), pp. 387–403. Edinburgh: University Press.

Hadziyev, D., & Steele, L. (1970). Dehydrated mashed potatoes – chemical and biochemical aspects. *Adv. Food Res. 25:* 55–136.

Hague, R., trans. (1955). *The Life of St. Louis by John of Joinville*. New York: Sheed & Ward.

Hakluyt, R. (1589). *The Principall Navigations, Voyages and Discoveries of the English Nation.* Cambridge: Hakluyt Society. Reprint, 1965.

Hakluyt, R. (1927/8). *The Principal Navigations, Voyages, Traffiques and Discoveries of the English Nation.* London: Dent.

Hales, S. (1727). *Vegetable Staticks.* London: Innys & Woodward.

Hall, A. R. (1962). *The Scientific Revolution 1500–1800.* 2nd ed. Boston, MA: Beacon Press.

Hall, M. (1820). On the acceptance of the term scorbutus and on the prevalency of the disease at different periods. *Edinburgh Med. Surg. J.* 16: 204–9.

Hallberg, L. (1981). Effect of vitamin C on the bioavailability of iron from food. In: *Vitamin C: Ascorbic Acid* (J. N. Counsell & D. H. Hornig, eds.), pp. 49–61. London: Applied Science Publishers.

Hammarsten, E. (1938). The Nobel Prize in Physiology and Medicine for the year 1937. In: *Les Prix Nobel en 1937*, pp. 45–8. Stockholm: Norstedt.

Hammond, R. J. (1954). *Food and Agriculture in Britain 1939–45. Aspects of Wartime Control.* Stanford, CA: Stanford University Press.

Hammond, W. A. (1853). Observations on the use of potash in the treatment of scurvy; with cases. *Am. J. Med. Sci.* [n.s.] 25: 102–5.

Hammond, W. A. (1865). *Scurvy, Report of a Committee of the Sanitary Commission, Washington.* 2nd ed. Washington, DC: McGill & Witherow.

Hanck, A. (1982). Tolerance and effects of high doses of ascorbic acid. *Int. J. Vitam. Nutr. Res.* [Suppl.] 23: 221–36.

Hansen, O. G. (1947). Food conditions in Norway during the war, 1939–45. *Proc. Nutr. Soc.* 5: 263–70.

Harden, A., & Zilva, S. S. (1918). The antiscorbutic factor in lemon juice. *Biochem. J.* 12: 259–69.

Harden, A., & Zilva, S. S. (1919). Experimental scurvy in monkeys. *J. Pathol. Bacteriol.* 22: 246–51.

Harden, A., Zilva, S. S., & Still, G. F. (1919). Infantile scurvy: the antiscorbutic factor of lemon juice in treatment. *Lancet i:* 17–18.

Harlan, G. P. (1917). Land scurvy in England. *Br. Med. J. ii:* 46.

Harris, J. (1705). *A Compleat Collection of Voyages and Travels*, vol. 1. London: Bennet.

Harris, L. J. (1933). Vitamins. *Ann. Rev. Biochem.* 2: 253–98.

Harris, L. J. (1934). Vitamins. *Ann. Rev. Biochem.* 3: 247–94.

Harris, L. J. (1935). *Vitamins in Theory and Practice.* Cambridge: University Press.

Hart, K. (1912). Über die experimentelle Erzeugung der Möller-Barlowschen Krankheit und ihre endgültige Identifizierung mit dem klassischen Skorbut. *Virchows Archiv.* 208S: 367–96.

Hartman, A. M., & Dryden, L. P. (1965). *Vitamins in Milk and Milk Products.* Champaign, IL: American Dairy Science Association.

Harvey, G. (1675). *The Disease of London or a New Discovery of the Scorvey.* London: Thackery.

Harvier, P. (1917). Une epidémie de scorbut. *Paris Méd.* 7: 394–8.

Hatton, R. M. (1968). *Charles XII of Sweden.* London: Weidenfeld & Nicolson.

Hawkesworth, J. (1773). *An Account of the Voyages Undertaken – for Making Discoveries in the Southern Hemisphere*, vol. 1. London: Strahan & Cadell.

Hawkins, R. (1847). *Voyage into the South Sea, in the Year 1593.* London: Hakluyt Society. Original edition, London: Jaggard, 1622.

Haworth, W. N. (1938). The structure of carbohydrates and of vitamin C. In: *Les Prix Nobel en 1937*, pp. 1–16. Stockholm: Nobelstiftelsen.

Haworth, W. N., & Hirst, E. L. (1933). Synthesis of ascorbic acid. *Chem. Ind. (London)* 52: 645–6.

Haworth, W. N., Hirst, E. L., & Zilva, S. S. (1934). Physiological activity of synthetic ascorbic acid. *J. Chem. Soc. ii:* 1155–6.

Heagerty, J. J. (1928). *Four Centuries of Medical History in Canada*. Toronto: MacMillan.

Henderson, A. (1839). On sea-scurvy. *Edinburgh Med. Surg. J. 52:* 1–17.

Herbert, R. W., Hirst, E. L., Percival, E. G. V., Reynolds, R. J. W., & Smith, F. (1933). The constitution of ascorbic acid. *J. Chem. Soc. (London)* 1270–90.

Hess, A. F. (1917). Infantile scurvy. A study of its pathogenesis. *Am. J. Dis. Child. 14:* 337–53.

Hess, A. F. (1918). The role of antiscorbutics in our dietary. *J. Am. Med. Assoc. ii:* 941–3.

Hess, A. F. (1920). *Scurvy Past and Present*. Philadelphia, PA: J. B. Lippincott.

Hess, A. F., & Fish, M. (1914). Infantile scurvy: the blood, the blood vessels and the diet. *Am. J. Dis. Child. 8:* 385–405.

Hess, A. F., & Unger, L. J. (1918). The scurvy of guinea pigs. I. The experimental dietary. *J. Biol. Chem.* 35: 479–86.

Heubner, O. (1903). Ueber die Barlow'sche Krankheit. *Dtsch. Med. Wochenschrift 29:* 109–10.

Hickman, J. (1888). The occurrence of scurvy among troops and its prevention. *Practitioner 40:* 392–400.

Hirsch, A. (1885). *Handbook of Historical and Geographical Pathology*, vol. 2, London: New Sydenham Society.

Hirschsprung, H. (1896). Die Moellersche Krankheit. *Jahrb. f. Kinderheilk. 41:* 1–43.

Hirst, E. L. (1953). The chemistry of vitamin C. In: *Lind's Treatise on Scurvy* (C. P. Stewart & D. Guthrie, eds.), pp. 413–24. Edinburgh: University Press.

Hoare, M. E., ed. (1982). *The Resolution Journal of Johann Reinhold Forster 1772–1775.* 4 vols. London: Hakluyt Society.

Hodges, R. E., Baker, E. M., Hood, J., Sauberlich, H. E., & March, S. E. (1969). Experimental scurvy in man. *Am. J. Clin. Nutr. 22:* 535–48.

Hodgson, R. W. (1967). Horticultural varieties of *Citrus*. In: *The Citrus Industry* (W. Reuther, L. D. Batchelor, & H. J. Webber, eds.), vol. 1. Berkeley, CA: University of California Press.

Hoerschelman, E. (1917). Zur Klinik der Skorbuts in der russischen Armee. *Dtsch. Med. Wochenschr. 43:* 1617–19.

Holliday, J. S. (1981). *The World Rushed In: The California Gold Rush Experience*. New York: Simon & Schuster.

Holst, A. (1907). Experimental studies relating to "ship-beri-beri" and scurvy. I. Introduction. *J. Hyg. (Cambridge) 7:* 619–33.

Holst, A. (1908). Discussion on the causation and treatment of scurvy. *Br. Med. J. ii:* 725.

Holst, A. (1911). The etiology of beri-beri. *Trans. Soc. Trop. Med. Hyg. 5:* 76–80.

Holst, A., & Frölich, T. (1907). Experimental studies relating to ship-beri-beri and scurvy. II. On the etiology of scurvy. *J. Hyg. (Cambridge) 7:* 634–71.

Holst, A., & Frölich, T. (1912). Uber experimentellen Skorbut. Ein Beitrag zur Lehre von dem Einfluss einer einseitigen Nahrung. *Z. f. Hyg. 72:* 1–120.

Holst, A., & Frölich, T. (1913). Über experimentellen Skorbut II. *Z. f. Hyg. 75:* 334–44.

Holst, A., & Frölich, T. (1920). On the preservation of the anti-scorbutic properties of cabbage by drying. *J. Trop. Med. Hyg. 23:* 261–3.

Holt, L. B. (1972). The demise of the acid intoxication theory of scurvy. *Proc. R. Soc. Med. 65:* 47–8.

Home, W. E. (1900). The etiology of scurvy. *Lancet ii:* 321–2.

Hopkins, F. G. (1912). Feeding experiments illustrating the importance of accessory factors in normal dietaries. *J. Physiol. 44:* 425–60.

Hoppner, K., McLaughlan, J. M., Shah, B. G., Thompson, J. N., Beare-Rogers, J., Sayed, J. E., & Schaefer, O. (1978). Nutrient levels of some foods of Eskimos from Arctic Bay, N.W.T., Canada. *J. Am. Diet. Assoc. 73:* 257–61.

Howard, M. E. (1961). *The Franco-Prussian War*. London: Hart-Davis.

Høygaard, A. & Rasmussen, H. W. (1939). Vitamin C sources in Eskimo food. *Nature 143:* 943.

Hughes, C., Dutton, S., & Truswell, A. S. (1981). High intakes of ascorbic acid and urinary oxalate. *J. Hum. Nutr. 35:* 274–80.

Hughes, R. E. (1973). George Budd (1808–1882) and nutritional deficiency diseases. *Med. Hist.* *17:* 127–35.

Hughes, R. E. (1975). James Lind and the cure of scurvy: an experimental approach. *Med. Hist.* *19:* 342–51.

Hughes, R. E. (1977). Use and abuse of vitamin C – a review. *Food Chem. 2:* 119–33.

Hughes, R. E. (1981a). *Vitamin C. Some Current Problems.* London: British Nutrition Foundation.

Hughes, R. E. (1981b). Recommended daily amounts and biochemical roles – the vitamin C, carnitine, fatigue relationship. In: *Vitamin C: Ascorbic Acid* (J. N. Counsell & D. Hornig, eds.), pp. 75–86. London: Applied Science Publishers.

Hughes, R. E., & Jones, P. R. (1971). Natural and synthetic sources of vitamin C. *J. Sci. Food Agric. 22:* 551–2.

Hulme, N. (1768). *A Proposal for Preventing the Scurvy in the British Navy.* London: Cadell.

Hulme, N. (1778). *A Safe and Easy Remedy Proposed for the Relief of the Stone and Gravel, the Scurvy, Gout etc.* London: Robinson.

Huntford, R. (1979). *Scott and Amundsen.* London: Hodder & Stoughton.

Hunziker, O. F. (1946). *Condensed Milk and Milk Powder.* 6th ed. La Grange, IL: Hunziker.

Hutchinson, R. (1907). Scurvy (scorbutus). In: *Osler's Modern Medicine,* pp. 893–907. Philadelphia, PA: Lea Brothers & Co.

Huxham, J. (1747). A method for preserving the health of seamen in long cruizes and voyages. *Gentleman's Mag. 17:* 467–9.

Huxley, E. (1979). *Scott of the Antarctic.* London: Weidenfeld & Nicolson.

Huxley, L., ed. (1913). *Scott's Last Expedition.* 2 vols. New York: Dodd, Mead.

Ihde, A. J. (1964). *The Development of Modern Chemistry.* New York: Harper & Row.

Ihde, A. J., & Becker, S. L. (1971). Conflict of concepts in early vitamin studies. *J. Hist. Biol. 4:* 1–33.

Irwin, M. I., & Hutchins, B. K. (1976). A conspectus of research on vitamin C requirements of man. *J. Nutr. 106:* 821–79.

Jackson, F. G. (1899). *A Thousand Days in the Arctic.* 2 vols. London: Harper Bros.

Jackson, F. G., & Harley, V. (1900). An experimental enquiry into scurvy. *Proc. R. Soc. Lond. 66:* 250–65.

Jackson, L., & Moody, A. M. (1916). Bacteriological studies on experimental scurvy in guinea pigs. *J. Infect. Dis. 19:* 511–14.

Jackson, L., & Moore, J. J. (1916). Studies on experimental scurvy in guinea pigs. *J. Infect. Dis. 19:* 478–510.

Jacusiel (1903). Diskussion ueber die Barlow'sche Krankheit. *Dtsch. Med. Wochenschr. 29:* 117.

Jalland, W. H. (1873). Scurvy in a child ten months old. *Med. Times Gaz. (London) i:* 248.

Jenness, D. (1922). *Report of the Canadian Arctic Expedition, 1913–18,* vol. 12: *The Life of the Copper Eskimos.* Ottawa: F. A. Acland.

Johnson, B. C. (1954). Axel Holst. *J. Nutr. 53:* 3–16.

Jones, E., & Hughes, R. E. (1976). Copper boilers and the occurrence of scurvy: an experimental approach. *Med. Hist. 20:* 80–1.

Jones, H. L., trans. (1917). *The Geography of Strabo,* vol. 7. London: Heinemann.

Joseph, H. (1964). *Shakespeare's Son-in-law: John Hall, Man and Physician.* Hamden, CT: Archon Books.

Judd, D. (1975). *The Crimean War.* London: Wm. Clowes & Sons.

Judson, C. F., & Gittings, J. C. (1902). *The Artificial Feeding of Infants.* Philadelphia, PA: J. B. Lippincott.

Jukes, T. H. (1974). Are recommended dietary allowances for vitamin C adequate? *Proc. Natl. Acad. Sci. U.S.A. 71:* 1949–51.

Kahane, E. (1978). *Parmentier ou la dignité de la pomme de terre.* Paris: Blanchard.

Kane, E. K. (1870). *Arctic Explorations.* Hartford, CT: Bliss.

Kark, R. M. (1953). Ascorbic acid in relation to cold, scurvy, ACTH and surgery. *Proc. Nutr. Soc.* 12: 279–93.

Keevil, J. J. (1957–8). *Medicine and the Navy 1200–1900*, vol. 1 (1200–1649); vol. 2 (1649–1714). Edinburgh: Livingstone.

Kellie, A. E., & Zilva, S. S. (1939). The vitamin C requirements of man. *Biochem. J. 33:* 153–64.

Kelly, W. (1852). *A Stroll through the Diggings of California*. London: Simms & McIntyre.

Kendall, E. J. C. (1955). Scurvy during some British Polar Expeditions, 1875–1917. *Polar Record* 7: 467–85.

Keuning, J., ed. (1938). *De Tweede Schipvaart des Nederlanders naar Oost-Indie onder Jacob Cornelisz. Van Neck en Wybrant Warwick 1598–1600*, vols. 1 & 2. 'S-Gravenhage: M. Nijhoff.

Kim, Y-K. Tannenbaum, S. R., & Wishnok, J. S. (1982). In: *Ascorbic Acid, Chemistry, Metabolism, and Uses* (P. A. Seib & B. M. Tolbert, eds.), pp. 571–85. Washington, DC: American Chemical Society.

King, C. G. (1939). The water-soluble vitamins. *Ann. Rev. Biochem. 8:* 371–414.

King, C. G. (1953). The discovery and chemistry of vitamin C. *Proc. Nutr. Soc. 12:* 219–27.

King, C. G. (1979). The isolation of vitamin C from lemon juice. *Fedr. Proc. 38:* 2681–3.

King, C. G., & Burns, J. J., eds. (1975). Second conference on vitamin C. *Ann. N.Y. Acad. Sci. 258* (entire volume).

King, C. G., & Waugh, W. A. (1932). The chemical nature of vitamin C. *Science 75:* 357–8.

King, C. G., & Waugh, W. A. (1934). The effect of pasteurization upon the vitamin C content of milk. *J. Dairy Sci. 17:* 489–96.

King, C. G., Musulin, R. R., & Swanson, W. F. (1940). Effects of vitamin C intake upon the degree of tooth injury produced by diphtheria toxin. *Am. J. Public Health 30:* 1068–72.

King, L. S. (1958). *The Medical World of the Eighteenth Century*. Chicago, IL: University of Chicago Press.

King, L. S. (1970). *The Road to Medical Enlightenment, 1650–1695*. London: MacDonald.

Kinglake, A. W. (1881). *The Invasion of the Crimea*, vol. 4: *The Winter Troubles*. New York: Harper & Bros.

Kirkup, J., ed. (1978). *The Surgions Mate by John Woodall, 1617*. Bath, UK: Kingsmead Press.

Kirwan, L. P. (1959). *The White Road: A Survey of Polar Exploration*. London: Hollis & Carter.

Klipstein, F. A., & Corcino, J. J. (1974). Seasonal occurrence of overt and subclinical tropical malabsorption in Puerto Rico. *Am. J. Trop. Med. Hyg. 23:* 1189–96.

Knox, J. (1914). *An Historical Journal of the Campaign in North America 1757–1700*, vol. 2. Toronto: Champlain Society.

Kodicek, E., & Young, F. G. (1969). Captain Cook and scurvy. *Notes Rec. R. Soc. London 24:* 43–63.

Koettlitz, R. (1902). The British Antarctic expedition. Precautions against scurvy in the victualling of the "Discovery." *Br. Med. J.* i: 342–3.

Kon, S. K., & Watson, M. B. (1936). The effect of light on the vitamin C of milk. *Biochem. J. 30:* 2273–90.

Krebel, R. (1866). *Der Scorbut*. Leipzig: Ed. Wartig.

Kuhn, T. (1970). *The Structure of Scientific Revolutions*. 2nd ed. Chicago, IL: University of Chicago Press.

Lamb, G. (1902). On the etiology and pathology of scurvy. *Lancet* i: 10–4.

Lamb, W. K., ed. (1984). *George Vancouver's Voyage of Discovery . . . , 1791–95*. 4 vols. London: Hakluyt Society.

Lancereaux, E. (1885). Le scorbut des prisons du Département de la Seine. *Ann. d'Hyg. Publ. et de Méd. Lég. [n.s.]* 13: 296–303.

La Pérouse, J. F. G. de (1807). *A Voyage Round the World*, vol. 3. London: Lackington, Allen.

Large, E. C. (1940). *The Advance of the Fungi*. London: Jonathan Cape.

Larrey, D. J. (1814). *Memoirs of Military Surgery*. Baltimore, MD: Cushing.

Lasègue, C., & Legroux, A. (1871). L'épidémie de scorbut dans les prisons de la Seine et à l'Hôpital de la Pitié. *Arch. Gén. de Méd. [n.s.] 18:* 5–33, 680–706.

Lamb, W. K., ed. (1984). *George Vancouver's Voyage of Discovery to the North Pacific Ocean and Round the World, 1791–1795.* 4 vols. London: Hakluyt Society.

Latham, P. M. (1825). *An Account of the Disease Lately Prevalent at the General Penitentiary.* London: Underwood.

Laughton, J. K., ed. (1911). *Letters and Papers of Charles, Lord Barham (1758–1813),* vol. III. London: Navy Records Society.

Laycock, T. (1847). Purpura or land scurvy. *London Med. Gaz. [n.s.] 4:* 573–6.

Leicester, H. M. (1956). *The Historical Background of Chemistry.* New York: Wiley.

Leicester, H. M. (1974). *Development of Biochemical Concepts from Ancient to Modern Times.* Cambridge, MA: Harvard University Press.

Léon, A. (1868). Contribution à l'étiologie du scorbut. *Arch. Méd. Navale (Paris) 9:* 290–7.

Lepper, E. H., & Zilva, S. S. (1925). The bicarbonate of the plasma and the hydrogen ion concentration of the blood of guinea pigs suffering from scurvy. *Biochem. J. 19:* 581–8.

Le Roy de Méricourt, A. (1874). Causes et nature de scorbut (response à M. Villemin). *Bull. de l'Acad. de Méd. (Paris) [n.s.] 3:* 956–89, 998–1037.

Le Roy de Méricourt, A. (1875). Discussion sur le scorbut. *Bull. Acad. Méd. (Paris) [n.s.] 4:* 679–710.

Lesch, J. E. (1984). *Science and Medicine in France. The Emergence of Experimental Physiology, 1790–1855.* Cambridge, MA: Harvard University Press.

Letters and Documents Relating to the Services of Nelson's Ships, Squadrons and Fleets (1780–1805). Manuscripts at the Wellcome Institute for the History of Medicine, London.

Levine, V. E. (1955). Scurvy in Nebraska. I. The epidemic of scurvy at Fort Atkinson 1819–20. *Am. J. Dig. Dis. 22:* 9–17.

Lewin, S. (1976). *Vitamin C: Its Molecular Biology and Medical Potential.* London: Academic Press.

Lewis, H. B., & Karr, W. G. (1916–17). Changes in the urea content of blood and tissues of guinea pigs maintained on an exclusive oat diet. *J. Biol. Chem. 28:* 17–25.

Lewis, H. E. (1972). State of knowledge about scurvy in 1911. *Proc. R. Soc. Med. 65:* 39–42.

Lewis, T. L., Karlowski, T. R., et al. (1975). A controlled clinical trial of ascorbic acid for the common cold. *Ann. N.Y. Acad. Sci. 258:* 505–12.

Leyden, E., & Munk, P. (1861). Nierenaffection bei Schwefelsaure – Vergiftung. *Virchows Arch. 22:* 237–41.

Lieb, C. W. (1929). The effects on human beings of a twelve months' exclusive meat diet. *J. Am. Med. Assoc. 93:* 20–2.

Liebig, J. von (1842). *Animal Chemistry.* London: Taylor & Walton.

Lind, J. (1753). *A Treatise of the Scurvy.* Edinburgh: Millar. [Reprint, see Steward, C. P. & Guthrie, D. (1953).]

Lind, J. (1754). The danger of using some earthen vessels. *The Scots Magazine* 16 (May): 227–9.

Lind, J. (1772). *A Treatise on the Scurvy.* 3rd ed. London: Crowder.

Lind, J. (1788). *An Essay on Diseases Incidental to Europeans in Hot Climates.* 4th ed. London: Murray.

Linghorne, W. J., & McIntosh, W. G. (1946). The relation of ascorbic acid intake to gingivitis. *Can. Med. Assoc. J. 54:* 106–19.

Lloyd, C. (1961). The introduction of lemon juice as a cure for scurvy. *Bull. Hist. Med. 35:* 123–32.

Lloyd, C., ed. (1965). *The Health of Seaman: Selections from the Works of Dr. James Lind, Sir Gilbert Blane and Dr. Thomas Trotter.* London: Navy Records Society.

Lloyd, C. C. (1981). Victualling of the fleet in the eighteenth and nineteenth centuries. In: *Starving Sailors* (J. Watt, E. J. Freeman, & W. F. Bynum, eds.), pp. 9–15. London: National Maritime Museum.

Lloyd, C., & Coulter, J. L. S. (1961). *Medicine and the Navy 1200–1900*, vol. III, *1714–1815*. Edinburgh: Livingstone.

Lloyd, C., & Coulter, J. L. S. (1963). *Medicine and the Navy 1200–1900*, vol. IV, *1815–1900*. Edinburgh: Livingstone.

Logan, T. S. (1850). Land scurvy. *Southern Med. Rep.* 2: 468–80.

Lonsdale, H. (1847). On scurvy in Cumberland. *Monthly J. Med. Sci. (Edinburgh)* 8: 97–106.

Lorenz, A. (1953). Some pre-Lind writers on scurvy. *Proc. Nutr. Soc.* 12: 306–24.

Lorenz, A. J. (1957). Scurvy in the Gold Rush. *J. Hist. Med.* 12: 473–510.

Lowry, O. H. (1952). Biochemical evidence of nutritional status. *Physiol. Rev.* 32: 431–48.

Lubbock, A. B., ed. (1934). *Barlow's Journal of His Life at Sea, 1659–1703*. London: Hirst & Blackett.

Lugg, J. W. H., & Weller, R. A. (1943). Germinating seeds as a source of vitamin C in human nutrition. *Aust. J. Exp. Biol. Med. Sci.* 21: 111–14.

McBride, A. (1863). Vinegar as an anti-scorbutic. *Am. J. Med. Sci.* 45: 267–8.

MacBride, D. (1764). *Experimental Essays on Medical and Philosophical Subjects*. London: Becket & Cadell.

MacBride, D. (1767). *An Historical Account of a New Method of Treating the Scurvy at Sea*. London: Thomas Ewing.

MacBride, D. (1776). *Experimental Essays on Medical and Philosophical Subjects*. 3rd ed. London: Becket & Cadell.

McCollum, E. V. (1918). The "vitamin" hypothesis and the diseases referable to faulty diet. *J. Am. Med. Assoc.* 71: 937–41.

McCollum, E. V. (1957). *A History of Nutrition: The Sequence of Ideas in Nutrition Investigations*. Boston, MA: Houghton Mifflin.

McCollum, E. V. (1964). *From Kansas Farm Boy to Scientist, an Autobiography*. Lawrence, KA: University of Kansas Press.

McCollum, E. V., & Davis, M. (1913). The necessity of certain lipins in the diet during growth. *J. Biol. Chem.* 15: 167–75.

McCollum, E. V., & Kennedy, C. (1916). The dietary factor operating in the production of polyneuritis. *J. Biol. Chem.* 24: 491–502.

McCollum, E. V., & Pitz, W. (1917). The "vitamine" hypothesis and deficiency diseases. A study of experimental scurvy. *J. Biol. Chem.* 31: 229–53.

McConville, S. (1981). *A History of English Prison Administration*, vol. I: *1750–1877*. London: Routledge & Kegan Paul.

McCord, C. P. (1959). Scurvy as an occupational disease. The Sappington Memorial Lecture. *J. Occup. Med.* 1: 315–18.

McCord, C. P. (1971). Scurvy as an occupational disease. *J. Occup. Med.* 13: 306–7, 348–51, 393–5, 441–7, 484–91, 586–92.

McDonald, D. (1954). Dr. John Woodall and his treatment of scurvy. *Trans. R. Soc. Trop. Med. Hyg.* 48: 360–5.

MacDonald, J. (1927). *Memoirs of an Eighteenth Century Footman*. London: Routledge.

McDonald, R. K. (1958). Problems in biological research in schizophrenia. *J. Chron. Dis.* 8: 366–71.

McKie, D. (1961). Joseph Priestley and the Copley Medal. *Ambix* 9: 1–22.

MacLean, J. D., & Kamath, K. R. (1970). Infantile scurvy in Malaysia. *Med. J. Malaysia* 24: 200–7.

McMillan, R. B., & Inglis, J. C. (1944). Scurvy: a survey of fifty-three cases. *Br. Med. J.* ii: 233–6.

MacRae, D. (1908). Notes on scurvy in South Africa, 1902–1904. *Lancet* 1: 1838–40.

Magnus, O. (1972). *Historia de Gentibus Septentrionalibus, Romae 1555*. Copenhagen: Rosenkilde & Bagger.

Mahé, J. (1880). Scorbut. In: *Dictionnaire encyclopédique des sciences médicales* (A. Dehambre, ed.). 3rd ser., vol. 8: 35–257. Paris: Masson & Asselin.

Maitland, C. B. (1900). The causation of scurvy. *Lancet ii:* 1164.

Major, R. H. (1932). *Classic Descriptions of Disease.* Springfield, IL: Charles C. Thomas.

Markham, A. H. (1880a). *The Great Frozen Sea.* London: Kegan Paul.

Markham, A. H., ed. (1880b). *The Voyages and Works of John Davis.* London: Hakluyt Society.

Markham, C. R. (1877). *A Refutation of the Report of the Scurvy Committee.* Portsmouth: Griffin.

Markham, C. R. (1881). *The Voyages of William Baffin, 1612–1622.* London: Hakluyt Society.

Markham, C. R. (1911). *Early Spanish Voyages to the Strait of Magellan.* London: Hakluyt Society.

Marroin, A. (1861). *Histoire médicale de la flotte française dans la mer noire, pendant la guerre de Crimée.* Paris: Baillière et fils.

Martin, F. de Vitré (1604). Traicte du scurbut. In: *Description du premier voyage faict aux Indes Orientals par les françois.* Paris: Sonnius.

Martin, H. E. (1931). Scurvy following an ulcer diet. *Lancet ii:* 293–4.

Maupin (1860). Quelques considérations sur le scorbut épidémique de l'Armée d'Orient. *Rec. de Méd. de Chir. et de Pharm. Milit. [3e ser.]* 3: 190–209.

May, J. M. (1967). *The Ecology of Malnutrition in Northern Africa. Studies in Medical Geography,* vol. 7. New York: Hafner.

May, M. T. (1968). *Galen on the Usefulness of the Parts of the Body.* New York: Cornell University Press.

Mead, R. (1762). *The Medical Works.* London: Hitch.

*Medical and Surgical History of the War of the Rebellion (1875–1888).* Washington, DC: Government Printing Office.

Medical Research Council (1932). *Vitamins: A Survey of Present Knowledge.* Medical Research Council Special Report Series, no. 167. London: H. M. Stationery Office.

Meiklejohn, A. P. (1954). The curious obscurity of Dr. James Lind. *J. Hist. Med. Allied Sci.* 9: 304–10.

Mettler, C. C., & Mettler, F. A. (1947). *History of Medicine.* Philadelphia, PA: Blakiston Co.

Meyer, E. (1896). Ueber Barlow'sche Krankheit. *Dtsch. Med. Wochenschr.* 22: 23–4.

Micheel, F., & Kraft, K. (1933). Constitution of vitamin C. *Nature* 131: 274–5.

Milman, F. (1782). *An Enquiry into the Source from Whence the Symptoms of Scurvy and of Putrid Fevers Arise.* London: Dodsley.

Milner, R. D. (1902). The cost of food as related to its nutritive value. *U. S. Dept. Agric. Year Book,* pp. 387–406.

Mirsky, J. (1948). *To the Arctic.* New York: Alfred A. Knopf.

Moertel, C. G., Fleming, T. R., Creagan, E. T., Rubin, J., O'Connell, M. J., & Ames, M. M. (1985). High-dose vitamin C versus placebo in the treatment of patients with advanced cancer who have had no prior chemotherapy. *N. Engl. J. Med.* 312: 137–41.

Moll, A. A. (1944). *Aesculapius in Latin America.* Philadelphia, PA: W. B. Saunders.

Morgan, J. (1864). On a new process of preserving meat. *J. R. Soc. Arts* 12: 347–53.

Morgan, R. B. (1855). East India Reports, no. 5. The occurrence of scurvy on board troop ships. *Med. Times Gaz. [n.s.]* 9: 586–7.

Morison, S. E. (1939). *The Second Voyage of Christopher Columbus (1939).* Oxford: University Press.

Morison, S. E. (1971). *The European Discovery of America,* vol. 1: *Northern Voyages.* New York: Oxford University Press.

Morison, S. E. (1974). *The European Discovery of America,* vol. 2: *The Southern Voyages.* New York: Oxford University Press.

Morse, J. L. (1918). A resumé of the literature of infantile scurvy during the past five years. *Boston Med. Surg. J.* 178: 160–4.

Moulin, J. (1959). Sur quelques cas de scorbut observés chez les nomades du Grand Erg Occidental. *Arch. Inst. Pasteur d'Algérie* 37: 312–14.

Moyle, J. (1702). *Chirurgus Marinus: or the Sea Chirurgion.* 2nd ed. London: Tracy.

Much, H., & Baumbach, K. (1917). Skorbut. *Munch. Med. Wochenschr.* 64: 854.

Muir, J. R. (1939). *The Life and Achievements of Captain James Cook.* London: Blackie.

Munro, H. N. (1964). The origin and growth of our present concepts of protein metabolism. In: *Mammalian Protein Metabolism* (H. N. Munro and J. B. Allison, eds.), vol. 1. New York: Academic Press.

Munsell, H. E., Williams, L. O., Guild, L. P., Troescher, C. B., Nightingale, G., & Harris, R. S. (1949–50). Composition of food plants of Central America. *Food Res.* 14: 144–64; 15: 34–52.

Murata, A., Morishige, F., & Yamaguchi, H. (1982). Prolongation of survival time of terminal cancer patients by administration of large doses of ascorbate. *Int. J. Vitam. Nutr. Res.* 23: 103–13.

Murray (1838–9). On scurvy at Cape Town. *London Med. Gaz. [n.s.]* 1: 292–6, 367–72.

Murray, J. A. H., ed. (1933). *Oxford English Dictionary,* vol. 9. Oxford: Clarendon Press.

Naber, S. P. L'H., ed. (1932). *Reisebeschreibungen von Deutsche Beamten und Kriegslenten in dienst der Niederlandischen. West-und Ost-Indischen Kompagnien. 1602–1797,* vol. XIII. The Hague: M. Nijhoff.

Nagy, S. (1980). Vitamin C contents of citrus fruit and their products: a review. *J. Agric. Food Chem.* 28: 8–18.

Nansen, F. (1897). *Farthest North.* 2 vols. London: Constable.

Nares, G. S. (1878). *Narrative of a Voyage to the Polar Sea during 1875–6.* 2 vols. London: Sampson Low, Marston, Searle & Rivington.

National Food Survey Committee (1951). *The Urban Working-Class Household Diet, 1940–1949.* London: H. M. Stationery Office.

National Research Council (1941). *Recommended Dietary Allowances.* Washington, DC: Federal Security Agency.

National Research Council (1953). *Recommended Dietary Allowances,* Revised. Washington, DC: National Research Council.

National Research Council (1974). *Recommended Dietary Allowances,* 8th ed. Washington, DC: National Academy of Sciences.

National Research Council (1980). *Recommended Dietary Allowances,* 9th ed. Washington, DC: National Academy of Sciences.

Neale, W. H. (1883). The etiology of scurvy. *Lancet i:* 363–4.

Neale, W. H. (1896). How to avoid scurvy in the Arctic regions. *Practitioner. [n.s.]* 3: 585–8.

Neatby, L. H. (1970). *The Search for Franklin.* New York: Walker.

Nelson, P. E., & Tressler, D. K. (1980). *Fruit and Vegetable Juice Processing Technology.* 3rd ed. Westport, CT: Avi Publishing Co.

Netter, M. (1902). Scorbut infantile et lait sterilisé. Influence de la stérilisation sur la disparition du pouvoir antiscorbutique du lait. *Bull. Soc. Pédiatr. Paris,* 4: 298–316.

Neumann, H. (1902). Bemerkungen zur Barlow'schen Krankheit. *Dtsch. Med. Wochenschr.* 28: 647–9.

Newby, E. P. (1975). *World Atlas of Exploration.* New York: Rand McNally.

Newman, G. (1926). The disciples of Boerhaave in Edinburgh. *Edinburgh Med. J. [n.s.]* 33: 401–31.

Nicol, B. M. (1958). Ascorbic acid in the diets of rural Nigerian peoples. *W. Afr. Med. J.* 7: 185–9.

Nicolaysen, R. (1980). Arctic nutrition. *Perspect. Biol. Med.* 23: 295–310.

Nixon, J. A. (1937). The East India Company and the control of scurvy. *Proc. R. Soc. Med.* 31: 193–8.

Noble, J., ed. (1904). *Records of the Court of Assistants of the Colony of Massachusetts Bay 1630–1692.* Boston, MA: County of Suffolk.

Nordenskiöld, A. E. (1881). *The Voyage of the Vega Around Asia and Europe*. London: MacMillan.

Norris, J. (1983). The "scurvy disposition": heavy exertion as an exacerbating influence on scurvy in modern times. *Bull. Hist. Med. 57:* 325–38.

Northrup, W. P., & Crandall, F. M. (1894). Scorbutus in infants. *New York Med. J. 59:* 641–6.

Nowell, C. E., ed. (1962). *Magellan's Voyage Round the World*. Evanston, IL: Northwestern University Press.

Ogden, M. S., ed. (1938). *Liber de Diversis Medicinis*. London: Early English Text Society.

O'Hara-May, J. (1977). *Elizabethan Dyetary of Health*. Lawrence, KA: Coronado Press.

Oliver, M. H. (1973). Germinated seeds as anti-scorbutics: Western use of an ancient Chinese botanical medicine. *Econ. Bot. 27:* 204–9.

Oliver, W. S. (1863). Scurvy: its cause. *Lancet i:* 61.

Olliver, M. (1954). Estimation of ascorbic acid. In: *The Vitamins* (W. H. Sebrell & R. S. Harris, eds.), vol. 1: 242–59. New York: Academic Press.

Osborne, T. B., & Mendel, L. B. (1913). The influence of butter fat on growth. *J. Biol. Chem. 16:* 423–7.

Oshima, H., & Bartsch, H. (1981). The influence of vitamin C on the *in vivo* formation of nitrosamines. In: *Vitamin C (Ascorbic Acid)* (J. N. Counsell & D. M. Hornig, eds.), pp. 215–24. London: Applied Science Publishers.

Packer, J. E., Slater, T. F., & Willson, R. L. (1979). Direct observation of a free radical interaction between vitamin E and vitamin C. *Nature 278:* 737–8.

Pagel, W. (1972). Van Helmont's concept of disease. *Bull. Hist. Med. 46:* 419–54.

Parkes, E. A. (1864). *A Manual of Practical Hygiene*. London: Churchill.

Parkes, S. (1830). *Chemical Essays*. 3rd ed. London: Baldwin & Cradock.

Parliamentary Papers (1858). *Medical and Surgical History of the British Army which served in Turkey and the Crimea*, vol. 2. London: H. M. Stationery Office.

Parry, W. E. (1824). *Journal of a Second Voyage for the Discovery of a North-West Passage*. London: Murray.

Partington, J. R. (1961–2). *A History of Chemistry*, vols. 2 & 3. London: Macmillan.

Paterson, D. (1795). *A Treatise on the Scurvy*. Edinburgh: Manners & Miller.

Pauling, L. (1968). Orthomolecular psychiatry. *Science 160:* 265–71.

Pauling, L. (1970). Evolution and the need for ascorbic acid. *Proc. Natl. Acad. Sci. U.S.A. 67:* 1643–8.

Pauling, L. (1976). *Vitamin C, the Common Cold, and the Flu*. San Francisco: W. H. Freeman.

Pelletier, O. (1975). Vitamin C and cigarette smokers. *Ann. N.Y. Acad. Sci. 258:* 156–68.

Pellham, E. (1974). *God's Power and Providence Shewed in the Miraculous Preservation and Deliverance of Eight Englishmen Left by Mischance in Greenland Anno 1630 Nine Months and Twelve Days*. In: *A Collection of Voyages and Travels* (J. Churchill, ed.), vol. 4:743–55, London: Lintet & Osborn.

Penzer, N. M., ed. (1926). *The World Encompassed and Analogous Contemporary Documents Concerning Sir Francis Drake's Circumnavigation of the World*. London: Argonaut Press.

Percival, T. (1774). Observations on the medicinal uses of fixed air. Appendix 3 in J. Priestley's *"Experiments and Observations on Different Kinds of Air."* London: Johnson.

Pereira, J. (1843). *A Treatise on Food and Diet*. London: Longman.

Perrin, M. (1858). On scorbutus as observed in the French Army in the Crimea. *Med. Times Gaz.* [n.s.] 16: 145–6.

Pinkerton, J. (1808) *A General Collection of Voyages and Travels*. London: Longman, Hurst, Rees and Orme.

Pinkerton, J. (1812). *Voyages and Travels in All Parts of the World*, vol. 2. London: Longman.

Pitz, W. (1918). Studies of experimental scurvy II. The influence of grains, other than oats, and specific carbohydrates on the development of scurvy. *J. Biol. Chem. 33:* 471–5.

Platt, H. (1607). Certain Philosophical Preparations of Foode and Beverage for Sea-men in their Long Voyages. (Broadsheet in the Wellcome Institute for the History of Medicine, London.)

Porter, I. A. (1963). Thomas Trotter, M.D., naval physician. *Med. Hist.* 7: 155–64.

Pound, R. (1963). *Evans of the Broke.* London: Oxford University Press.

Poupart, F. (1708). A relation of some strange and wonderful effects of the scurvy which happened at Paris in the year 1699. *Philos. Trans. R. Soc. London* 26 (no. 318): 223–32.

Praslow, J. (1939). *The State of California: A Medico-Geographical Account, 1857* (F. C. Cordes, trans.). San Francisco, CA: John J. Newbegin.

Pratt, E. L. (1984). Historical perspectives: food, feeding and fancies. *J. Am. College Nutr.* 3: 115–21.

Press, J. C., ed. (1979). *American Men and Women of Science. Physical and Biological Sciences.* 14th ed. New York: R. R. Bowker.

Priestley, J. (1772). On different kinds of air. *Philos. Trans. R. Soc. London* 62: 147–264.

Pringle, J. (1750). Some experiments on substances resisting putrefaction. *Philos. Trans. R. Soc. London.* 46: 480–8; 525–34; 550–8.

Pringle, J. (1753). *Observations on the Diseases of the Army, with an Appendix Containing Some Papers of Experiments.* 2nd ed. London: Millar.

Pringle, J. (1776). *A Discourse upon Some Late Improvements of the Means for Preserving the Health of Mariners.* London: The Royal Society.

Purchas, S. (1906). *Purchas His Pilgrimes,* vols. 18 & 19. Glasgow: Hakluyt Society.

Quartermain, L. B. (1967). *South to the Pole.* London: Oxford University Press.

Quinn, D. B. (1977). *North America from Earliest Discovery to First Settlements.* New York: Harper & Row.

Rajalakshmi, R., Deodhar, A. D., & Ramakrishnan, C. V. (1965). Vitamin C secretion during lactation. *Acta Paediatr. Scand.* 54: 375–82.

Rae, J. (1883). Discussion on the etiology of scurvy. *Lancet* i: 363–5, 406–8.

Ranken, M. D. (1981). The use of ascorbic acid in meat processing. In: *Vitamin C (Ascorbic Acid)* (J. N. Counsell & D. H. Hornig, eds.), pp. 105–22. London: Applied Science Publishers.

Ralfe, C. H. (1877). Inquiry into the general pathology of scurvy. *Lancet* i: 868–71; ii: 81–3.

Ransom, W. B. (1902). Should milk be boiled? *Br. Med. J.* i: 440–3.

Ravenstein, E. G. (1898). *A Journal of the First Voyage of Vasco da Gama, 1477–1499.* London: Hakluyt Society.

Rawson, C. H. (1862). Health and hospitals in Mississippi. *Am. Med. Times* 5: 42, 125.

Reals, W. J. (1949). Scurvy at Fort Atkinson, 1819–20. *Bull. Hist. Med.* 23: 137–54.

Redpath, W. (1901). Some remarks on scurvy. *Lancet* ii: 1444–5.

Rees, J. (1854). Report on the scurvy which appeared in the Black Sea fleet in May, 1854. *Med. Times Gaz.,* 233–4.

Reichstein, T. (1984). Geschichten zur Geschichte der Vitamin-C-Synthese. *Roche Magazin* (no. 21): 10–15. Hoffman-La Roche AG, Basel, Switzerland.

Reichstein, T., Grussner, A., & Oppenheimer, R. (1933). Synthese der d- und l-Ascorbinsäure (C-vitamin). *Helvet. Chim. Acta* 16: 1019–33.

Reid, G. M. (1983). Scurvy: old disease – new insight. *Med. Hypotheses* 12: 167–9.

Reilly, J., & Rae, W. N. (1939). *Physico-Chemical Methods,* vol. I: *Measurement and Manipulation.* New York: Van Nostrand.

Renbourn, E. T. (1960). The natural history of insensible perspiration: a forgotten doctrine of health and disease. *Med. Hist.* 4: 135–52.

Reuler, J. B., Broudy, V. C., & Cooney, T. G. (1985). Adult scurvy. *J. Am. Med. Assoc.* 253: 805–7.

Rey, H. (1867). Étude analytique et critique sur le traité du scorbut de Lind. *Arch. de Méd. Nav.* (Paris) 7: 33–62, 216.

Rich, E. E., ed. (1946). *Minutes of the Hudson Bay Company 1679–1684.* Toronto: Champlain Society.

Rich, E. E. (1958). *The History of the Hudson's Bay Company 1670–1870*, vol. 1. London: Hudson's Bay Record Society.

Ritchie, C. (1847). Contributions to the pathology and treatment of scorbutus which is at present prevalent in various parts of Scotland. *Monthly J. Med. Sci.* 8: 38–49, 76–86.

Roddis, L. H. (1950). *James Lind, Founder of Nautical Medicine*. New York: Henry Schuman.

Rogers, A. F. (1974). The death of Chief Petty Officer Evans. *Practitioner* 212: 570–80.

Rolleston, H. D. (1915). James Lind, pioneer of naval hygiene. *R. Nav. Med. Serv. J.* 1: 181–90.

Rolleston, H. D. (1916). Sir Gilbert Blane, M.D., F.R.S. an administrator of naval medicine and hygiene. *R. Nav. Med. Serv. J.* 2: 72–81.

Rolleston, H. D. (1919). Thomas Trotter, M.D. *R. Nav. Med. Serv. J.* 5: 412–19.

Rouffear, G. P., & Ijzerman, J. W., eds. (1925). *De Eerste Schipvaart der Nederlanders Naar Oost-Indie onder Cornelis de Houtman 1595–1597*. 'S-Gravenhage, Holland: Martinus Nijhoff.

Rouppe, L. (1772). *Observations on Diseases Incidental to Seamen*. London: Carnan & Newbery.

Rousseau, J. (1953). The Anneda mystery. *Proc. XIX Congr. Int. Physiol.* Montreal, pp. 117–29.

Russell, W. H. (1858). *The British Expedition to the Crimea*. London: Routledge.

Rusznyák, S., and Szent-Györgyi, A. (1936). Vitamin P: flavonals as vitamins. *Nature* 138: 27.

Salaman, R. N. (1949). *The History and Social Influence of the Potato*. Cambridge: University Press.

Salmenpera, L. (1984). Vitamin C nutrition during prolonged lactation. *Am. J. Clin. Nutr.* 40: 1050–6.

Sato, T., & Nambu, K. (1908). Zur Pathologie und Anatomie des Skorbuts. *Virchows Arch.* 194: 151–81.

Sato, P. & Udenfriend, S. (1978). Studies on ascorbic acid related to the genetic basis of scurvy. *Vitam. Horm.* 36: 33–52.

Savours, A., & Deacon, M. (1981). Nutritional aspects of the British Arctic (Nares) Expedition of 1875–76 and its predecessors. In: *Starving Sailors* (J. Watt, E. J. Freeman, and W. F. Bynum, eds.), pp. 131–62. London: National Maritime Museum.

Sawtelle, C. M. (1876). *Pioneer Sketches*. Ms. in Bancroft Library, University of California, Berkeley.

Scarborough, H. (1945). Observations on the nature of vitamin P and the vitamin P potency of certain foodstuffs. *Biochem. J.* 39: 271–8.

Scheele, C.-W. (1966). *Chemical Essays*. London: Dawson Reprint Series.

Schilder, G. G., ed. (1976). *De Ontdekkingsreis van Willem Hesselz de Vlamingh in de Jaren 1696–1697*. 2 vols. 'S-Gravenhage, Holland: Nijhoff.

Schlegel, J. U. (1975). Proposed uses of ascorbic acid in prevention of bladder carcinoma. *Ann. N.Y. Acad. Sci.* 258: 432–6.

Schoute, D. (1937). *Occidental Therapeutics in the Netherlands East Indies During Three Centuries of Netherlands Settlements (1600–1900)*. Netherlands Indies Public Health Service.

Scott, E. L. (1970). "The Macbridean doctrine" of air: an eighteenth century explanation of some biochemical processes including photosynthesis. *Ambix* 17: 43–57.

Scott, R. F. (1905). *The Voyage of the 'Discovery.'* 2 vols. London: Smith, Elder.

Scoutten (1847). Épidémie de scorbut. *Arch. Gen. de Méd. [n.s.]* 14: 505–6.

Seib, P. A., & Tolbert, B. M. (1982). *Ascorbic Acid: Chemistry, Metabolism and Uses*. Washington, DC: American Chemical Society.

Severs, D., Williams, T., & Davies, J. W. (1961). Infantile scurvy – a public health problem. *Can. J. Public Health* 52: 214–20.

Shapiro, L. R., Samuels, S., Breslow, L., & Camacho, T. (1983). Patterns of vitamin C intake from food and supplements: survey of an adult population in Alameda County, California. *Am. J. Public Health* 73: 773–8.

Shapter, T. (1847). On the recent occurrence of scurvy in Exeter and the neighbourhood. *Provincial Med. Surg. J.*, pp. 281–5.

Shaw, R. C. (1896). *Across the Plains in '49.* Farmland, IN: W. C. West.

Sherlock, P., & Rothschild, E. O. (1967). Scurvy produced by a Zen macrobiotic diet. *J. Am. Med. Assoc.* 199: 794–8.

Sherwen, J. (1798). Scurvy caused by common culinary salt. *Gentleman's Magazine* 68: 105–8, 192–5.

Shipley, P. G. (1929). Our fathers and the scorby. *J. Am. Diet. Assoc.* 5: 1–10.

Sibbald (1847). Epidemic scurvy. *Provincial Med. J.*, p. 413.

Sick and Hurt Board (1786). Letter dated 28 March 1786, with copy of letter from Stephen Matthews dated 16 December, 1784. *ADM.FP/29*, National Maritime Museum, Greenwich, London, SE10 9NF.

Siegel, R. E. (1960). Hippocratic description of metabolic diseases in relation to modern concepts. *Bull. Hist. Med.* 34: 335–64.

Singer, D. W. (1949–50). Sir John Pringle and his circle. *Ann. Sci.* 6: 127–80, 229–61.

Smith, A. (1880). *An Inquiry into the Nature and Causes of the Wealth of Nations,* 1784 ed., vol. 1. Oxford: Clarendon Press.

Smith, A. H. (1918). Beer and scurvy. *Lancet ii:* 813–15.

Smith, A. H. (1919). A historical inquiry into the efficacy of lime juice for the cure of scurvy. *J. R. Army Med. Corps.* 32: 93–116, 188–208.

Smith, L. (1883). Second voyage of the 'Eira' to Franz-Josef Land. *Proc. R. Georg. Soc. [n.s.]* 5: 204–20.

Smith, T. (1895–6). Swine erysipelas or mouse-septicaemia bacilli from an outbreak of swine disease. *Ann. Rep. Bureau of Animal Industry,* Washington, DC: U. S. Department of Agriculture, pp. 166–79.

Solomons, N. W., & Viteri, F. E. (1982). Biological interaction of ascorbic acid and mineral nutrients. In: *Ascorbic Acid: Chemistry, Metabolism, and Uses* (P. A. Seib & B. M. Tolbert, eds.), pp. 551–69, Washington, DC: American Chemical Society.

Somerville, B. (1934). *Commodore Anson's Voyage into the South Seas and Around the World.* London: Heinemann.

Spencer, H. (1879). *The Study of Sociology.* New York: Appleton.

Spencer, W. G. (1935). *Celsus de Medicina,* vol. I. London: Heinemann.

Spevack, M. (1973). *The Harvard Concordance to Shakespeare.* Cambridge, MA: Harvard University Press.

Stamm, W. P., MacRae, T. F., & Yudkin, S. (1944). Incidence of bleeding gums among R.A.F. personnel and the value of ascorbic acid in treatment. *Br. Med. J. ii:* 239–41.

Stansfield, D. A. (1984). *Thomas Beddoes, M.D., 1760–1808.* Dordrecht, Holland: D. Reidel.

Starnes, de W. T., and Leake, C. D., eds. (1945). *A Profitable and Necessary Booke of Observations by William Clowes, 1596.* New York: Scholars Facsimiles and Reprints.

Steele, L., Jadhav, S., & Hadziyev, D. (1976). The chemical assay of vitamin C in dehydrated mashed potatoes. *Lebensm. Wiss. u. Technol.* 9: 239–45.

Stefansson, V. (1918). Observations on three cases of scurvy. *J. Am. Med. Assoc.* 71: 1715–18.

Stefansson, V. (1946). *Not By Bread Alone.* New York: MacMillan.

Steiner, P. E. (1968). *Disease in the Civil War.* Springfield, IL: Charles C. Thomas.

Stewart, C. P. (1953). Scurvy in the nineteenth century and after. In: *Lind's Treatise on Scurvy* (C. P. Stewart & D. Guthrie, eds.), pp. 404–12. Edinburgh: University Press.

Stewart, C. P., & Guthrie, D., ed. (1953). *Lind's Treatise on Scurvy.* Edinburgh: University Press.

Stiff, W. P. (1847). Remarks on the scurvy endemic at Nottingham. *Med. Times (London)* 16: 392.

Stille, C. J. (1866). *History of the United States Sanitary Commission.* Philadelphia, PA: J. B. Lippincott.

Stinson, B. (1966). Scurvy in the Civil War. *Civil War Times Illustrated* 5: 19–25.

Stockman, R. (1926). James Lind and scurvy. *Edinburgh Med. J. [n.s.]* 33: 329–50.

Stone, I. (1966). Hypoascorbemia: the genetic disease causing the human requirement for exogenous ascorbic acid. *Perspect. Biol. Med.* 10: 133–4.

Stone, I. (1972). *The Healing Factor. Vitamin C Against Disease.* New York: Grosset & Dunlap.

Svirbely, J. L., & Szent-Györgyi, A. (1932). Hexuronic acid as the antiscorbutic factor. *Nature* 129: 576.

Szent-Györgyi, A. (1928). Observations on the function of the peroxidase systems and the chemistry of the adrenal cortex. Description of a new carbohydrate derivative. *Biochem. J.* 22: 1387–409.

Szent-Györgyi, A. (1963). Lost in the twentieth century. *Annu. Rev. Biochem.* 32: 1–14.

Tanner, J. R., ed. (1926). *Private Correspondence and Miscellaneous Papers of Samuel Pepys 1679–1703*, vol. 1. London: Bell.

Tayler, W. H., & Tayler, J. W. (1869). On the treatment of scurvy by the binoxalate of potash. *Lancet i:* 777–8.

Taylor, G. (1916). *With Scott: The Silver Lining.* New York: Dodd, Mead.

Technical Commission on Nutrition, League of Nations (1938). Report on the work of third session. *Bull. Health Org.* 7: 460–98.

Temkin, O. (1973). *Galenism.* Ithaca, NY: Cornell University Press.

Temple, R., & Anstey, L. M., ed. (1932). *The Life of the Icelander Jon Olaffson.* London: Hakluyt Society.

Thomas, D. P. (1969). Experiment versus authority: James Lind and Benjamin Rush. *N. Engl. J. Med.* 281: 932–3.

Thompson, B. (Count Rumford) (1800). *Essays, Political, Economical and Philosophical.* 5th ed., vol. I. London: Cadell & Davies.

Thompson, D. (1977). *Scott's Men.* London: Allen Lane.

Thomson, F. (1790). *An Essay on the Scurvy Showing Effectual and Practicable Means for Its Prevention at Sea.* London: Robinson.

Thomson, J. (1859). *An Account of the Life, Letters and Writings of William Cullen, M.D.,* vol. 1. Edinburgh: Blackwood.

Thomson, T. (1830). *The History of Chemistry,* vol. 1. London: Colburn & Bentley.

Tickner, F. J., & Medvei, V. C. (1958). Scurvy and the health of European crews in the Indian Ocean. *Med. Hist.* 2: 36–46.

Tolbert, B. M., Downing, M., Carlson, R. W., Knight, M. K., & Baker, E. M. (1975). Chemistry and metabolism of ascorbic acid and ascorbate sulfate. *Ann. N.Y. Acad. Sci.* 258: 48–69.

Torrey, J. C., & Hess, A. F. (1917–8). The relationship of the intestinal flora to the scurvy of guinea pigs and of infants. *Proc. Soc. Exp. Biol. Med.* 15: 74–8.

Travis, J. (1762). A letter tending to show that the use of copper vessels in the navy is one of the principal causes of the sea scurvy. *Med. Obs. Enquiries* 2: 1–16.

*Treatment of Prisoners of War by the Rebel Authorities* (1869). Rep. no. 45. House of Representatives, 3rd sess., 40th Congress, Washington, DC: U.S. Government Printing Office.

*Trial of Henry Wirz* (1868). Exec. Document no. 23. House of Representatives 2nd sess., 40th Congress, Washington, DC: U.S. Government Printing Office.

Tripler, C. S. (1858). The causes, nature and treatment of scurvy. *Cincinnati Lancet and Observer* 7: 129–48.

Trotter, T. (1786). *Observations on the Scurvy with a Review of the Theories Lately Advanced on that Disease.* Edinburgh: Elliott.

Trotter, T. (1792). *Observations on the Scurvy: A New Theory Defended.* 2nd ed. London: Longman.

Trotter, T. (1795). *Medical and Chemical Essays.* London: Jordan.

Trotter, T. (1800). On citric acid. *Med. Physical J (London)* 4: 154–6.

Trotter, T. (1804). *Medicina Nautica,* 2nd ed., vol. 1. London: Longman.

Truswell, A. S. (1976). A comparative look at recommended nutrient intakes. *Proc. Nutr. Soc.* 35: 1–14.

Tuderman, L., Myllylä, R., & Kivirikko, K. I. (1977). Mechanisms of the prolyl hydroxylase reaction. *Eur. J. Biochem.* 80: 341–8.

Turnbull, A. (1902). Discussion on the prevention of scurvy. *Br. Med. J. ii:* 1023–4.

Turnbull, H. W., ed. (1959). *The Correspondence of Isaac Newton,* vol. 1: *1661–1675.* Cambridge: Royal Society.

Turner, E., Pitt, D., & Thomson, R. (1959). Scurvy yesterday and today. *Med. J. Aust.* 2: 243–6.

Tyson, J. L. (1955). *Diary of a Physician in California, 1850.* Oakland, CA: Biobooks.

U.S. Surgeon-General (1897). Barlow's disease. In: *Index Catalogue to the Library of the Surgeon-General's Office [ser. 2]* 2: 105–6. Washington, DC: Government Printing Office.

U.S. Surgeon-General (1920). Barlow's disease. In: *Index Catalogue to the Library of the Surgeon-General's Office [ser. 3]* 2: 351–5.

Van Ingen, P., & Taylor, P. E., eds. (1912). *Infant Mortality and Milk Stations.* New York: The New York Milk Committee.

Vander, A. J. (1981). *Nutrition, Stress, and Toxic Chemicals.* Ann Arbor, MI: University of Michigan Press.

Vassal, P.-A. (1956). D'ou vient le mot "scorbut"? *Rev. Path. Gén. Physiol. Clin.* no. 680: 1279–83.

Vaughan (1850). Scurvy on board temperance vessels. *Med. Times (London)* 21: 269.

Veith, I. (1958). Preface to L. S. King's *The Medical World of the Eighteenth Century.* Chicago: University of Chicago Press.

Villemin, J. A. (1874). Causes et nature du scorbut. *Bull. Acad. Natl. Méd. (Paris) [n.s.]* 3: 680–732, 738–818.

Villemin, J. A. (1875). Discussion sur le scorbut. *Bull. Acad. Natl. Méd. (Paris) [n.s.]* 4: 590–636, 650–68, 710–4.

Vilter, R. W., Woolford, R. M., & Spies, T. D. (1946). Severe scurvy: a clinical and hematological study. *J. Lab. Clin. Med.* 31: 609–30.

Wagner, H. R. (1929). *Spanish Voyages to the North West Coast of America in the Sixteenth Century.* San Francisco: California Historical Society.

Wallis, H. (1965). *Carteret's Voyage Round The World 1766–1769.* 2 vols. Cambridge: Hakluyt Society.

Walter, R. (1748). *A Voyage Round the World by George Anson, Esq.* 4th ed. London: Knapton.

*War of the Rebellion: Official Records of the Union and Confederate Armies (1880–1902).* Washington, DC: U.S. Government Printing Office.

Watt, J. (1979). *Medical Perspectives of some Voyages of Discovery.* Lettsomian Lecture. London: Medical Society of London.

Watt, J. (1981). Some consequences of nutritional disorders in eighteenth-century British circumnavigations. In: *Starving Sailors* (J. Watt, E. J. Freeman, & W. F. Bynum, eds.), pp. 51–71. London: National Maritime Museum.

Watt, J. (1982). Nutrition in adverse environments. 1. Forgotten lessons of maritime nutrition. *Hum. Nutr. (Appl. Nutr.)* 36A: 35–45.

Watt, J. (1983). James Lind (1716–1794). *University of Edinburgh J.* 31: 37–9.

Waxell, S. (1952). *The American Expedition.* London: Hodge.

Wesley, J. (1751). *Primitive Physick.* 2nd ed. London: Woodfall.

Whelan, W. S., Fraser, D. Robertson, E. C., & Tomczak, H. (1958). The rising incidence of scurvy in infants. *Can. Med. Assoc. J.* 78: 177–81.

White, J. (1712). *De recta Sanguinis Missione.* London: Brown.

Whorton, J. C. (1982). *Crusaders for fitness. The History of American Health Reformers.* Princeton, NJ: University Press.

Wilcox, L. A. (1969). *Anson's Voyage.* New York: St. Martin's Press.

Will, G., & Murdoch, W. R. (1960). Megaloblastic anemia associated with adult scurvy. *Postgrad. Med. J.* 36: 502–4.

Willcox, W. H. (1920). The treatment and management of diseases due to deficiency of diet: scurvy and beri-beri. *Br. Med. J. i:* 73–7.

Williams, G. (1967). *Documents Relating to Anson's Voyage Round the World 1740–1744.* Greenwich, UK: Navy Records Society.

Williams, R. J., & Deason, G. (1967). Individuality in vitamin C needs. *Proc. Natl. Acad. Sci. U.S.A. 57:* 1638–41.

Wilson, E. A. (1905). The medical aspects of the Discovery's voyage to the Antarctic. *Br. Med. J. ii:* 77–80.

Wilson, E. A. (1966). *Diary of the Discovery Expedition.* London: Blandford Press.

Wilson, H. K., Price-Jones, C. D., & Hughes, R. E. (1976). The influence of an extract of orange peel on the growth and ascorbic acid metabolism of young guinea-pigs. *J. Sci. Food Agric. 27:* 661–6.

Wilson, L. G. (1975). The clinical definition of scurvy and the discovery of vitamin C. *J. Hist. Med. Allied Sci. 30:* 40–60.

Wiltshire, H. W. (1918). A note on the value of germinated beans in the treatment of scurvy. *Lancet ii:* 811–13.

Winslow, C.-E. A., & Duran-Reynals, M. L. (1948). Jacme D'Agramont and the first of the plague tractates. *Bull. Hist. Med. 22:* 747–65.

Winslow, C.-E. A., & Duran-Reynals, M. L., trans. (1949). Regimen of protection against epidemics or pestilence and mortality. *Bull. Hist. Med. 23:* 57–94.

Wood, E. (1895). *The Crimea in 1854 and 1894.* London: Chapman & Hall.

Woodall, J. (1617). *The Surgions Mate.* London: Griffin. [Reprinted under the editorship of J. Kirkup (1978).]

Woodham Smith, C. (1962). *The Great Hunger: Ireland 1845–9.* London: Hamish Hamilton.

Wrench, E. M. (1867). An outbreak of scurvy. *Med. Times Gaz. i:* 317–18.

Wright, A. E. (1897). On a simple method of measuring the alkalinity of the blood. *Lancet ii:* 719–21.

Wright, A. E. (1900). On the pathology and therapeutics of scurvy. *Lancet ii:* 565–7.

Wright, A. E. (1904). Discussion on the etiology of scurvy. *Trans. Epidemiol. Soc. (London),* pp. 94–7, 108–9.

Wright, R. T. (1886). Notes on the prevention and treatment of scurvy in peace and war. *Ind. Med. Gaz. 21:* 33–6, 70–4, 142–3, 285.

Wyatt, H. V. (1976). James Lind and the prevention of scurvy. *Med. Hist. 20:* 433–8.

Yüceöglu, M. (1949). Beobachtungen über die Schwankungen des vitamin C in der Frauen-milch. *Annales Paediatrici 173:* 142–50.

Zilva, S. S. (1932). Hexuronic acid as the antiscorbutic factor. *Nature 129:* 690.

Zuckerman, A. (1976–7). Scurvy and the ventilation of ships in the Royal Navy; Samuel Sutton's contribution. *Eighteenth Cent. Stud. 10:* 222–34.

# Index